Second Edition

The Process of Community Health Education and Promotion

Eva I. Doyle
Baylor University

Susan E. Ward
Espinoza Ward Solutions and Texas Woman's University

Jody Oomen-Early
Walden University

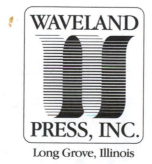

WAVELAND

PRESS, INC.

Long Grove, Illinois

For information about this book, contact:
Waveland Press, Inc.
4180 IL Route 83, Suite 101
Long Grove, IL 60047-9580
(847) 634-0081
info@waveland.com
www.waveland.com

Cover photo credits:
Top left, Jody Oomen-Early; middle, Eva I. Doyle; lower right, Eva I. Doyle.

Chapter opener photo credits:
Page 3, Teoman Alemdar; page 23, AP Photo/Michael Dwyer; page 47, AP Photo/Miguel Tovar; page 101, AP Photo/The Hawk Eye, John Lovretta; page 179, Public Health Image Library, Centers for Disease Control and Prevention; page 205, © 2008 Jim West/The Image Works; page 255, Public Health Image Library, Centers for Disease Control and Prevention; page 289, AP Photo/Los Angeles County Dept. of Public Health, Rene Macura; page 307, Fred Weissman; page 339, AP Photo/ Sayyid Azim.

We dedicate this book to our families and students.
You are our source of encouragement and inspiration.

Contents

Part I
Health and Community Perspectives   1

Part II
The Process of Health Programming　125

Part III
Communicating Needs and Managing Resources   231

11   Communicating Health Information

Preface

This textbook provides an introductory overview of information, perspectives, and competencies needed to effectively promote health and quality of life in community health education and health promotion, public health, and health-care settings. Our discussion in chapter 1 about emerging professional paradigms in these health professions and the powerful impact of boundary-crossing partnerships across disciplines is indicative of our philosophy and intended audience for this book. We invite all who are interested in the health and quality of life of individuals and whole communities to engage in the experiential learning approach that lies at the heart of this textbook.

A Recommended Learning Perspective

This book was written by three individuals who view learning as a journey rather than a destination. In fact, we confess that we actually *enjoy* the learning process. This is probably because life experience has taught us that change is inevitable and constant, and that we all learn through this ongoing change process whether we like it or not. We use the word "enjoy" loosely because experiences in which true learning occurs are often as demanding and exhausting as they are exhilarating. That is the experience we wish for our readers. We are by no means implying that merely reading this book will demand, exhaust, and exhilarate. We are, however, suggesting that its application in the real world of community health promotion can contribute to your lifelong learning experience in ways that can be significant and worth the effort.

We invite you to view this book as more than a required reading assignment in a college course. If you only read it to memorize facts to regurgitate on an exam, you will have missed its intent. Instead, we encourage you to think of it as a tool for action. Because people learn by doing (more so than by reading, listening, or taking notes), we encourage you to consider the following recommendations as you read this book.

1. *Ask "so what?"* When you read a passage, ask yourself why you would need to know that information. Think about how that knowledge or developed skill could be of value to you in your current or future practice as a health professional. There is a rationale and intended use for each chapter section. Reading with the intention of discovering this practical use can enhance your learning and application.

2. *Seek second opinions.* Don't just take our word for it. Though we have worked to present accurate and current information and to discuss issues from differing viewpoints, we encourage you to further explore alternative perspectives.

Learning from varying perspectives can broaden and enrich your understanding of the profession.

3. ***Apply it and customize it.***   Test the textbook information and recommended approaches in the real world at every opportunity. (See "Textbook Highlights" for suggestions.) Your real-world experimentation will breathe life into your learning experience and will help you master the ability to adapt textbook content for a variety of situations and uses.

About Professional Competencies

Chapter 1 contains a brief description of emerging professional paradigms and a rationale for forging boundary-crossing partnerships across health disciplines. The chapter also contains brief descriptions of some core knowledge and competency frameworks for public health and health education, as well as a *For Your Information* box (FYI 1.1) of suggested textbook readings that are associated with the current *seven areas of responsibility* of an entry-level certified health education specialist (CHES). These competency frameworks evolve as part of the natural growth and adaptation of a profession to an ever-changing world. We urge you to become actively involved in professional organizations, seek and maintain professional certification, and remain abreast of these evolving frameworks throughout your professional career.

Textbook Highlights

Each chapter of this textbook is designed to engage you in thought, discussion, and action. Where possible, we use examples about real people, illustrations that relate to common elements of life, practical questions, a conversational tone, and even a little humor to engage you in a personal way. We also include special features to help you explore ideas, test recommended approaches, and develop knowledge and competencies that will inform your health promotion efforts. We highlight these features below and provide more in-depth information for the course instructor in an accompanying Instructor's Guide.

For Your Information

Every chapter contains *For Your Information* (FYI) boxed features that provide nutshell descriptions, how-to guidelines, checklists, and examples that complement and expand on chapter content. In some cases, the FYI material serves as a prompt for or example of information you can use in a course project (see "Course Project") or as a self-directed learning activity.

For Your Application

You will find the *For Your Application* (FYA) feature at the end of each chapter. The FYAs contain instructions for recommended activities that can be undertaken on your own if they haven't already been assigned by the instructor. Some FYA activities can occur totally within the confines of a classroom. Others may require you to visit a local neighborhood or community organization for a stronger real-world experience. Moreover, some FYA activities can reinforce your work on a course project if one is assigned (see "Course Project") or further develop your professional résumé or portfolio. In all cases, FYA activities are designed to engage you in discussion and application of the knowledge and competencies described in that chapter.

Course Project

One of the most basic responsibilities for those working in community health is to assess the actual and perceived needs of communities. Therefore, the major project for this course is a *Community Assessment* (see Appendix B). Steps in the assessment process are outlined succinctly in chapter 6. You will find that many of the FYA activities throughout each chapter are components of this project. A Project Guide is included in Appendix B.

Web Resources

The *Web Resources* in Appendix A are a useful tool as you seek additional information and expand your knowledge about a variety of health-related organizations and information sources. Your course instructor has access to a Web Link file that allows direct linkage to the Web site(s) if you are online.

Learning Objectives and Review Questions

The learning objectives at the beginning of each chapter and the review questions at the end will help you highlight and organize your reading and notes around targeted learning concepts. The chapter content that addresses each objective/question not only provides key definitions and concepts but is designed to help you understand those concepts as they are applied in real-world settings.

To the Instructor

We believe the accompanying Instructor's Guide CD will be a valuable resource as you design and teach your course. It offers a wealth of materials and the flexibility to adapt them to various teaching styles and preferences. On the CD you will find an overview of the changes between the first and second editions; teaching tips linked to specific features of this text; a test bank and answer key; chapter-specific PowerPoints; Web Links; and a Professional Portfolio Guide, Project Guide, and Resource Inventory in formats that allow you to adapt them to your course needs.

Acknowledgments

The concept that "it takes a village" could be applied to this project. We thank the multitude of students whose input identified the need for and shaped the content of this book. We also thank a variety of colleagues whose encouragement and honest critique helped us reach our goal. We would like to especially acknowledge the assistance of Dr. Ashley Walker and Ms. Ivory Johnson, who helped us organize some of the PowerPoints for the Instructor's Guide; Jessica Hartman, who helped us update our Web Resources; and Teoman Alemdar, a gifted photographer who allowed us to use his beautiful images from around the world. We also extend our gratitude to those instructors and students who have used our text and have sent us feedback. We welcome comments, suggestions, and personal stories about applying these concepts in the field; your insights will help us keep future editions of this textbook current and meaningful.

PART I

Health and Community Perspectives

CHAPTER
one

Health and Quality of Life

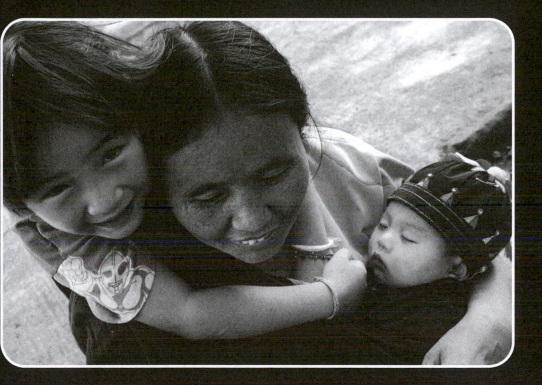

The elderly woman leans back in her chair and absentmindedly pushes her glasses back up on her nose. She gives you a knowing, tolerant look and says, "Honey, I ain't never had a need for that before. Don't see why I should start now." She's talking about the low-fat diet you just described to her. You knew before you started that it would be a tough sell—in some ways tougher than explaining the complexities of her diabetic condition. Now you're compelled to discuss changes in eating habits, habits that developed over a lifetime for a person who has overcome more of life's challenges than you may ever face. How do you convince her that such a drastic lifestyle change could make a difference in her health and quality of life?

CHAPTER OBJECTIVES

1. Describe varying perspectives on and definitions of health and quality of life.
2. Describe the historical development of professional concepts related to health, wellness, and quality of life.
3. Name immediate and global factors that influence health and quality of life.
4. Explain the reciprocal relationships between social conditions, health, and quality of life.
5. Describe the basic concepts of the socio-ecological approach.
6. Describe emerging professional paradigms and approaches in health care, public health, and health education.
7. Define and explain the benefits of boundary-crossing partnerships in community health education and promotion.

Health and Quality of Life

Imagine yourself as a talk-show host who goes out on the street to conduct an informal survey. Your quest is to capture the "average" person on national television with a microphone in his face as he tries to think of intelligent answers. Your first question seems harmless enough: "How do you define health?" Your victim scratches his head and blurts out an answer. You look knowingly into the camera, repeat his answer, and try not to laugh. Then you ask with a smug look on your face, "What is quality of life?" Now he's really stumped. He stammers as he tries to form a coherent response. You grin and the camera cuts back to the studio.

Few health professionals would ever intentionally interview someone in the condescending manner just described. Yet, experienced health professionals sometimes feel like the talk-show host who can't believe what she is hearing. The overarching goal of most health professionals is to enhance the health and quality of life of individuals and communities. But they often find it difficult to accomplish this goal given the imprecise array of health-related definitions and perspectives among clients, community leaders, and even other professionals. If you want to accomplish your professional goal of promoting healthy lifestyles, you have to know how people define health. To gain a clear understanding of your goals as a developing health professional, we invite you to examine some diverse and evolving perspectives about health and quality of life.

Common Viewpoints about Health

Take a moment to jot down words or concepts that come to mind when you think of the word *health*. Try to avoid textbook or professional definitions. Instead, think of your childhood experiences and how your family, friends, and others shaped your ideas about what it means to be healthy. Think of older adults that you know who are approaching the later stages of life, or think of someone who is challenged with a disability, and imagine how that person may define health.

The point of this exercise is to help you remember that the definition of what it means to be healthy can differ from person to person, and that some individuals you will encounter as a health professional have no clear understanding of the professional definitions presented in this textbook. These differing health views can significantly impact a person's life and your ability to help. The woman in this chapter's introductory story is a diabetic patient. A change in her eating habits and other behaviors could mean the difference between a life of relative wellness and one racked with health complications. Her calm rejection of a healthier diet could be driven by the belief that she is "healthy enough"—a viewpoint that could eventually cost her dearly.

To develop a better understanding of common views about health, we interviewed 393 children, parents, and elementary school teachers in a local community to learn how they defined *health*. Listed below are responses from a few of our participants:

- "Health is seeing the dentist and doctor regularly and particularly if you are sick." (Kyle, age 13)
- "It's not feeling sick, not having a cold." (Mary, age 7)
- "Health is how you feel. How your body works and how your systems work. The way you eat—not eating too much junk food. What activities you do, like swimming and running." (Katie, age 9)

Like Kyle and Mary, many of our participants thought health was related to illness. Some, like Katie, thought health had something to do with the actions we take or the activities in which we participate. Several elementary school teachers added dimensions beyond physical well-being such as "coordination of mind and body;" "skills to perform effectively in life—socially, emotionally, and academically;" "mind, body, and spirit;" and "keeping safe, avoiding anything damaging, feeling good about self, and [having] socialization skills." One said, "Health is a whole host of things from exercise to religion." Despite these few holistic perspectives, the majority confined their health definition to a physical state marked by the absence of disease. These findings serve as a sobering reminder that despite gains in health education and promotion, health professionals have more work to do to promote health awareness in all of its dimensions.

Evolving Professional Concepts

It's not surprising that people hold different views about health: Even health professionals can't agree on a single definition, and literally hundreds of definitions and descriptions of health can be found in the professional literature. These differing professional views may be partially due to the natural evolution of information and concepts that occurs in most professions. Newly discovered health information and technologies, shifting population demographics, evolving cultures, historical events at global and local levels, and a host of other factors have contributed to an ongoing demand for health professionals to adapt to a changing world.

To remain abreast of these constant changes, students enrolled in university degree programs are often encouraged to continue to attend professional conferences, read journals, and stay connected to the profession long after they graduate. It is also important for students and their instructors to examine the prevailing professional philosophies and approaches of the present within the context of the past; in other words, how those philosophies and approaches evolved. Mastering this historical perspective will help you effectively integrate proven approaches and further refine them in the future. Without a sense of the profession's history, you could inadvertently repeat mistakes of the past or contribute to a complacent acceptance that "we now know all there is to know." A good place to begin developing this historical perspective is with some of the early definitions of health used by recognized health organizations and leaders.

In 1947, the World Health Organization (WHO, 1947) told the world that **health** is "a state of complete physical, mental, and social well-being, and not merely the absence of disease and infirmity" (pp. 1–2). That declaration may not seem like earth-shattering news as you read it now. But prior to 1947, the prevailing view of health among many health leaders had mirrored what we learned through our recent survey of students, parents, and teachers: Health had been largely viewed as the absence of infectious diseases.

There were good reasons for a focus on infectious diseases at that time in history. The classic story of smallpox eradication (Henderson, 2006) illustrates this point. In the early 1900s, smallpox was a widespread killer in the United States. Though outbreaks of its severest form had declined by 1929, a 1947 outbreak in New York City resulted in the immunization of 6 million city residents. Smallpox continued to claim lives around the globe for decades, but a declaration by the World Health Assembly in 1958 led to the launching in 1967 of a global WHO campaign to eradicate smallpox. That goal was finally achieved in 1980. Thus, a definition of health as the absence of smallpox resulted in millions of lives saved.

The need for vigilance over infectious diseases is still an important component of public health (Curran, 2006). Newly identified diseases such as SARS, avian flu, and the Ebola virus; a resurgence of tuberculosis; and growing rates of HIV infection and antibiotic-resistant illnesses currently demand the attention of many health professionals (Coque et al., 2008; Curran, 2006; Lashley & Durham, 2007; Longtin et al., 2008; Verhoef et al., 2008). Yet, impressive strides in infectious-disease control have made a positive impact to the extent that only 25% of physician visits in the U.S. and just under one fourth of deaths worldwide have been recently attributed to infectious diseases (Curran, 2006).

As the overall impact of infectious diseases became less pronounced, attention turned to emerging health issues of a more chronic nature, such as cancer and heart disease. By 1970, the U.S. Communicable Disease Center had changed its name to the Center for Disease Control (currently, the Centers for Disease Control and Prevention) to reflect a broader scope that included chronic disease control and health promotion (Keck, 2006). During this time, the traditional epidemiology model (agent, host, and environment) gave way to an early version of the **social-ecological model** (Morris, 1975; Figure 1.1) because the latter included social and behavioral factors as part of the complex web surrounding chronic health issues. Similarly, the Canadian Ministry of Health and Welfare's **health field concept** (Lalonde, 1974) encompassed the four areas or types of factors that contribute to health: human biology (bodily systems, genetics, maturation, etc.), environment (climate, economics, community structure, social norms, etc.), lifestyle (controllable choices and behaviors), and the health care system (factors related to health care delivery).

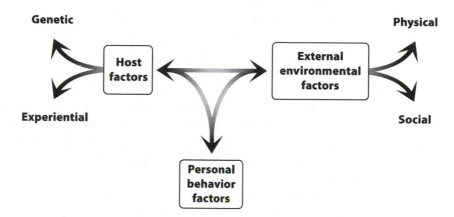

Figure 1.1   The social-ecological model (early version).
From *Uses of Epidemiology*, 3rd ed., by J. N. Morris, 1975, Edinburgh: Churchill Livingstone. Used with permission.

By the early 1980s, the U.S. government had embraced a massive undertaking that changed the course of how health is viewed and addressed by health professionals. The effort was launched by the publication of two landmark reports. In the first report, *Healthy People: The Surgeon General's Report on Health Promotion and Disease Prevention* (U.S. Public Health Service, 1979), the surgeon general described the health status of Americans and announced national goals for preventing premature deaths and promoting healthy lifestyles. A follow-up report in 1980, *Promoting Health/Preventing Disease: Objectives for the Nation*, contained more than 200 targeted health objectives designed to help Americans achieve the *Healthy People* goals by 1990 (U.S. Department of Health and Human Services [USDHHS], 1980). The U.S. government has been tracking and reporting *Healthy People* achievements related to those goals and objectives since 1980, and updated goals and objectives are announced at the beginning of each new decade. (See chapter 2 for more information about current community-based *Healthy People* goals and activities.)

We can examine the evolution of the *Healthy People* initiative to illustrate how views about health have changed over the past several decades. The initial 1979 and 1980 reports marked a significant shift from a traditional **medical model** perspective (Friedson, 1988), which emphasized "fixing a problem" through diagnosis and treatment, to a **wellness** perspective that focused on moving toward a positive state of health and well-being. This shift in perspective compelled health professionals to learn more about what wellness can mean for a person who is not currently ill and to devise programs to help people achieve wellness. By the mid-to-late 1990s, it was generally accepted that wellness is influenced by the multidimensional interplay of physical, emotional, spiritual, environmental, social, and interpersonal factors (Insel & Roth, 1994). Five commonly accepted dimensions of personal wellness include:

- *Physical wellness.* A physical state that enables a person to perform daily activities that lower the risk of preventable disease and are conducive to high levels of wellness in the other four dimensions, and to carry out such activities at levels that are personally satisfying.

- *Intellectual wellness.* A cognitive state that enables a person to apply sound critical-thinking processes when gathering information, forming opinions, making decisions, solving problems, and communicating with others.

- *Emotional wellness.* An emotional state that enables a person to recognize and understand, and effectively manage and express, feelings and emotions.

- *Social wellness.* An interactive state that enables a person to interrelate with others in ways that are mutually satisfying, supportive, and/or productive.

- *Spiritual wellness.* A communal state that enables a person to develop a sense of life purpose and meaning and/or a sense of connectedness with a higher power.

Total wellness describes an integrated or holistic combination of these five dimensions. As illustrated in the illness-wellness continuum (Figure 1.2), total wellness is dynamic in that it can fluctuate back and forth along a range from premature death to high-level wellness (Insel & Roth, 2000).

The concepts of wellness and equality were addressed jointly in *Healthy People 2000* (USDHHS, 1990), which advanced the goals of increasing life spans, reducing

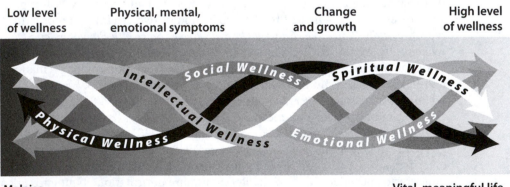

| Low level of wellness | Physical, mental, emotional symptoms | Change and growth | High level of wellness |

Malaise   Vital, meaningful life

Figure 1.2   The illness-wellness continuum.
Personal wellness is composed of five interrelated dimensions, all of which must be developed in order to achieve total wellness. Adapted from *Core Concepts in Health*, by P. M. Insel and W. T. Roth. © 2000. Used with permission of the McGraw-Hill Companies.

health disparities, and increasing access to preventive services for all Americans. The national data generated through earlier *Healthy People* efforts had demonstrated that all Americans were *not* equal in terms of health status and service access. That meant that health professionals needed to work with others to address a wide variety of environmental factors (e.g., social, financial, political, cultural, physical) that contribute to imbalances across groups.

By the time the *Healthy People 2010* goals (USDHHS, 2000) were announced, yet another important health-related concept had emerged, quality of life. The hard work of health professionals throughout the country had resulted in the good news that many Americans were living longer than previous generations. However, it had also become evident that living longer did not necessarily mean that Americans were living healthy and well throughout their life span. And though important progress had been made to address health disparities, some groups in America continued to suffer at disproportionate levels. For these reasons, the two overarching goals for *Healthy People 2010*, "to increase quality and years of healthy life" (p. 8) and "to eliminate health disparities" (p. 11) were used to establish quality of life as a critical component of health and to focus efforts on marginalized groups.

Quality of life became a concept used by health professionals to refer to an individual's or a group's perceptions about physical and mental well-being over time (Detmar et al., 2002; National Center for Chronic Disease Prevention and Health Promotion [NCCDPHP], 2007). Quality of life indicators include levels of perceived life satisfaction and the ability to perform day-to-day activities, and the term **health-related quality of life** (HRQOL) was coined to refer to the impact of health problems and health promotion on these levels (NCCDPHP, 2007). HRQOL also became a useful criterion for measuring disparities in health and well-being across groups.

As you can see, the evolution of health perspectives since 1947 has followed an interesting path. The traditional emphasis on disease-causing agents for infection control gave way to a new focus on chronic health problems and a wide spectrum of influences. Medical model perspectives were overshadowed by a more positive orientation toward wellness and prevention. Quality of life became the motivator for making healthy choices and the benchmark for comparing health status across individuals and whole communities. The prevailing viewpoint about health, shared by health professionals from a wide array of subdisciplines, is that the health of individuals can only be effectively understood within the context of entire communities and broader environments, meaning that efforts to promote health and quality of life must encompass both individual and community-wide strategies.

Personal Wellness, Quality of Life, and Broad Social Issues

The visual in Figure 1.3 was designed to illustrate the reciprocal interplay between personal wellness, quality of life, and broader social and environmental issues. We represent these three areas of concern as separate wheels (center of diagram) because that is how some professional efforts address them—as separate entities. Two examples of these isolated approaches include health care treatments that are designed to promote personal wellness without consideration of the patient's real or perceived quality of life

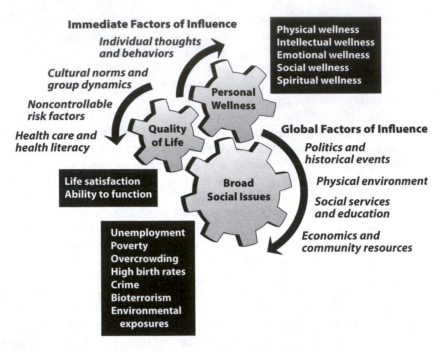

Figure 1.3   Wellness, quality of life, and broad social issues.
Wellness, quality of life, and broad social issues are connected through reciprocal relationships. Both immediate concerns and global factors influence all three directly or indirectly through their influence on any one component.

and political efforts to combat crime (a social issue) without consideration of how quality of life issues may contribute to violent behavior. We placed cogs on the wheels and arrows around them to symbolize how a change in any one area, either positive or negative, can impact conditions in the other two areas. This mutually influencing relationship is referred to by Bandura (1977) as **reciprocal determinism**.

In the black boxes linked to each wheel we provide dimensions or factors that would commonly be addressed within that area of concern. The close proximity of the wheels representing quality of life and personal wellness illustrates the connections between these two entities on an individual basis. In the sections that follow we describe some immediate factors than can influence a person's level of wellness and quality of life. We then turn to the third wheel of the diagram, broad social issues and global factors of influence.

Immediate Factors of Influence

The list of immediate factors in Figure 1.3 includes those that can directly impact individuals and members of their immediate groups (e.g., families, neighbors, local churches, social or work groups). Individual behavior is a strong determinant of health and quality of life. It is often influenced by individual thoughts (knowledge, attitudes, beliefs, values) and the thoughts and behaviors of significant people in one's life (cultural norms and group dynamics). **Noncontrollable risk factors,** such as age, gender, and genetics, can impact the type and severity of health and quality of life issues.

Quality health care can immediately improve a person's health and quality of life; conversely, the lack of quality care can destroy both. But the presence of skilled health professionals and up-to-date facilities is no guarantee that all eligible clients know how to access and fully benefit from these services. Complex systems, confusing forms, medical jargon, and rushed appointments are a few of the factors that can confuse and discourage those in need of care. **Health literacy** is a term often used to describe knowledge and skills levels needed to navigate the health care system and obtain quality care. It is technically defined as "the capacity of an individual to obtain, interpret, and understand basic health information and services and the competence to use such information and services in ways that are health enhancing" (Gold & Miner, 2002, p. 6). Being health literate and having access to health care are thus important determinants of your personal wellness and quality of life.

Social Issues and Global Influences

The United Nations (UN, 2007a) tracks the developmental status of countries around the globe through 12 social indicators (see FYI 1.1 on the following page). **Social indicators** are "statistics, statistical series, and all other forms of evidence that enable us to assess where we stand and are going with respect to our values and goals, and to evaluate specific programs and determine their impact" (Bauer, 1967, p. 1). A social indicator can be a partial measure of the physical environment in which people live, such as the degree to which safe and adequate housing, drinking water, and sanitation are available. Other social indicators can measure the social environment (for example, childbirth rates, crime, and education). In some instances, these environmental factors have a direct and readily detectable impact on health. For example, in their *2007/2008 Human Development Report* (Watkins, 2007), UN leaders noted that ongoing climate changes and droughts directly contribute to malnourishment. This direct impact has been particularly evident in Ethiopia, where children aged 5 or younger who were born in a drought season were reportedly 36% more likely to be malnourished and 41% more likely to suffer from stunted growth patterns.

Though many direct links between the environment and health exist, physical and social elements also impact the health of individuals and communities through indirect routes that are not always obvious. In Figure 1.3 we included global factors that indirectly influence personal wellness and quality of life through their effect on social conditions. For instance, political decisions and other historical events like financial recessions and natural disasters have, through time, contributed to unemployment rates and poverty throughout the world. Widespread poverty and lack of community resources in turn force individuals to live in crowded, substandard housing where exposure to infectious diseases and environmental hazards is high. The inability to afford health care and limited access to healthy foods can in turn lead to long-term health complications. Poor education and few opportunities for personal development can impact quality of life and contribute to poor behavioral choices, high birth rates, and crime. It is easy to see how these consequences of unemployment and poverty can become part of the vicious cycle that sends some societies into a down-

FYI 1.1   United Nations Social Indicators

Social indicators are statistical measures of environmental factors (physical and social) that serve as evidence of a community's health and well-being.

Child-Bearing
- Adolescent fertility rate
- Total fertility rate
- Maternal mortality ratio

Child and Elderly Populations
- Percentage of total population under 15 years
- Percentage of male population aged 60+
- Percentage of female population aged 60+
- Sex ratio (men/100 women) of population aged 60+

Contraceptive Use
- Contraceptive prevalence among married women of childbearing age, any method and modern methods

Education
- School life expectancy (in years), primary to tertiary education, total and by sex

Health
- Life expectancy at birth, by sex
- Infant mortality rate
- Under-five mortality rate

Housing
- Average number of persons per room for total, urban, and rural areas

Human Settlements
- Population distribution, by urban and rural residence
- Annual rate of population change, by urban and rural residence

Income and Economic Activity
- Per capita GDP ($US)
- Adult (15+) economic activity rate, total and by sex

Literacy
- Adult (15+) literacy rate, total and by sex
- Youth (15–24) literacy rate, total and by sex

Population
- Estimated population (in thousands), total and by sex
- Sex ratio (men per 100 women)
- Annual population growth rate

Unemployment
- Adult (15+) unemployment rate, total and by sex

Water Supply and Sanitation
- Improved drinking water coverage, total and by urban/rural area
- Improved sanitation coverage, total and by urban/rural area

From *Social Indicators*, United Nations, 2007 (December): http://unstats.un.org/unsd/demographic/products/socind/statistics.htm

ward spiral. In contrast, strong political and professional efforts to bring about positive changes in the social and physical environment can promote high levels of wellness and quality of life for individuals and communities.

Picture trying to put out a raging house fire with a single glass of water, or imagine painting a gigantic mural on the side of an office building using only a Q-tip. With these images in mind, you can begin to grasp the difficulty of bringing about meaningful change in a society that is beset by the complex web of factors we have described. In order to approach community health education and promotion on this scale, we need a model that incorporates both the immediate and the far-reaching effects of people's social and physical environments. Figure 1.4 provides one such model. The **socio-ecological model** (Ammerman et al., n.d.; McLeroy, Bibeau, Steckler, & Glanz, 1988; Partnership for Prevention, 2008a) provides a visual conceptualization of the broad approach needed to truly impact health and quality of life for individuals within the context of their environments. This model helps health professionals and community partners visualize how health and quality of life are impacted by ever-widening layers of influence. These factors or levels of influence include interpersonal groups such as friends and family, organizations or institutions that provide needed support, community organizations and social groups, and public policies that influence the availability and quality of health services and other needed resources. We

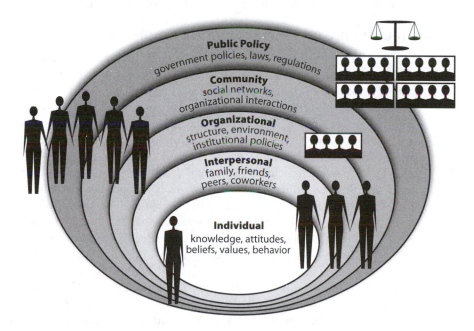

Figure 1.4   The socio-ecological model.
The socio-ecological model provides a tool for conceptualizing how the health and quality of life of individuals are impacted by ever-widening layers of influence from interpersonal groups, individual organizations or institutions, community networks, and public policies. Source: "An Ecological Perspective on Health Promotion Programs," by K. R. McLeroy, D. Bibeau, A. Steckler, and K. Glanz, 1988, *Health Education Quarterly 15*(4), pp. 351–377.

will discuss in chapter 2 some concepts and processes of community health promotion as they relate to the socio-ecological approach. Before you read that discussion, it may be useful to consider some related perspectives and approaches that shape how health and quality of life are addressed by health professionals.

Emerging Professional Perspectives

To complete our discussion in this chapter about health and quality of life concepts, we have included here a brief description of some evolving professional paradigms within the health professions. We define a **professional paradigm** as the philosophical or theoretical framework and related practices of a profession. A professional paradigm contains the rationale for *why* and *how* members of that profession use certain approaches in their work. Professional paradigms are usually evident in a profession's stated mission and goals, theoretical constructs and evidence-based methods, and professional competencies and skills taught and used in that profession. Evolving professional paradigms in health care, public health, and health education can have a profound impact on the health and quality of life of the individuals and communities served by these professions. That is why we have included a brief description of differences and connections across these professions.

Health Care and Public Health Paradigms

The health care profession plays a critical role in health and quality of life issues for reasons that are probably obvious. The diabetic woman in our introductory story would be less likely to have known she was diabetic had it not been for the health care professionals who diagnosed her condition, and the interventions offered to manage her diabetes can make a huge difference in her quality of life. The health care profession saves lives because of a commitment to quality diagnosis and treatment within its professional paradigm.

Yet, the isolated focus on individual diagnosis and treatment is no longer considered sufficient for addressing the health needs of our society (Institute of Medicine [IOM], 2007; Navarro et al., 2007; WHO, 2006b). The leaders of such major health organizations as the World Health Organization, Institute of Medicine, Centers for Disease Control, and the U.S. Department of Health and Human Services have called for a more collaborative, community-wide approach that combines health care, humanitarian actions, and the promotion of healthy lifestyles (CDC, 2007b; IOM, 2000, 2003; Partnership for Prevention, 2008a; USDHHS, 2000; WHO, 2006b).

In a landmark report called *Who Will Keep the Public Healthy?* (IOM, 2003), leaders of the Institute of Medicine recommended that medical and nursing schools include public health training as part of their curriculum and that health care professionals become part of collaborative teams to address the health of entire communities. In a follow-up study mandated by the U.S. Congress, the IOM (2007) recommended an integrated approach that would prepare *all* physicians (through medical schools and professional development programs) to some degree to work with whole populations (the public health approach) while providing specialty training in public health to those who choose to become public health physicians. This movement in the medical field toward population-based health care (in contrast to traditional individual practice) is a primary reason for the growing focus on the paradigm of public health.

For an interesting and interactive way to learn about public health, we invite you to visit a Web site called What Is Public Health? (Association of Schools of Public Health [ASPH], n.d.). This site contains the "Public health is . . ." statements provided in FYI 1.2. The public health paradigm focuses on the protection and improvement of community health with a primary goal of preventing health problems (rather than treating illnesses). This goal calls for a multidisciplinary approach to public health services that has traditionally included five core areas: behavioral sciences/health education, biostatistics, environmental health sciences, epidemiology, and health services administration (ASPH, 2001). Trained public health professionals should have a basic understanding of all five areas and some earn specialization degrees specific to one of these five areas (Council on Education for Public Health [CEPH], 2008). Collaboration across specialty areas is central to the public health paradigm because the collective knowledge and skills has a greater capability to produce needed changes at a variety of community levels.

These professionals are also expected to master additional cross-cutting competencies or skill sets that have been proven effective in public health practice. Public health leaders are currently in the process of refining these competencies as they relate to analysis/assessment, policy development/program planning, communication, cultural competency, community dimensions of practice, public health science, financial planning and management, and leadership and systems thinking (Council on Linkages between Academia and Public Health Practice, 2008). The National Board of Public Health Examiners (n.d.) established in 2008 a certification exam for public health professionals to become **certified in public health** (CPH) based on the five core areas of public health and these cross-cutting competencies.

FYI 1.2   **What Is Public Health?**

- Public health is the science and art of protecting and improving the health of communities through education, promotion of healthy lifestyles, and research for disease and injury prevention.

- Public health helps improve the health and well-being of people in local communities and across our nation.

- Public health helps people who are less fortunate to achieve a healthier lifestyle.

- Public health works to prevent health problems before they occur.

- Public health professionals achieve true job satisfaction by knowing they are making the world a better place.

From *What Is Public Health?*, Association of Schools of Public Health, n.d. Retrieved August 15, 2008, from http://www.whatispublichealth.org/

Many professionals from the health care and public health traditions have embraced the emerging trend of working in collaborative partnerships to improve human conditions. They understand that, to impact the health and quality of life of individuals and communities, they must develop perspectives and skills that allow them to connect and work with partners from a broad array of perspectives, experiences, and professional disciplines. Doctors, nurses, and other health professionals are now considered part of the public health workforce:

> The most common professional disciplines within the U.S. public health workforce are nurses, physicians, environmental specialists, laboratorians, health educators, disease investigators, outreach workers, and managers. Public health also includes dentists, social workers, nutritionists, anthropologists, psychologists, economists, political scientists, engineers, information technology specialists, public health informaticians, epidemiologists, biostatisticians, and lawyers. Any professional whose primary function is to improve health can be considered part of the public health workforce. (Keck, 2006, p. 217)

The ASPH (2008) describes the public health workforce as follows:

> Employed by governmental public health agencies, community-based service organizations, academic and research institutions, private organizations, hospitals, health plans and medical groups, these professionals function broadly, with activities including health surveillance, protection, promotion, planning, regulation, and health services organization, delivery, and evaluation. (p. 1)

The professional paradigms and workplace settings that once distinguished health care from public health are beginning to blur in ways that could positively influence the health and quality of life of individuals and communities.

Health Education and Health Promotion Paradigms

The professional paradigm of health education is framed by a broad mission: to promote healthy lifestyles and environments that enhance health, wellness, and quality of life for individuals and communities. We include *health* and *wellness* in this mission statement because of the tendency for some to think of health as merely the absence of disease. Though disease prevention is often one of the targeted outcomes of health education, it is not the primary focus. Health education is "a discipline of applied social-behavioral sciences" (Woodhouse, Auld, Livingood, & Mulligan, 2006, p. 260) that is well-grounded in research related to the psychosocial aspects of health behavior. This research points to quality of life goals as a primary incentive for adopting healthy lifestyles and improving environments among individuals, organizations, and communities. We present a detailed discussion of evidence-based theories and models needed for this work in chapter 5. In our discussion here we want to stress that health and wellness are considered means of achieving quality of life goals and are not just measures of success in disease prevention.

You probably noticed that health educators were listed in the previous section as part of the public health workforce. So you probably would not be surprised to learn that the professional paradigms of health education and public health share some common elements. The socio-ecological model and multidisciplinary approaches to community-based health promotion are valued in both paradigms. In fact, the processes of health promotion and health education have received considerable attention in recent years as key elements of collaborative health initiatives (Bureau of Labor Statistics [BLS], 2007a; Navarro et al., 2007). The Joint Committee on Terminology for Health Education and Promotion (2001) provided the following definitions for these two processes:

> **Health promotion:** Any planned combination of educational, political, environmental, regulatory, or organizational mechanisms that support actions and conditions of living conducive to the health of individuals, groups, and communities. (p. 101)

> **Health education:** Any combination of planned learning experiences based on sound theories that provide individuals, groups, and communities the opportunity to acquire information and the skills needed to make quality health decisions. (p. 101)

Health education and promotion have become valued components of the socio-ecological approach to promoting health and quality of life in communities and populations (IOM, 2000, 2003; Liburd & Sniezek, 2007; Navarro et al., 2007). Health education is a recognized component of the traditional public health core in behavioral sciences (ASPH, 2001), and community health education is a growing area of specialization in public health settings (CEPH, 2008; Woodhouse et al., 2006). For that reason, concepts relating to how the health education paradigm is applied in work settings is an important part of our discussion in this chapter.

One way to learn more about the role of health educators is to consult the Bureau of Labor Statistics' *Occupational Outlook Handbook* (BLS, 2007a). In an earlier version of its online handbook, the description provided for the standard classification code for "health educators" was as follows:

> Promote, maintain, and improve individual and community health by assisting individuals and communities to adopt healthy behaviors. Collect and analyze data to identify community needs prior to planning, implementing, monitoring, and evaluating programs designed to encourage healthy lifestyles, policies, and environments. May also serve as a resource to assist individuals, other professionals, or the community, and may administer fiscal resources for health education programs. (BLS, 2001, para. 1)

As is the case for the public health profession described in a previous section, health educators work in a wide variety of settings that include public health agencies, non-governmental organizations (NGOs), health care facilities, businesses, universities, and schools (BLS, 2007a; Teixeira, 2007). The common denominator of health education work across these settings lies in the application of specific professional competencies that have been clearly defined by the health education profession.

We previously indicated that a professional paradigm contains the rationale for the *why* and *how* of the methods they use. Professional competencies are also part of a professional paradigm because they represent *what* members of that profession should be able to do. A **professional competency** is a measure of ability or a standard of performance in a specific skill area that is needed to effectively practice in a profession. Professional competencies often serve as a guide for developing education and training programs, certification and licensure exams, performance standards, and job descriptions and hiring practices in a profession.

An example of how competencies are linked to professional paradigms can be illustrated using the concept of total wellness. In the professional paradigm of health education, total wellness is considered an important conceptual framework and motivational tool for helping individuals and communities reach their health and quality of life goals. The ability to effectively use evidence-based techniques and strategies to promote total wellness is part of the professional competencies of the health education profession.

In FYI 1.3 we provide a list of the **seven areas of responsibility** that frame the professional competencies of health educators (National Commission for Health Education Credentialing [NCHEC], Society for Public Health Education [SOPHE], and American Association for Health Education [AAHE], 2006). We also reference the chapters in our textbook that contain information related to each area of responsibility. These recommended readings are by no means an exhaustive list of all of the information needed to master each area. We encourage you to visit the NCHEC Web site (see Appendix A) for a complete list of the competencies and subcompetencies that define these seven areas.

FYI **1.3**   **Health Education Areas of Responsibility and Related Textbook Information**

Area of Responsibility	Type of Information	Chapter
Area I: Assess individual and community needs for health education	Definitions/factors that influence health and quality of life	1
	Epidemiological assessments	3
	Population-specific health issues and perspectives	4
	Assessment design and methods	**6***
Area II: Plan health education strategies, interventions, and programs	Concepts about community-based capacity building	2
	Identifying needed program focus	3, 4, 6
	Theories and models used in program goals and design	5
	Planning concepts, strategies, and methods	**7**
Area III: Implement health education strategies, interventions, and programs	Cultural competence needed for implementation	2
	Logic model components that guide implementation	7
	Implementation concepts, strategies, and methods	**8**
	Process evaluation of implementation activities/methods	9
	Accessing resources for implementation	13
Area IV: Conduct evaluation and research related to health education	**Epidemiological aspects of research**	**3**
	Special population considerations	4
	Theory and models as guides for designs and measures	5
	Assessment measures for use in of evaluation and research	6
	Evaluation and research concepts, strategies, and methods	**9**

Area of Responsibility	Type of Information	Chapter
Area V: Administer health education strategies, interventions, and programs	Emerging partnership approaches across health professions	1
	Assessment and programming elements of administration	6–9
	Administration concepts, strategies, and methods	**10**
	Communication and advocacy elements of administration	11, 12
	Resource management of administration	13
Area VI: Serve as a health education resource person	Information sources for professional paradigms/competencies	1
	Epidemiological data sources	3
	Information sources for special populations and issues	4
	Resource concepts, strategies for access and use, and links	**13**
Area VII: Communicate and advocate for health and health education	Community-based partnerships as opportunities for advocacy	2
	Culture-based considerations in communication	2, 3
	Communication concepts, strategies, and methods	**11**
	Advocacy concepts, strategies, and methods	**12**

Seven Areas of Responsibility of an Entry Level Health Educator from the National Commission for Health Education Credentialing (NCHEC, http://www.nchec.org/).

*Bold type denotes an entire chapter devoted to this topic. All others listed are partial information or perspectives implied/embedded in the focal topic of that chapter. This is a *selected* list (not an *exhaustive* list) of competency-related sources within the textbook.

These health education competencies are used by the National Commission for Health Education Credentialing as a framework for the national certification exam that an eligible health education professional can take to become a **certified health education specialist** (CHES). They are also used by the SOPHE/AAHE Baccalaureate Program Approval Committee (SABPAC) to evaluate undergraduate degree programs in colleges and universities. Health education degrees and the CHES credential represent a recognized standard of professional preparation for the health education workforce (BLS, 2007a).

As we write this chapter, a national health education job analysis is in progress as part of the profession's ongoing efforts to remain abreast of professional practice trends. When completed, results of that study and any ensuing competency updates will be posted on the NCHEC Web site. We also encourage you to visit the Web site of the National Implementation Task Force for Accreditation in Health Education (see Appendix A) to learn about additional discussions and activities related to degree program accreditation.

Crossing Boundaries to Common Ground

Though professional schools of preparation and licensure/certification for specialized health practice still (and should) clearly define some specific roles, the need for partnered approaches to address broader health concerns has begun to draw these health disciplines together in a more unified effort. Leaders of the Institute of Medicine (IOM, 2002) and the Centers for Disease Control and Prevention (CDC, 2006a; Slonim et al., 2007) have called for interdisciplinary collaboration and community-based partnerships that involve public and private sectors in integrated approaches to health programming and research. These leaders have intensified efforts to support cross-cutting research and interdisciplinary innovations that address the *Health Protection Goals* developed at the CDC (2007g): healthy people across all stages of life; healthy places and communities; preparedness against infectious, occupational, environmental, and terrorist threats; and improved global health.

The widening acceptance of the socio-ecological model across these health professions is providing common ground for partnered approaches that link health care, public health, and health education. The potential success of any partnership is enhanced when each partner understands and appreciates the abilities and contributions of other partners. Yet, some would argue that simply appreciating other disciplines while continuing to work within the boundaries of one's own discipline is a missed opportunity (Tsui & Law, 2007). "It is no longer sufficient for an individual to acquire expertise within the boundary of one's own discipline or profession nor is it possible for one to know everything, even in one's own field of expertise" (Tsui & Law, 2007, p. 1289). "While the core of a practice is a locus of expertise, radically new insights and developments often arise at the boundaries between [professional] communities" (Wenger, McDermott, & Snyder, 2002, p. 153).

Please allow us to paraphrase what you just read: You *cannot* know everything and, despite what some may tell you, you cannot find all the answers within your chosen profession. Exciting and innovative ideas can be generated when people push themselves outside the boundaries of their professional comfort zones and try something in a different way. We call this effort **boundary crossing**. Boundary-crossing partnerships are essential to the socio-ecological approach. It is our intent with this textbook to help members of these boundary-crossing partnerships find common ground in the process of community health education and promotion.

In Conclusion

Promoting health and quality of life for individuals and communities can be a challenge, especially when your clients and professional and community partners think differently about what those concepts mean and how to promote them. The socio-ecological perspective, emphasizing the interplay between health and wellness, quality of life, and broad social issues, can help you better prepare for your role as a health professional. We encourage you to participate in boundary-crossing partnerships that can more effectively impact the lives of those you serve.

REVIEW QUESTIONS

1. Define health and quality of life.
2. Describe the five dimensions of wellness and the illness-wellness continuum.

3. Explain how general professional concepts about health have changed through the years as they relate to the medical model, total wellness, and the socio-ecological approach.

4. List some social indicators and explain how they are connected to health.

5. Explain the reciprocal relationships between health, wellness, and broad social issues; and name some factors that influence these relationships.

6. Describe the professional paradigms of health care, public health, and health education.

7. Explain the nature and utility of boundary-crossing partnerships in community health education and promotion.

☛ FOR YOUR APPLICATION

Mapping Your Philosophy

Examine your personal philosophy about health through this cognitive mapping exercise. You'll need 1–2 sheets of paper, a pencil, and small self-adhesive sticky notes (if available). In the middle of one sheet of paper write the word *health*. Draw a small circle around it. Ask yourself: *What factors can affect a person's health?* Write every factor you can think of in the space surrounding your *health circle* (or write each factor on a separate sticky note and place it on the paper.) Work quickly and generate as many factors as possible. When finished, look for patterns in the factors you generated. Group them by categories (connect similar factors with lines or cluster sticky notes). Example categories include behaviors (hand-washing, smoking), attitudes (sense of humor, hate exercise), people (supportive family, stressful employer), circumstances (educational opportunities, unemployment), environments (social connectedness, air pollution), and services/programs (high quality, nonexistent). Were you more likely to name factors people can control (attitudes, behaviors) or factors not easily controlled (the economy)? Did you name more *illness-causing* (stress) or *wellness-promoting* (exercise) factors? Based on this exercise, what would you say is your personal philosophy about health and wellness? What can be done to promote health and quality of life? Write your observations on a second piece of paper and use them to create your professional philosophy for inclusion in your portfolio (see Appendix C). You can also adapt and use this exercise to interview members of a community to learn more about their health perspectives and philosophies (see community assessment project guide, Appendix B).

Community and Cultural Concepts

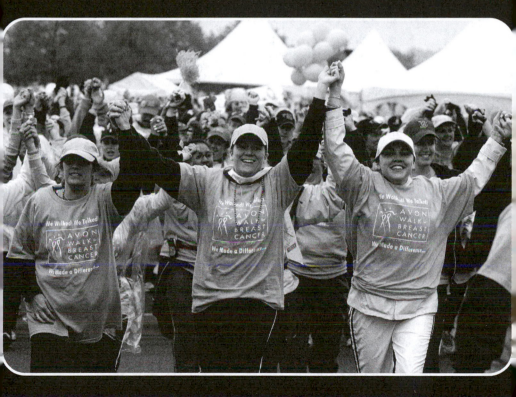

You didn't mean to take that wrong turn back there. This part of town can be a little dangerous after dark. The shabby buildings with bars on the windows make you feel a little uneasy. Is that a person lying over there next to the garbage can? A block later, a ball bounces out of nowhere into the street and you slam on your brakes—just missing the little girl who ran after it and the teenager who ran after the little girl. The teenager scoops up the girl and the ball and turns toward an apartment building where an elderly woman stands waiting for them with her hands on her hips. This neighborhood looks weary—the people, the buildings, the dirty streets. You feel guilty for being glad you don't have to wake up to this every morning. But what about the people who do?

CHAPTER OBJECTIVES

1. Describe the characteristics and actions of a healthy community.

2. Describe the components of community structure and capacity.

3. Explain the connections between Maslow's hierarchy of needs, heritage consistency, and social connectedness.

4. Describe concepts and recommended approaches to community capacity building.

5. Describe settings in which community health promotion happens and how public health agencies and nongovernmental organizations are involved.

Healthy People in Healthy Communities

On the current Web site of the *Healthy People* initiative described in chapter 1 is a section titled *Be a Healthy Person*. That section begins with the statement: "Take every opportunity to improve your own health, the health of your loved ones, and the health of your community" (USDHHS, n.d., *Be*). This sentence embodies the concepts of the socio-ecological model in a way that can personalize it for you—the health professional—and the individuals you serve. It implies that we all play a role in the health of our communities, and that role begins with your personal health and the health of those you care about. It also implies that community members and the professionals who work in those communities should understand the strong connections between individual and community health.

Healthy People in Healthy Communities (USDHHS, 2001) is the vision statement for the *Healthy People* initiative. It articulates the viewpoint held by health professionals from a wide spectrum of subdisciplines: the health of individuals can only be effectively understood within the context of whole communities and broader environments, and efforts to promote health and quality of life must encompass both individual and community-wide strategies (Minkler, 2005; USDHHS, 2007c). The following quote from *Healthy People 2010* (USDHHS, 2000) further explains this integrated perspective.

> Over the years, it has become clear that individual health is closely linked to community health—the health of the community and environment in which individuals live, work, and play. Likewise, community health is profoundly affected by the collective beliefs, attitudes, and behaviors of everyone who lives in the community. Indeed, the underlying premise of *Healthy People 2010* is that the health of the individual is almost inseparable from the health of the larger community and that the health of every community in every state and territory determines the overall health status of the Nation. That is why the vision for *Healthy People 2010* is "Healthy People in Healthy Communities." (p. 3)

At this writing, the *Healthy People 2020* goals and objectives are currently under development. It is expected that the ecological approach to promoting healthy communities will remain a priority.

Now that we have established the connection between the health of individuals and communities, the next logical step is to gain an understanding of what it means to be healthy as an individual and as a community. The discussions about health, wellness, and quality of life in chapter 1 provide a firm foundation for conceptual understanding. In the chapters that follow we provide details about the processes and resources used to assess and promote individual and community health. But what standards will you use to work, and motivate others to work with you, toward the goal of healthy individuals in healthy communities? In other words, how do you know when an individual or a community is healthy?

Healthy Individuals

The U.S. Department of Health and Human Services (n.d., *Leading*) has identified 10 **leading health indicators** to measure the health of the nation (Figure 2.1 on the following page). These indicators were selected because they contribute in significant ways to the health of individuals and whole populations. They serve as a guide for developing *Healthy People* goals and objectives (USDHHS, 2000), strategies for health promotion, and standards for measuring success in those efforts. They also serve as a guide for targeting risky behaviors and promoting healthy lifestyles. According to data provided through the CDC's Behavioral Risk Factor Surveillance System (BRFSS), a national system used to track the health-related behaviors of Americans, an individual can improve health and reduce health risk by engaging in appropriate levels of regular exercise, maintaining a healthy weight, using seat belts, and getting adequate preventive medical care such as flu shots, mammograms, and other health screenings (USDHHS, 2008a).

A number of quality resources exist for health professionals and individuals who are interested in learning more about individual health, how it is measured, and the steps a person can take to improve it. We recommend you start by visiting the CDC's Web site (see Appendix A) to take advantage of the wide array of information provided there about healthy living and other health topics. For the purposes of our discussion here about healthy individuals in healthy communities, we point out that the 10 leading health indicators for individuals and communities are influenced by both individual choices and community resources and support for healthy living.

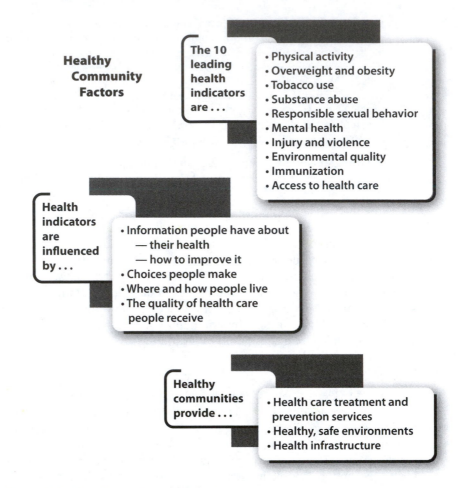

Figure 2.1   Healthy community factors.

Sources: *Leading Health Indicators: Priorities for Action*, USDHHS, n.d.; *Healthy People 2010: Understanding and Improving Health*, USDHHS, 2000, Washington, DC: U.S. Government Printing Office; *Healthy People in Healthy Communities*, USDHHS, 2001, Washington, DC: U.S. Government Printing Office.

Healthy Communities

"A **healthy community** is one that embraces the belief that health is more than merely an absence of disease; a healthy community includes those elements that enable people to maintain a high quality of life and productivity" (USDHHS, 2001, p. 1). You probably recognized the total wellness and quality of life concepts we described in chapter 1. Though access to quality health care services is an important component of what healthy communities provide, it is only one of several essential ingredients for community health. As illustrated in Figure 2.1, a community's leading health indicators are also shaped by information access, behavioral choices, and living conditions which, in turn, compel a community to provide quality treatment and prevention services, healthy and safe environments, and healthy infrastructures (USDHHS, n.d. *Leading*).

Healthy infrastructures provide community members with opportunities to pursue education, work, and recreation within safe environments, and also motivate residents to help maintain those environments. An important first step in motivating people to become stakeholders in their communities and equipping health professionals to promote healthy communities is to make sure that all involved understand how communities are structured and generally function.

Community Structure and Capacity

When you hear the word *community*, what comes to mind? If you picture a small midwestern town where neighbors are friendly and most children grow up in one place, you can probably understand why the term seems to have lost its meaning in some parts of America. In some communities, low-income apartment buildings stand next to factories while, blocks away, high-income apartments are built near business districts. In the suburbs, residents may commute long hours to work or school, and life moves at a fast pace. For these and other reasons, communities aren't necessarily well-defined by geographic boundaries alone.

Instead, we invite you to think of communities in terms of their structure and capacity. In using the word *structure*, we aren't necessarily referring to the physical buildings of a community, though physical structures do partially define a community. But a community's structure can also be defined in terms of social, cultural, and even political networks that bond individual community members into unified groups. These bonds can be viewed as assets that shape a community's capacity to be a healthy community.

People in Communities

Communities are usually defined by what people have in common. The common link may be structural, as in a shared neighborhood, workplace, or school. Or it may reflect common values, interests, or incomes. Age, ethnicity, and sexual orientation can bond individuals into a community. Followers of a particular religion or spiritual belief may function as a community. Even members of the same civic organization or social club can function as a community when goals, interests, and activities are shared. Regardless of the common link, people are the heart of a community.

People interact with one another for many reasons. You may, for example, interact with university professors to meet a desired career goal or with family members to satisfy needs for emotional or financial support. Abraham Maslow (1954), a well-known American psychologist, would argue that people are motivated to act (and we would add "to interact with others") based on five levels of human need that are often referred to as **Maslow's hierarchy of needs** (Figure 2.2 on the following page). We believe this hierarchy explains why individuals bond into communities.

According to Maslow's hierarchy, physiological needs (food, water, oxygen) and the need for physical safety are the most basic and influential motivators of human behavior. You may never have experienced an intense physiological or safety crisis that led to desperate action. Yet you can likely understand why a starving person

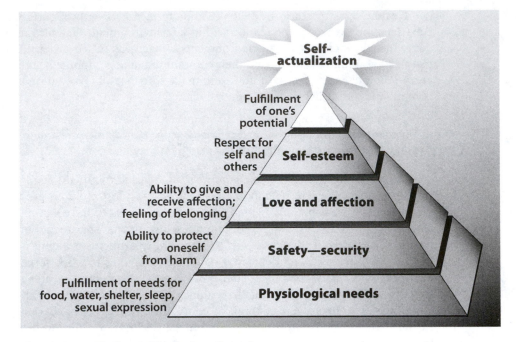

Figure 2.2   Maslow's hierarchy of needs.
Maslow reminds us that a community's basic physiological and safety needs must be met before efforts can focus on higher level needs such as self-actualization. Adapted from *Motivation and Personality*, by A. Maslow, 1954, New York: Harper & Row.

would resort to stealing food or an abused teenager would choose to live on the streets. When safety and physiological needs are at stake, nothing else seems to matter. That's why it is sometimes necessary for community health efforts to address these basic needs first before attempting to tackle less crisis-oriented health issues.

On a higher level of Maslow's hierarchy, the need for love, acceptance, appreciation, and respect can motivate people to join formally structured groups (churches, clubs, etc.) and informal social networks. Though gang membership and other negative relationships can result from this need, the more positive connections can help an individual advance to the highest level of the hierarchy. **Self-actualization** is characterized by emotional and spiritual health in which a person accepts oneself and others, optimizes personal capabilities, and possesses a keen sense of fulfillment and purpose in life. Individuals at this level may become active in community organizations, work on college degrees, or choose a specific profession or interest area because these challenges provide opportunities for self-improvement and the chance to make a difference to society.

Maslow's hierarchy explains why, within any given community, you will likely find smaller subgroups of individuals bound together by need. At lower hierarchy levels, individuals may join support groups to deal with addictions, disease, or other problems. Some community volunteers working in these programs may do so because they have been personally touched by the problem and wish to make a difference for someone else. At higher hierarchy levels, individual community members who seek to connect with others and to perhaps pursue self-actualization may become valuable partners in your effort to promote community health.

Cultural Connections

Our previous discussion about the human need for acceptance sets the stage for an examination of how culture and ethnicity shape communities. Though culture and ethnicity share some common elements, these concepts represent different and equally important characteristics of a community. To clarify these differences, we will describe the concept of **heritage consistency,** which represents the degree to which a person's lifestyle reflects his or her traditional culture or cultural roots (Spector, 2004). This is an important concept because individual members of a cultural group or ethnic community may adhere to different levels of heritage consistency, which impacts the depth and nature of community connections.

Spector (2004) proposed a model of heritage consistency in which a person's worldview is shaped by three intrinsically linked elements—culture, ethnicity, and religion. **Culture** encompasses the knowledge, beliefs, practices, values, customs, and norms of a group of people that are passed from one generation to the next. It is learned from family and community members and shaped by traditional religion, the environment, and historical events. Culture can serve as the framework that bonds individuals within a close-knit community. It is a powerful shaper of human behavior and often dictates how people interact. **Ethnicity** is distinguished from culture in this model as the degree to which a person deliberately chooses to identify with and embrace the practices and beliefs of an ethnic group. This distinction allows for the possibility that individuals may be shaped by their cultural roots without openly embracing an ethnic identity.

Religion, the third component of the model, is defined as "a set of beliefs, values, and practices based on the teachings of a spiritual leader" (Office of Minority Health, 2001, p. 132). Despite shifting patterns in religious beliefs and practices in the United States, religion remains a powerful predictor of ethnicity (Abramson, 1980; Eck, 2001; Spector, 2004). Religious teachings often provide the framework for ethnicity-specific values and norms, and are particularly influential in shaping ethics, purpose, and life meaning. These religious teachings and other bonds of heritage consistency can positively impact a community's environment.

Community Environments

As we stated in chapter 1, the socio-ecological model reminds us that individuals, groups, and whole communities are impacted by a variety of environmental factors. **Environmental health** is one of the five core areas of public health and is particularly relevant in terms of the health risks associated with the physical environment (ASPH, 2001). Economic, political, and social environments are also important components of a community's structure and capacity. A clear understanding of these environmental dimensions is essential to your ability to promote community health.

The Ministry of Social Development of New Zealand (MSD, 2007a) describes the **physical environment** as "land, air, water, plants and animals, buildings and other infrastructure, and all of the natural resources that provide our basic needs and opportunities for social and economic development" (*Introduction*, para. 1). Common environmental health issues around the world include the provision of safe drinking water, clean air, and protection from toxic elements. The physical environment is central to the emergence of **healthy community design**, the process of planning and designing communities where physical activity and social interaction are part of the daily routine, and adults can continue to live in the community as they grow older and lose physical abilities (National Center for Environmental Health, 2008).

A community's **economic environment** undeniably impacts its health. Low-income communities struggle with unemployment and low wages, poor housing conditions and insufficient infrastructure, limited access to quality health care, and numerous other challenges to quality of life that are intertwined with complex social issues. A community's **political environment** plays a significant role in the extent to which leaders can obtain needed assistance; for example, becoming a designated **medically underserved area** (MUA) or **medically underserved population** (MUP) and thereby eligible for government assistance (U.S. Health Resources and Services Administration, n.d). Political leaders impact community health through decisions related to water quality, wastewater treatment, landfills, industry zoning laws, and support of police and fire departments. The availability and quality of city parks and recreational areas, schools and libraries, and community centers also affect health because they offer opportunities to exercise mind and body, develop social skills, and enhance quality of life.

The state of a community's **social environment** is often measured by such indicators as literacy rates, housing quality, and other factors that draw attention to community shortcomings (see FYI 1.1). The term *social connectedness* is useful because it is a measure of the degree to which "people [join] together to achieve shared goals that benefit each other and society as a whole" (MSD, 2007b, *Introduction*, para. 1). When social connectedness is high in a community, members enjoy positive social roles and relationships that "give people support, happiness, contentment, and a sense they belong and have a role to play in society" (para. 1). Social connectedness fulfills a need for acceptance, enhances health and well-being, and compels people to think of others. Communities with high levels of social connectedness are usually healthier communities.

Community Capacity

The health of a community is measured not only by its current health status but also by what it is doing to enable its members to enjoy high quality of life (USDHHS, 2001). In other words, a community's ability to take action on its own behalf is an essential characteristic of a healthy community. For you to be able to promote a community's ability to take action, you must first be able to measure the community's capacity to do that.

In the health promotion profession, **community capacity** is often defined as "the characteristics of communities that affect their ability to identify, mobilize, and address social and public health problems" (Goodman et al., 1999, p. 259). So, what *are* those capacity characteristics? A multidisciplinary team from sociology, urban planning, psychology, and social work created a conceptual framework for understanding community capacity (Chaskin, Brown, Venkatesh, & Vidal, 2001). According to this framework (2001, p. 16), the four characteristics of community capacity are:

- a sense of community (connectedness among members and recognition of mutual circumstances),
- commitment to the community among its members (assumed responsibility and a willingness to act),
- an ability to solve problems ("to translate commitment into action"), and
- access to resources ("economic, human, physical, and political within and beyond the community").

This framework has been used in health promotion and public health (Kegler, Norton, & Aronson, 2008; Kieffer & Rieschmann, 2004; Sotomayor, Pawlik, & Dominguez, 2007) and other disciplines (Díaz, 2007; Hardcastle, Powers, & Wenocur, 2004; Stith, 2007; Weil & Reisch, 2005). Community capacity "is what makes well-functioning communities function well" (Chaskin et al., 2001, p. 7). It is built through the interaction of human capital (leadership, skills, etc.), organizational resources, and social capital.

The concept of social capital is emerging as a theory of community health education. For now we will define **social capital** as "relationships and structures within a community that promote cooperation for mutual benefit" (Minkler & Wallerstein, 2005, p. 35). The World Bank measures social capital in six dimensions: (a) the existence of supportive groups and networks, (b) a cohesive sense of trust and solidarity, (c) collective action and cooperation for working together, (d) inclusion of the marginalized for social cohesion, (e) empowerment and political action, and (f) communication that promotes access to information (Dudwick et al., 2006; Grootaert et al., 2004). When social capital is combined with human capital, needed resources, and effective organization, a community's capacity for action increases.

Capacity-Building Concepts

A number of communities in the United States and other parts of the world possess at least some characteristics of a healthy community. But others could hardly be defined as *communities* in terms of social connectedness, social capital, and other capacity elements. In most areas, some form of capacity building is needed.

Concept Model for Capacity Building

Figure 2.3 illustrates how some elements of capacity described in the previous section fit within the concept of capacity building. Social connectedness, social capital, and community action share common elements that often take root in the beginning stages of capacity building. The sequence in Figure 2.3 illustrates a snowball effect with growth in each component contributing to the development of other components. For example, social connectedness, which begins with shared needs, interests, and/or heritage consistency, can develop into stronger connections of trust and social cohesion (social capital dimensions). As these connections deepen, stronger networks are developed and enable the community to communicate and work cohe-

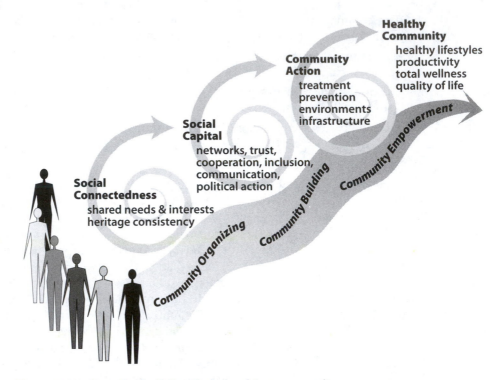

Figure 2.3   Capacity building for a healthy community.

Sources: *Healthy People in Healthy Communities*, U.S. Department of Health and Human Services, 2001, February, Washington, DC: U.S. Government Printing Office; *Overview: Social capital*, World Bank, 2008, Washington, DC: Author. Retrieved July 30, 2008, from http://go.worldbank.org/C0QTRW4QF0

sively on a common cause that can include political or social actions (other social capital dimensions). This developed social capital, which combines relationship links with a capacity for organized effort, can launch the kinds of community action described in Figure 2.1 that result in healthy communities: quality health care treatment and prevention services, healthy environments, and healthy infrastructures. The ultimate goal of this effort is to establish a community that enables its members to live healthy and productive lives and enhances their well-being and quality of life.

Community Building and Empowerment

Has anyone ever "helped" you in a way that wasn't really helpful? In some communities, your offer to help may be welcomed by some and viewed suspiciously by others. Though they may trust your sincerity, they may be skeptical about your ability to maintain long-range commitments; or they may simply be uncomfortable with the idea of *needing* help. As noted public health educator Dr. Larry Green explains, "Many communities have grown weary . . . with yet another . . . initiative seeking to point out their needs, which usually translate as deficiencies embarrassingly catalogued and publicized, often without solution" (Gilmore & Campbell, 2005, p. vii).

We encourage you to consider the meaning of the word *help* within the context of three terms often used when discussing community capacity building. The challenge in describing these terms is that varying definitions and uses have sometimes blurred their distinctions. To avoid confusion, we urge you to consult the discussion of these concepts by Minkler (2005); Minkler, Wallerstein, and Wilson (2008); and Chaskin et al. (2001). Meanwhile, we have provided some basic information that begins with operational descriptions from Minkler et al. (2008):

> **Community organizing:** A process through which communities are helped to identify common problems or goals, mobilize resources, and in other ways develop and implement strategies for reaching their goals they have collectively set. (p. 287–288)

> **Community empowerment:** A social action process by which individuals, communities, and organizations gain mastery over their lives in the context of changing their social and political environment to improve equity and quality of life. (p. 295)

> **Community building:** An orientation to community that stresses community assets and shared identity, whether or not task-oriented organizing takes place. (p. 289)

Notice that community organizing and empowerment are described above as *processes* while community building is called an *orientation to community* (a perspective or way of thinking about a community).

Community organizing (or community organization) has evolved since the late 1800s into a broad approach to helping communities achieve goals. Multiple models have been developed to focus on the processes and/or tasks needed to help communities solve problems (Minkler et al., 2008). However, this original emphasis on community collaboration to address deficiencies is viewed by some as being too outsider- and problem-focused to foster real community leadership toward positive goals (Chaskin et al., 2001; Minkler, 2005; Minkler et al., 2008).

We certainly are *not* suggesting that you should hesitate to help a community get organized and accomplish needed processes and tasks. Community organizing efforts can help "identify and mobilize key individuals and groups to develop or maintain a health promotion program" (Glanz, Rimer, & Viswanath, 2008, p. 26). As illustrated in Figure 2.3, this process can contribute to social connectedness and social capital. However, we *are* encouraging you to embrace the concepts of community building and empowerment as the primary guides for how you view and work with communities. In contrast to the traditional problem-focused orientation of community organizing, the community-building approach (Minkler et al., 2008) focuses on community assets and strengths and blends "community identity and autonomy with the dimensions of community planning" and "community action" (p. 292). And, instead of the outsider/organizer-led work of some community-organizing efforts, community empowerment fosters *community-led* initiatives to reach *community-defined* goals.

Thus, the community building and empowerment perspectives contribute to capacity building by shifting the focus from *doing for* the community to *working with* the community in partnerships that enable the community to *do for itself.* A healthy community can emerge when community members develop social capital and invest it in health-promoting actions (see Figure 2.3). We use these concepts throughout this textbook to talk about such processes as assets mapping (chapter 6), coalition building (chapter 7), and community-based participatory research (chapter 9).

Partnership Development

Capacity building that is based on the principles of community building and empowerment necessitates the development of strong community-based partnerships. Your partnership-building objective should be to nurture a shared vision that connects community goals to the services and actions you can help develop. The strategies for partner development listed in FYI 2.1 may help you achieve your objective.

FYI **2.1   Strategies for Partnership Development**

Community-Based Goals: Emphasize community goals rather than agency objectives. Clearly state agency objectives and activities but frame them as partnership contributions toward community goals.

Strength-Focused Discussions: Focus on community strengths, assets, and capacities rather than shortcomings.

Shared Power: Involve community members as true partners. Share decision-making power, responsibilities, and credit. Whenever possible, be flexible and follow their lead.

Realistic Expectations: Be cautious and realistic about promised contributions, planned activities, and expected outcomes. Establish clear understandings about roles, limitations, and expectations for all partners. Be consistent and follow through.

Celebrate Accomplishments: Celebrate every stage of accomplishment. Be willing to adapt to changing needs and capacities over time.

Sources: *Community Capacity and Capacity Building*, by R. J. Chaskin, P. Brown, S. Venkatesh, and A. Vidal, 2001, Hawthorne, NY: Aldine; *Health Behavior and Health Education: Theory, Research, and Practice*, 4th ed., by K. Glanz, B. K. Rimer, and K. Viswanath (Eds.), 2008, San Francisco: Jossey-Bass; *Community Organizing and Community Building for Health*, 2nd ed., by M. Minkler (Ed.), 2005, New Brunswick, NJ: Rutgers University Press.

A true community-based partnership is evident when the community commits to identifying its own needs, creating community-based goals, and using its own strengths to achieve those goals. Though we understand that your role in the partnership must in some way match the goals of your work setting, these goals should be presented to the community as a guide for how *you* can partner with *them* to achieve *their* goals. Discussions that emphasize community strengths and capacities can help avoid the unintended implication that the community needs to be rescued by you. Identifying community assets can facilitate a shared power approach that engages community members as true partners in decisions and responsibilities.

All partners engaged in the effort must maintain realistic expectations. One way to accomplish this is through clear communication about the expected roles of each partner. Open discussions about expectations, progress, and anticipated outcomes will help avoid misunderstandings. You will likely find that a sincere, ongoing effort to be true to your word and to follow through may strengthen the community's trust in you; but be patient. Community trust-building takes time and consistent effort.

As you and your community partners work toward community goals, we encourage you to celebrate each progressive step in the work, no matter how small it may seem (celebrated accomplishments). Community building and partnership development require hard work, and observable outcomes seldom happen quickly. Well-designed goals and objectives (see chapter 7) should measure incremental progress, and can therefore serve as milestones of success. And nothing contributes to the momentum of capacity building quite like the celebration of success.

Cultural Competence

We would be remiss if we did not caution you about the potential challenges of partnership development and capacity building. Your level of cultural competence within the community you serve could facilitate or destroy your chances of success. Imagine attempting to establish a partnership with a community that you know nothing about, and having to rely on what you *think* you know about that community based upon what you *think* you know about its culture.

Consider, for example, the case of a health professional who mistakenly assumed that all Latina women in a community adhered to traditional Catholic views about using birth control, and shaped recommendations for community health promotion accordingly. Or the health professional who suspected an eating disorder when an adolescent female consistently refused to eat when others were eating (Mayo Clinic, 2008), only to discover the young female was observing Ramadan, the Islamic month for prayer and spiritual cleansing, and could only eat after sundown and before sunrise (F. Youssefi, personal communication, April 4, 2000). As in these cases, you may discover a tendency to act on stereotypes (oversimplified and distorted images or descriptions of a group) or faulty assumptions that can cause you to inadvertently misinterpret, misadvise, and impede trust in the community you wish to serve. That is why health professionals must develop cultural competence as an essential component of capacity building.

Cultural competence in community health education and promotion has been defined as "the ability of an individual to understand and respect values, attitudes, beliefs, and mores that differ across cultures, and to consider and respond appropriately to these differences in planning, implementing, and evaluating health education and promotion programs and interventions" (Gold & Miner, 2002, p. 4). This definition integrates **cultural awareness** (gaining descriptive knowledge about cultural norms and practices) with **cultural sensitivity** (understanding and respecting the values and beliefs that shape those norms and practices). Cultural awareness and sensitivity, coupled with basic guidelines for effective cross-cultural communication, can lead to cultural competence (see chapter 11).

Cultural competence begins with an awareness of differences between one's personal cultural perspectives and those of community members, and progresses to a respectful insight into the reasons behind those differences. As adults, these differences can sometimes be shaped by our **cultural luggage.** The influence of culture has been described as mental programs or ways of assigning meaning that a person learns during childhood from caregivers/families, schools, and communities (Hofstede, 2001). These mental programs are the cultural "luggage that each of us carries around for our lifetime" (Spector, 2004, p. 9). This cultural influence can shape the way an individual interacts and connects with others. For example, if you were taught as a child that direct eye contact with a person of authority is disrespectful, you may automatically misinterpret the behavior of a person who was taught that direct eye contact is a way of showing respect. A culturally competent response to eye contact, or the lack of it, can then be based on an understanding of and appreciation for the culture-based reasons behind that behavior.

When we use the word *luggage*, we do not mean to imply that these ways of thinking are negative. Most cultural luggage contains both positive and negative elements. The utility of this term is that it serves as a reminder that most individuals, including health professionals, are influenced by the cultural luggage they still carry as adults, even if they are aware that it exists. When you are in the early stages of learning how to appropriately interact in a culture that is different from your own, you will likely make some mistakes along the way. A teachable attitude and a willingness to apologize when those mistakes happen (cultural humility) will positively impact your trust-building efforts in the community.

Be patient and realistic in your expectations when working to become culturally competent in a community of interest. Because true cultural competence in all contexts is virtually impossible to achieve, it is more accurately described as a developmental process rather than an arrival point. It often takes months to begin to gain some basic understandings of a particular culture group and years to develop a significant level of competence in effectively working with that group. True cultural competence is a life-long developmental process. You will know that you are moving in a positive direction toward cultural competence if you:

- Engage in ongoing self-analysis to identify and address your personal perspectives and any existing cross-cultural biases.

- Actively seek to view life through the eyes of others and, through that, develop a greater level of sensitivity for the values and life challenges of other groups.

- Participate in hands-on training opportunities for practice and feedback that can help you master new skills and refine existing techniques that enhance cultural competence.

- Seek opportunities to engage in cross-cultural interactions in all aspects of life. (Doyle, 2008, p. 165)

In general, your ability to identify and appreciate a community's collective heritage (culture, ethnicity, religion) as a source of social capital will enable you to interact from a culturally competent standpoint. Self-identified ethnic communities or subgroups often have a strong sense of pride and community identity that can be a valuable capacity-building asset.

Community Health Partnerships and Settings

We began this chapter by explaining that a healthy community enables its members to maintain quality of life and productivity through health care treatment and prevention services, healthy and safe environments, and healthy infrastructure

(USDHHS, 2001). We followed with descriptions of community structure, community capacity, and capacity-building concepts to help you develop a conceptual framework for community health. We offer in this final section a brief introduction to organizations and settings in which community health partnerships often occur. We invite you to visit the Web sites of organizations and programs mentioned in this chapter, and those listed in Appendix A, to learn more about current community health partnerships and settings.

The *Healthy People* Framework

The *Healthy People* initiative (USDHHS, 2007c) is a good place to begin learning about community health partnerships and settings. The two primary goals of *Healthy People 2010*, to increase quality and years of healthy life and eliminate health disparities, serve as a road map for community health promotion. The *Healthy People* plan for educational and community-based programs encompasses a comprehensive socio-ecological approach to promoting community health through four settings: schools, worksites, health care facilities, and communities (USDHHS, 2000, 2007c). Figure 2.4 on the following page illustrates these four settings, the 2010 objectives created for each setting, and some national initiatives designed to address or monitor progress toward achieving those objectives.

School Setting

In the United States, the school setting (see Figure 2.4) includes public and private educational institutions for kindergarten through 12th grade (K–12) as well as colleges and universities. Although the extent to which health is part of the K–12 curriculum differs from state to state, most states include health in the public school curriculum at some learning level. But school health includes more than what happens in the classroom. The CDC's National Center for Chronic Disease Prevention and Health Promotion promotes school health through its Division of Adolescent and School Health (DASH). Examples of DASH-supported efforts include the Youth Risk Behavior Surveillance System (YRBSS), a national database of priority health-risk behaviors; the School Health Index, a self-assessment and planning tool that schools use to enhance health-related policies and programs; and capacity-building support for nongovernmental organizations (NGOs) to help prevent HIV infection and other priority health problems in schools and high-risk youth populations.

DASH leaders also develop Coordinated School Health Programs (CSHPs) that engage community members and organizations as partners with local schools to create a more comprehensive health promotion approach. The eight-component CSHP model includes planned and sequential curricula for the health education and physical education classrooms; three components that promote coordinated health, nutrition, and counseling and psychological services for students; a healthy school environment component that addresses physical and psycho-social safety and well-being; a health promotion for staff component for school employees; and a family/community involvement component that promotes school-parent-community partnerships. According to the *Healthy People 2010: Midcourse Review* (USDHHS, 2007c), a report on the progress made toward *Healthy People 2010* objectives by the halfway (5-year) point, the CSHPs and partnerships with school nursing associations are largely responsible for successful objective achievements in this setting.

Student health on college and university campuses is another *Healthy People 2010* priority in the school setting. Through DASH, the CDC partnered with the American College Health Association (ACHA) to develop a manual, *Healthy Campus 2010: Mak-*

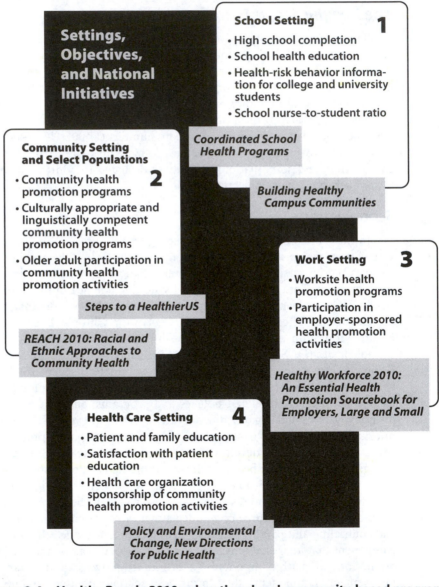

Figure 2.4   Healthy People 2010, educational and community-based programs.

Source: *Healthy People 2010: Midcourse Review*, U.S. Department of Health and Human Services, 2007, Washington, DC: U.S. Government Printing Office.

ing It Happen (ACHA, 2002), and to launch the Building Healthy Campus Communities Project to enhance the capacity of health professionals who work in campus health centers to address health-risk behaviors among college students and promote healthy campus environments.

The midcourse review of *Healthy People 2010* (USDHHS, 2007c) noted that mechanisms to assess health-risk behavior information provided to college and university students are not yet in place. This reminds us of a useful principle for capacity building. The objectives created to reach your community's long-term goals will likely be in a constant state of development and readjustment over time. Don't panic if some of your original objectives are not addressed or achieved. This is a normal part of long-range community health promotion. We will provide more information about developing goals and objectives in chapter 7.

Work Setting

Worksite health promotion and employee wellness programs are another important setting for promoting healthy communities. Business leaders who support these programs often do so to reduce employee absenteeism, increase productivity and job satisfaction, and lower insurance and health care costs. The following worksite health promotion terms (Partnership for Prevention, 2001, p. 4) may be of use if you engage in worksite health promotion:

- *work promotion* and *health and productivity management:* terms used to describe, promote, and track links between employee health and productivity
- *demand management* and *medical self-care:* terms that relate to appropriate use of health services and self-care practices
- *health risk appraisals* (HRAs): measures of health risk based on behaviors and genetic history
- *population health management:* the use of HRA databases as health assessment and programming tools
- *virtual wellness:* technology-based health promotion

Worksite health promotion programs vary greatly. Some companies initiate their own programs, while others contract out for part or all of their health promotion efforts. Common health education classes include stress management, fitness, smoking cessation, nutrition, weight management, parenting, and drug abuse prevention; programs in cancer and cardiovascular disease awareness and prevention are also common. Health fairs, screenings, and HRAs are regular components of most programs. Some programs consist of after-work and weekend recreation activities that involve employees and their families in friendly sports competitions. Company picnics, marathons, ropes courses for professional development, and other one-time events may also fall under the worksite health promotion umbrella in some settings. Management of facilities, equipment, and personnel is part of the job in larger programs.

Based on results of the *1999 National Worksite Health Promotion Survey* (Association for Worksite Health Promotion, 1999), at least 34% of organizations employing 50 or more employees, and 50% of those with 750 or more employees, offered comprehensive worksite health promotion programs; 90% of worksites surveyed provided at least one employee health promotion activity. Those findings prompted the development of *Healthy People* objectives to increase to 75% both the percentage of worksites offering comprehensive programs and employee participation levels in employer-sponsored health promotion activities.

Though progress toward these worksite objectives has been mixed (Linnan et al., 2007; USDHHS, 2007c), a number of initiatives are underway to promote worksite health. For example, CDC's Healthier Worksite Initiative and Worksite Safety and Health Web pages (www.cdc.gov/niosh) contain resources, program models, and other information that can be used for worksite health promotion. Partnership for Prevention, a national membership organization that promotes evidence-based efforts for health promotion and disease prevention, provides information linking employee health to business-related benefits (2001) and an action guide that encourages employers to help reduce tobacco use and exposure and promote cancer screenings, physical activity, and healthy eating among their employees (2008b).

Health Care Setting

Health care providers are in a unique position to improve the health of individuals in several ways. The most obvious avenue of influence is through diagnosis and treatment that can help an individual move away from illness on the illness-wellness continuum (chapter 1). However, as we explained, healing and recovery to the point of the absence of illness is not the full definition of health. There is much more that can be done in health care settings to contribute to high levels of wellness, holistic health, and quality of life. Teachable moments arise when patients interact with health care providers about specific health conditions. The influence of health care providers on health behavior can be powerful (USDHHS, 2000).

An organization called The Alliance for the Healthiest Nation, a collaboration of individuals and organizations committed to accelerating improvements in America's health system, called for a commitment "to rebalancing our nation's health system and making sure that our investments prioritize health promotion, prevention of poor health, and preparedness for new threats—just as much as they prioritize access to affordable quality medical care for these conditions once they do occur" (2008, para. 1). The CDC-supported Guide to Community Preventive Services, an online source of information for health care and prevention, asserts that health care professionals are "ideally situated to promote partnerships between practitioners and community groups to address such issues as physical activity, nutrition, vaccination coverage, and tobacco use" (2009, para. 1). Recommendations for improving the U.S. health system include training health care professionals to work in multidisciplinary teams and community partnerships for "better prevention and management of chronic diseases to enhance quality of life" (Commonwealth Fund, 2008, p. 10; IOM, 2003, 2007).

The *Healthy People 2010* goals for health care settings originally included patient and family education as well as health care organization sponsorship of community health promotion activities (Figure 2.4). Though these objectives had to be dropped at the midpoint review due to lack of sufficient data to address them (USDHHS, 2007c), a number of professionals in health care settings are nevertheless engaging in partnerships that promote healthy communities (Keck, 2006; IOM, 2007). It is likely that efforts in this area will be reviewed and included in the 2020 objectives.

Community Setting

It may seem a bit confusing to talk about *community* settings as one of four distinct areas in which community-based programs occur, especially when the other three settings (schools, worksites, and health facilities) are also considered channels to the broader community. Our earlier statement about how communities are defined by what people have in common may be helpful in understanding the rationale. Health promotion programs implemented in the other three settings impact three loosely defined groups in America: working adults, school- and college-aged young people, and medical patients who are eligible for and need health care services. However, those three channels of access do not reach all members of the broader American community. That is why a community setting, one that allows for a wide variety of approaches to community-based programming, is needed.

In the *Healthy People* framework, the community setting includes "public facilities; local government and agencies; and social service, faith, and civic organizations that provide channels to reach people where they live, work, and play" (USDHHS, 2000, sect. 7). A major contributor to these community-based efforts is the **public health system**. Though both public and private organizations are considered part of this system, governmental health agencies are the backbone of public health (IOM, 2002, 2003; National Association of County and City Health Officials [NACCHO], 2006). The 10 **essential public health services** listed in FYI 2.2 serve as a guide for U.S. public health agencies at the national/federal, state, and local levels (Public Health Functions Steering Committee, 1994). The U.S. government also engages in international public health efforts (Merson, Black, & Mills, 2006). However, we will begin our

FYI **2.2**   **Essential Public Health Services**

1. **Monitor health status** to identify and solve community health problems.
2. **Diagnose and investigate** health problems and health hazards in the community.
3. **Inform, educate, and empower people** about health issues.
4. **Mobilize community partnerships** and action to identify and solve health problems.
5. **Develop policies and plans** that support individual and community health efforts.
6. **Enforce laws and regulations** that protect health and ensure safety.
7. **Link people** to needed personal health services and assure the provision of health care when otherwise unavailable.
8. **Assure competent** public and personal health care **workforce.**
9. **Evaluate effectiveness, accessibility, and quality** of personal and population-based health services.
10. **Research for new insights** and innovative solutions to health problems.

Source: *The Essential Public Health Services*, Centers for Disease Control (n.d.). Retrieved August 15, 2008, from http://www.cdc.gov/od/ocphp/nphpsp/essentialphservices.htm

description of community-based public health efforts with a description of local health departments; that is, the units most likely to actively engage as partners in your community-based health promotion efforts.

Local Health Departments

According to NACCHO, **local health departments** (LHDs) are the "foundation of the public health system" (2006, p. 2) because they are primarily responsible for public health promotion in local communities. LHD jurisdictions or service areas can encompass a single county or city, a combined city-county jurisdiction, or a district or region of multiple counties or cities. Most of their funds come from a mixture of local county/city governments and state and federal sources, but some portion can come from private foundations and fees charged to local residents. We mention this to point out that LHDs aren't solely government funded; local community partnerships are important.

An essential component of LHD services includes the ability to respond to disease outbreaks, environmental hazards, natural disasters, and, since the 2001 terrorist attacks on the World Trade Centers and other targets, emergency preparedness for threats of bioterrorism (NACCHO, 2006). Though specific services and activities vary, many LHDs provide (or partner with other organizations to provide) adult and child immunizations, communicable/infectious disease surveillance and screenings (for example, tuberculosis and sexually transmitted diseases/infections), chronic disease surveillance and prevention (high blood pressure and cancer screenings, tobacco use prevention, exercise and healthy eating promotion, etc.), food service inspections and food safety education, and environmental health surveillance and protection. Maternal and child health services are offered by a large number of LHDs, while a smaller number also offer behavioral/mental health services, substance abuse services, oral health care, home health care, and primary health care and treatment services (NACCHO, 2006).

"The role of every LHD is to intentionally coordinate all public health activities in a community, regardless of which organization may take the lead in a particular area" (NACCHO, 2006, p. 43). So whether you work in a nongovernmental organization or government agency, the LHD that serves your community of interest will be a critical ally in your community health education and promotion efforts. This is true not only because of LHD connections with local community groups but also because LHDs are often linked to available information and resources from state and federal health agencies.

State Health Departments

The Association of State and Territorial Health Officials (ASTHO) is the national nonprofit organization that represents U.S. state public health agencies (also U.S. territories and the District of Columbia). "State public health functions may be assigned to a single health agency, to several divisions within an umbrella agency, or among a number of independent state agencies" (ASTHO, 2007, p. 2). But despite this variance in structure, most state health departments (SHDs) engage in health promotion and protection efforts related to chronic and infectious disease, emergency and disaster preparedness, environmental health and safety, health care delivery, maternal and child health, mental health and substance abuse, and injury control (ASTHO, 2007). Some SHDs provide community-specific health data (by county, city, or zip code) and support for capacity-building projects (for example, funding, training, informa-tion/materials, or technical assistance).

Federal Health Agencies

In addition to local and state efforts, the federal government promotes commu-nity-based programs through the **U.S. Department of Health and Human Services** (USDHHS). The USDHHS (2008b) protects health and provides basic human ser-vices for U.S. citizens. It sponsors over 300 programs, including the *Healthy People* ini-tiative; health insurance programs for the elderly and disabled (Medicare) and low-income individuals (Medicaid); and **Head Start**, a preschool education and ser-vices program for low-income children. The public health service agencies within the USDHHS (see Appendix E) are highly visible and active agents for community health promotion. Among them is the Centers for Disease Control and Prevention (CDC), the primary agency for national public health initiatives. The CDC's mission is "to promote health and quality of life by preventing and controlling disease, injury, and disability," embodied in its vision for the 21st century: "Healthy People in a Healthy World—Through Prevention" (CDC, n.d., *About,* para. 1). In addition to the office of the director, the CDC consists of the National Institute for Occupational Safety and Health, and coordinating centers/offices for environmental health, health information and service, health promotion, infectious diseases, global health, and terrorism preparedness and emergency response (CDC, 2007c; see chart, Appendix E). In each of these subunits, "CDC seeks to accomplish its mission by working with partners throughout the nation and the world to:

- monitor health
- detect and investigate health problems
- conduct research to enhance prevention
- develop and advocate sound public health policies
- implement prevention strategies
- promote healthy behaviors
- foster safe and healthful environments
- provide leadership and training" (CDC, 2006c)

The USDHHS and CDC promote the empowerment of communities through a number of successful programs and initiatives. One example is the *Steps to a Healthier US Initiative* (Steps) established in 2003 to promote health and prevent chronic disease in U.S. communities (USDHHS, n.d., *Steps*). This national program focuses on diabe-tes, obesity, and asthma with a specific emphasis on promoting physical activity and nutrition and preventing tobacco use. Funding is provided to local communities in urban areas, rural counties (through state health departments), and tribal groups (CDC, 2008k). Steps program partners also include several nongovernmental organi-zations at the national level. For example, the YMCA of the USA has worked to dis-tribute mini-grants to fund local community Steps projects, and the Robert Wood Johnson Foundation and the University of North Carolina School of Public Health are linked to the Steps program through the Active Learning by Design program.

The Steps program supports similar boundary-crossing partnerships at the local community level by "reaching beyond the public health community and bringing together a wide range of disciplines—including business, transportation, and city planning—to help improve the health of local communities" (CDC, 2008k, p. 5). Funded community partners have established community-based walking programs, weight management and exercise programs for kids and parents, health assessments in tribal communities, public service announcements about healthy behaviors, fitness programs in faith-based centers, and other projects in school, worksite, and health care settings. A Steps program action guide, *The Community Health Promotion Handbook: Action Guides to Improve Community Health* (CDC, 2008d) is a valuable online resource for communities of all sizes.

Another CDC-sponsored program with a capacity-building focus is the Racial and Ethnic Approaches to Community Health Across the U.S. (REACH U.S.) program (CDC, 2007a). REACH U.S. is specifically designed to eliminate health disparities among ethnic groups through Action Communities (ACs), "community-based programs implementing evidence-based programs and approaches to eliminate disparities in a selected health problem. ACs are particularly attentive to cultural and environmental influences on health status and behaviors" (para. 3). REACH U.S. funds are also used to support Centers of Excellence in the Elimination of Disparities (CEEDs), national and regional centers through which culturally competent experts mentor "communities in processes of community mobilization, community-based participatory research, and program development and evaluation" (para. 2).

We encourage you to visit the Web sites of the national health agencies listed in Appendix A and develop a general familiarity with their contribution to community health promotion.

Other Health Organizations

NGOs are also part of the community setting targeted by *Healthy People* objectives. These largely nonprofit organizations often serve as essential partners in community-based programs because of the health-related expertise, cultural competence, community connections, and funding support they can provide. For example, **voluntary health agencies** (VHAs) such as the American Heart Association and the American Cancer Society contribute to community health through public education, patient services, research, and advocacy related to a specific health issue or special population.

Faith-based organizations and other **nonprofit community organizations** with established roots in, or connections to, a local community can open doors for you, both literally and figuratively, to establish community partnerships. Local community residents who work or volunteer in these organizations, and the professionals who work with them, can help shape the program in ways that meet community interests and needs in a culturally appropriate format.

Private and grant-making **foundations** (Appendix A) not only provide needed funds for NGOs and public health agencies, but also can provide expertise and support to community-based partnership groups. The Robert Wood Johnson Foundation (RWJF) mentioned earlier and the W.K. Kellogg Foundation (WKKF) are examples of grant-making foundations that actively support community-based health promotion programs and other community empowerment initiatives. The RWJF (2008) funds a variety of health-related initiatives including childhood obesity, vulnerable populations, and various aspects of public health and health care. The WKKF (n.d.) promotes capacity-building efforts that improve the lives of vulnerable children (and their families and communities) in the United States, southern Africa, South America, and the Caribbean.

A commitment to global health is evident in the activities of several U.S. organizations and agencies. For example, the USDHHS **Office of Global Health Affairs** maintains a Web site called globalhealth.gov (Appendix A) and collaborates with other agencies and governments to address international and refugee health issues (USDHHS, 2007a). The CDC maintains a global health Web page called Healthy People in a Healthy World (CDC, n.d., *Healthy*) and partners with the World Health Organization on a variety of global health initiatives. The **World Health Organization** (WHO), part of the United Nations system, leads the world in global health promotion. WHO's (2008f) socio-ecological approach to global health is evident in its six-point agenda: two health objectives (health security and health systems), two strategic needs (socioeconomic development and research-related efforts), and two operational approaches (partnerships and organizational efficiency/effectiveness). WHO is headquartered in Geneva, Switzerland, with six regional offices strategically placed around the world. The Pan American Health Organization (PAHO), headquartered in Washington, DC, serves as the WHO regional office to the Americas. We encourage you to become familiar with WHO and other global health organizations (Appendix A). As we discuss in chapter 14, you will likely discover a global health connection to your work, even if you never work outside of the United States.

In Conclusion

Health professionals from a wide variety of disciplines are working in community-based partnerships to build capacities, empower communities, and promote the concept of *healthy communities*. Your ability to develop cultural competence and form strong partnerships will impact your level of success in the community you serve. A number of public health organizations (both government and nongovernment) are working toward solutions to community health needs. A community's ability to assume leadership and provide health-enhancing opportunities for its members is the true key to becoming a healthy community. We invite you to consider the perspectives and processes described in subsequent chapters in light of the community and cultural concepts presented here.

 REVIEW QUESTIONS

1. Define healthy communities and describe what they do for their community members.

2. Describe Maslow's hierarchy of needs and the model of heritage consistency and explain how they contribute to social connectedness.

3. Define community capacity and describe its elements (social connectedness, social capital, environmental components).

4. Define community empowerment, community building, and community organizing and explain their importance in community health promotion.

5. Describe the model for community capacity building and recommended approaches to community partnership development.

6. Define cultural competence, cultural luggage, and cultural humility and explain their impact on community partnership development and capacity building.

7. Describe the four settings in which the *Healthy People* initiative has targeted efforts to establish educational and community-based programs. Identify some accomplishments and challenges associated with each.

8. Describe the role of public health agencies at the local, state, and national levels. What role do nongovernmental organizations play in community health partnerships?

☛ FOR YOUR APPLICATION

Neighborhood Windshield Tour

Conduct a windshield tour or a walk-through in a local low-income neighborhood. (Be sure to find out about neighborhood safety before you go and take needed precautions.) Go with a friend who can help you note the condition of store fronts, housing, and automobiles; existing and missing resources (food stores, gas stations, banks, health clinics) and access to private (cars) and public transportation (buses, taxis, subways); the nature and content of prominent signs and/or graffiti; and the types of activities and interactions of people who live and work there. Visit the neighborhood at different times of the day and on different days of the week to note the ebb and flow of community life. If possible, sit in a local eatery or public place and observe patterns of activity. Then, drive through a more economically developed neighborhood and note similarities and contrasts. Create a list of your impressions for both types of neighborhoods. Identify factors that contribute to these neighborhood differences and any health-related implications.

Epidemiological Considerations

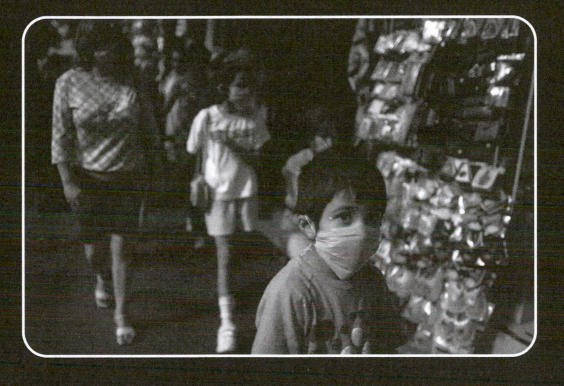

You have just started a new job at the local public health department. The director notifies you that a local physician has reported a case of measles (a disease that is preventable through vaccination). He says that he and other health officials are concerned about the potential for an epidemic. You are not absolutely sure what he means or how they will know an epidemic has started. In fact, even through measles is a disease almost everyone has heard about, you can't remember many specifics of its causes, transmission, or symptoms. You wonder what role you will play if there is an epidemic.

CHAPTER OBJECTIVES

1. Describe the epidemiological approach to understanding patterns of disease and disease-related behaviors among humans.
2. List the purposes of epidemiology.
3. Compare current and historical life expectancies in the United States.
4. Identify measures of mortality and morbidity.
5. Classify causes of disease.
6. Describe the factors that influence morbidity.
7. List sources of epidemiologic data.
8. Describe concepts related to infectious disease, such as agent, host, environment, mode of transmission, and spectrum of disease.
9. Identify concepts related to noninfectious disease, such as acute illness, chronic illness, and web of causation.

The Epidemiological Approach in the Community

The word *epidemiology* originally comes from Greek. If you have studied medical terminology, you know that the suffix *ology* means "study of" and the prefix *epi* means "among or upon." The root word *deme* means "commune or group of people." Therefore, the literal definition would be "the study of groups of people." We think a good working definition of **epidemiology** is the study of disease, the determinants of health, and the behaviors that prevent or cause disease or injury among groups of people. This definition implies that epidemiology serves many purposes. Some of these purposes are to

- study past or current trends in health status or level of disease
- identify causes of death
- establish **etiology** (cause) of disease
- define risk factors and determinants of disease
- determine need for health services

- identify feasible disease-prevention and health promotion strategies
- suggest need for future research in health and disease
- predict future disease outbreaks

An **epidemiologist** is a specialist in **epidemics**, or outbreaks of disease. In a sense, epidemiologists are detectives. They seek answers. In general, epidemiologists consider the population as a whole, or the community, in their investigations. They ask questions of individuals so that they can understand the disease or prevention strategy in the group. You may not be preparing to be an epidemiologist; however, you will need to understand their work. You may be part of a team that studies specific issues related to health or you may use an epidemiologist's report to support your work in prevention. In any case, basic knowledge of the field is imperative to your success.

If you were responsible for gathering information about diseases, and there was an outbreak of a disease in your community, how would you start your investigation? Some obvious questions might be "How many people are sick now?" and "How quickly is it spreading?" With our hypothetical case of measles, you would first find out as much as possible about measles. Even if you already knew a lot about the disease, you would find out if new information had been discovered. Next, you would talk with the girl who had measles, her physician, and family. Other people with similar symptoms would be interviewed to determine if more cases of measles were present in the community. The long-term purpose of your investigation would be to protect the community from an epidemic.

Even if you weren't yet sure of the name of the disease or its cause, you would probably start with questions like "How many cases?" and "How fast is it spreading?" to determine the incidence and prevalence. You may have heard the words before, but they are sometimes used incorrectly even in professional literature. **Incidence** is the number of new cases of a specific disease among a specific group of people in a specific period of time. For example, in 2006 there were 56,300 new cases of AIDS in the United States (CDC, 2007d). **Prevalence** is the total number of cases (not just the new ones) of a specific disease among a specific group of people in a specific period of time.

As the investigating health professional, you should determine prevalence and incidence in order to make decisions about whether an outbreak, or epidemic, of a disease is present. That's important because an epidemic is an increase in the normal incidence of a disease. You might plot an epidemic curve to assist in the decision-making process. The epidemic curve would illustrate the first infection (**index case**) and the number of new cases at selected intervals in time until there are no further new cases. In our measles example, the case reported to the health department would be the index case. Any others that were found during interviews would be plotted. Historical incidence rates for measles in the community would be compared to the current rate. If the current rates are higher, an outbreak is occurring. If people die as a result of a disease outbreak, you might also determine disease-specific death rates early in the investigation.

Mortality

Of course, you would want to move as quickly as possible in collecting epidemiological information to minimize risk of mortality. **Mortality** means death. Epidemiologists compute crude mortality, or death, rates in order to get an overall picture of the level of death in a community. Mortality rates are computed by dividing the number of deaths in a specific place by the number of people in the population at a given period of time. FYI 3.1 lists formulas commonly used in epidemiology. A **crude mortality rate** cannot be used to estimate the degree of risk an individual has of dying in a community because many factors have powerful influences on death rates. The most powerful is age. If the community you are investigating has a large number of older individuals, it will have a higher mortality rate than a community with many young individuals—not because it is a riskier place to live, but because older people are more likely to die.

What if you suspect that a disease outbreak is specific to a particular age group? To test your assumption, you can compute rates. Sometimes epidemiologists will compute **age-specific mortality** rates in order to study the frequency of death among people of a selected age group. This mortality rate is computed by dividing the num-

---

FYI 3.1   Formulas for Selected Rates and Ratios Used in Epidemiology

Rates and ratios play important roles in epidemiology. They are not difficult to use when you know the formulas. Some of the most common are listed here.

Morbidity

$$\text{Incidence} = \frac{\text{Number of new cases of a disease}}{\text{Total number of people at risk}} \text{ over a period of time } \times 100{,}000$$

$$\text{Attack Rate} = \frac{\text{Number of people sick}}{\text{Number of people both sick and well}} \text{ during a period of time } \times 100$$

$$\text{Prevalence} = \frac{\text{Total number of people with a disease}}{\text{Average number of people}} \text{ during a period of time } \times 100{,}000$$

Mortality

$$\text{Crude mortality} = \frac{\text{Number of deaths in a selected year}}{\text{Number of people in the population}} \times 100{,}000$$

$$\text{Infant mortality*} = \frac{\text{Number of infant deaths during a year}}{\text{Number of live births during a year}} \times 1{,}000$$

$$\text{Disease-specific mortality} = \frac{\text{Number of deaths due to a specific disease}}{\text{Number in population}} \times 100{,}000$$

$$\text{Age-specific mortality} = \frac{\text{Number of deaths in a specific age group}}{\text{Number of people in the same age group}} \times 100{,}000$$

*Infant deaths are defined as deaths among babies from 0 to 365 days old.

ber of deaths among people in a specific age group (for example, 13–18 year olds) by the number of people in the age category at a specific period of time. You can also compute the mortality for other age groups to compare across groups. Performing calculations to remove age influences on crude mortality rates makes it more feasible to compare risk of death between communities because you have removed the effect of the factor that influences rates the most.

Morbidity

Morbidity means illness. We've already stated that incidence and prevalence are morbidity rates commonly used by epidemiologists and other health professionals to determine the level of illness in a community. The morbidity rates of different types of diseases that affect communities vary over time, according to the place, and with the characteristics of the people. If you review Figure 3.1 (on the following page) you will note shifts in the types of disease that caused death in the 20th century. As you can see, the types of disease that were the leading causes of death early in the 20th century are completely different than the leading causes of death early in the 21st century.

Major causes of morbidity come from two categories of disease, infectious and noninfectious. Infectious diseases such as tuberculosis (TB), pneumonia, and gastroenteritis were more common causes of death in the early 1900s than were noninfectious diseases (Friis & Sellers, 1999). Today, noninfectious diseases like heart disease, cancer, and stroke are the most common causes of death (National Center for Health Statistics, 2007b), although we may see another shift if infectious diseases like avian flu become prevalent in the United States. Morbidity and mortality influence both life expectancy and quality of life, which are two issues that make the understanding of epidemiology imperative for health educators.

Life Expectancy

Fluctuations in morbidity and mortality rates in a community will, of course, affect the life expectancy of its residents. **Life expectancy** refers to the average number of years groups of people are expected to live. Life expectancy rates have changed over time. Advances in available treatments, prevention methods, and healthier lifestyles have contributed to the change. In 1900 the life expectancy in the United States was 47.3 years, whereas in 2005 the U.S. life expectancy was 77.8 (Kung, Hoyert, Xu, & Murphy, 2008). In 2006, preliminary data indicated that life expectancy at birth had risen to a record high of 78.1 years (Heron, Hoyert, Xu, Scott, & Tejada-Vera, 2008a), but final data put that number at 77.7 (Heron, Hoyert, Murphy et al., 2009). Figure 3.2 (on p. 53) graphs life expectancies for men and women and Blacks and Caucasians in the United States. The reasons behind the differences in genders and ethnic groups are not easy to understand; however, it is imperative to both seek the causes of the differences and actively address them.

According to Marmot and Wilkinson (2006), differences in life expectancy are directly related to poverty. Low socioeconomic status influences insurance coverage, which in turn, influences access to medical care. Even if medical care is accessible, poor people may not be able to afford nutritious food or even enough food. Their housing may be inadequate and safety may be a major issue. Education may not be

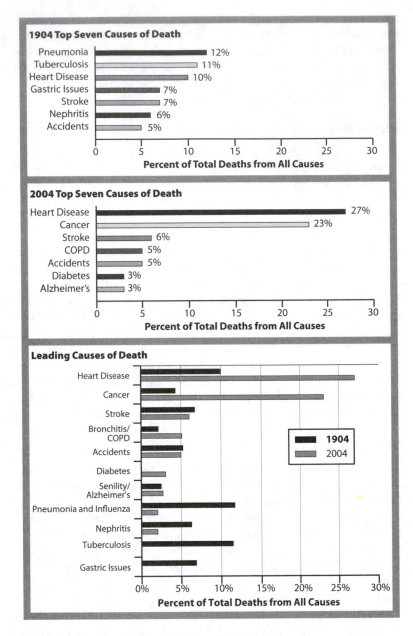

Figure 3.1   Shifts in causes of death from 1904 to 2004.

As you can see from these graphs, the types of diseases that cause death have shifted over time. Even though we are currently seeing some infectious diseases, such as tuberculosis, becoming more prevalent today, the major causes of death are related to lifestyle choices.

Sources: "Deaths, Percent of Total Deaths, and Death Rates for the 15 Leading Causes of Death: United States and Each State, 1999–2004," Centers for Disease Control and Prevention, 2007. Retrieved April 12, 2008, from http://www.cdc.gov/nchs/data/dvs/LCWK9_2004.pdf; "Deaths and Death Rates for Leading Causes of Death: Death Registration States, 1900–1940." Retrieved April 12, 2008, from http://www.cdc.gov/nchs/data/dvs/lead1900_98. pdf.

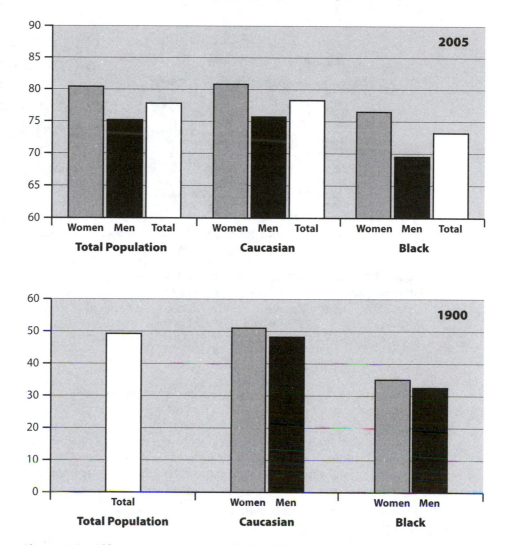

Figure 3.2   Life expectancy charts, United States, 1900 and 2005.
Life expectancy has increased dramatically over time for all people in the United States; however, disparities still exist between people of different ethnicities. These charts illustrate both the increase in life expectancy and some of the disparities.
Sources: "United States Life Tables," by E. Arias, 2007, *National Vital Statistics Reports*, 56(9); "Deaths: Final Data for 2005," by H. Kung, D. Hoyert, J. Xu, and S. Murphy, 2008, *National Vital Statistics Reports*, 56(10).

attainable; and this problem alone influences all of the aforementioned. Poverty and its influence on health will be discussed in more detail in later chapters.

Figure 3.3 illustrates the life expectancies of people in selected regions of the world. Note the differences in life expectancies and try to identify some of the reasons they exist. Life expectancy rates sometimes differ as a result of the level of development of a country or region. Some regions just don't have the technology to address

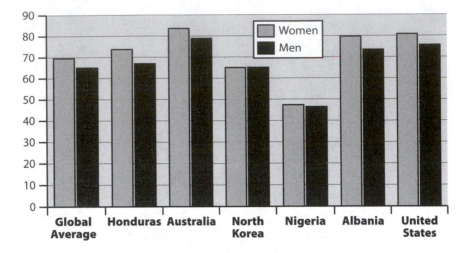

Figure 3.3   Life expectancies for selected regions.
Life expectancies have not increased for all regions of the world. As you can see from this chart, some countries fall well below the United States and other developed countries.
Source: "Field Listing—Life Expectancy at Birth," CIA Fact Book, 2008. Retrieved August 12, 2008, from https://www.cia.gov/library/publications/the-world-factbook/fields/2002.html

medical problems that is available to developed countries. Other regions have environmental problems or cultural practices that influence life expectancies. For example, a nuclear power plant accident could cause dramatic increases in several types of cancer. Health professionals have an opportunity to broaden the scope of their work in communities by seeking answers to root causes of death and disease. In order to do so, they must understand where to get information about how disease impacts the population.

Sources of Data

Prevention efforts should begin with the collection of health-related data or epidemiological research. Plans for health education programs of all types should be based on assessment of relevant information. There are two major places from which information can be gathered for the epidemiological investigation. These include primary and secondary sources.

Primary Sources

Using primary sources of data involves the active process of collecting specific information through research. In our example, you would need to collect data on how many individuals have measles; their ages; the disease status of their families, friends, and associates; and immunization status of the community. This strategy helps you accomplish two things. The most obvious is that it can provide accurate, community-specific data about the problem and potential solutions. If conducted appropriately, the process can also help you establish important relationships with community members.

In primary data collection efforts, epidemiologists use four major types of studies to discover patterns, compare numbers, and establish causation. These study types include cross-sectional, cohort, case-control, and experimental designs. We will learn more about the research process itself in chapter 9, but for now let's examine these four study designs.

Cross-Sectional Studies

These studies involve a "snapshot" of a group of people. A **cross-sectional study** is a one-time data-collection effort (by survey or some other means) that often uses a self-report format. **Self-report** simply means that no clinical or official measurement is made; rather, people report information about themselves. This type of study is also called a *prevalence study* if the researcher is studying the presence of a disease. Why would a cross-sectional study determine prevalence? Review the definition of prevalence given earlier in the chapter if you have difficulty answering this question. The title of the study (cross-sectional) describes the sample; a cross section of the population is selected to participate in the study. Many types of information can be gathered during the data-collection process, from health behaviors to attitudes and beliefs.

Cross-sectional studies can identify relationships; for example, if you conducted a survey in an urban community, you might find that many people report a concern about pollution and many people also recycle trash. You can compute a type of statistic called a **correlation** to see if there is a mathematical relationship between the number of people who have concern about pollution and the number who recycle. Unfortunately, if there is a mathematical relationship, it does not prove that having a concern about pollution causes a person to recycle or vice versa. It just means there is a relationship of some sort. Let's look at another example that will make this easier to understand. If you went to a very small town, a medium size town, and a large city and counted both the number of churches and the number of crimes, what do you think you would find? If you computed a correlation, you would find that there is a mathematical relationship (high correlation) between the number of churches and the number of crimes; where there are more churches, there are more crimes. So, should we hold a news conference and declare that churches cause crime? Absolutely not! All we found from our study is that there is a relationship in the numbers—when one number goes up so does the other. Why do you think we would find more crime in places where there are more churches? Hopefully, you realized immediately that when there are more people there will be both more churches and more crimes. We could just have easily counted the number of grocery stores and crimes and discovered the same correlation. Although cross-sectional studies can provide you with a lot of information about relationships, you must be careful not to make unwarranted assumptions about cause and effect.

Cohort Studies

These studies are sometimes called *incidence studies*. As you know, the frequency of new cases of a disease is used to compute an incidence rate. In a **cohort study**, a cohort of healthy people is followed through time to see if they develop a specific disease of interest. Other information is also collected, such as health behaviors, beliefs, and exposures. As a result, the incidence rate for the disease of interest can be computed. Cohort studies allow comparisons of incidence rates between people who report a specific behavior (such as exercise) and those who report they do not engage in the specific behavior (in this case, exercise).

A **cohort** is any group whose members have something in common. The commonality might be age, place or location, gender, occupation, or virtually any other characteristic. Cohort studies cost more than other types of studies because they are carried out over a long period of time. These studies are also referred to as *longitudinal studies* because of the length of time they take, or *prospective studies* because they are future-oriented. One of the classic cohort studies was the Framingham study, in which more than 5,000 people in one community were assessed and followed over many years. The study provided some outstanding information about risk factors for heart disease.

The U.S. Department of Defense began a large cohort study in 2001 because of concerns regarding the long-term health effects of serving in the military. The project currently has 150,000 participants who were randomly selected for the sample. The study will address issues such as posttraumatic stress disorder, depression, alcohol misuse, respiratory illnesses, and brain injuries (Naval Health Research Center, n.d.). Data will be collected every three years until 2022. Some important information has already been identified; for example, "Service members who had experienced prior violent or sexual assault in their lives were more vulnerable to posttraumatic stress disorder after deployment. It was also found that exposure to actual combat rather than deployment itself was a factor in the onset of PTSD symptoms" (Force Health, 2008 p. 4).

Case Control Studies

In **case control** studies, a specific disease is generally the focus of the research. In the most common use of case control, a group of people with the disease is selected to be *cases* in the study. A second group, without the disease but otherwise very similar to the first in regard to characteristics like age, gender, ethnicity, and socioeconomic status, is selected to be *controls*. Researchers ask people in both groups to recall behaviors or health determinants from the past, or they use retrospective (past) medical records to study how the two groups differ. The objective is to discover how and/or why the disease occurs.

D'Souza and associates (2007) conducted a case-control study with 100 oropharyngeal cancer patients and 200 controls. They sought evidence that the human papillomavirus (HPV) played a role in oropharyngeal cancer. They determined that even when cancer patients did not smoke or use alcohol, there was a strong association between infection with HPV and the presence of oropharyngeal cancer.

Experimental Studies

A true scientific experiment is the only type of study from which researchers can determine the cause of a disease or the effectiveness of treatments. In an **experimental study**, participants are randomly selected from the population of interest. A computerized process, much like throwing every person's name into a hat and drawing out the number needed, is used to randomly choose those who will be in the study. This **random selection** process gives each person the same chance of being in the study. In other words, one type of person won't be over- or underrepresented in the study. Participants are also randomly assigned to either the intervention or control group. Participants in the control group will not receive the treatment or intervention but will be treated the same in every other way. Differences in the groups will be analyzed in order to determine the efficacy of the intervention.

The U.S. Food and Drug Administration (USFDA, 2007) conducted an experimental study to determine if the type of health message on food products impacted participants' perceptions and intent to purchase the food. This study was actually conducted via the Internet, which is an increasingly popular method for communicating with study participants. The participants were not randomly selected from the total U.S. population, but the study was still experimental in nature because a legitimate sampling technique was used and an intervention occurred. An experimental study must have an intervention. In the FDA study the findings showed that if a food product had a label giving both the name of a nutrient and the positive health effect to be expected, participants were more likely to consider buying it. Participants were least likely to consider buying a food product that had a label with only a nutrient content message.

Secondary Sources

Secondary data consists of information that has already been collected by national, state, or local sources. Going back to our measles example, it would be wise to identify data that had been collected by other cities regarding measles cases. Secondary data helps you determine how your outbreak compares to those of other communities who face similar issues. You can learn about effective and ineffective approaches attempted in other places and may gain some insight otherwise missed. You can then consider the specific characteristics and needs of your community and adapt what you learned from those secondary sources.

The World Health Organization is a good source of secondary data because it assesses the burden of disease across the globe. The first assessment, sponsored by the World Bank with the help of the Harvard School of Public Health, was conducted in 1993. At that time the project goals, still in use today, were detailed (Murray, Lopez, Mathers, & Stein, 2001). This complex data-collection process is a great example of the use of numerous sources of data. The WHO sources include epidemiologic research (primary data collection) and disease registries, population surveys, and health facility data (secondary data sources).

Disease Registries

Disease registries involve databases that list numbers of new cases of diseases. Certain diseases that occur in the United States are considered notifiable. Physicians or other health care providers who diagnose these illnesses are required to record and report the diseases to the state in which they practice (CDC, 2008f). The state officials then compile and report the numbers to the CDC. As you can see in FYI 3.2, measles is on the notifiable list for 2008. Changes in the specific diseases that require notification occur as new infections emerge or as the incidence declines dramatically over a long period of time.

FYI 3.2   **National Notifiable Infectious Diseases, United States 2008**

Acquired Immunodeficiency
  Syndrome (AIDS)
Anthrax
Arboviral neuroinvasive and
  non-neuroinvasive diseases
Botulism
Brucellosis
Chancroid
Chlamydia trachomatis, genital infections
Cholera
Coccidioidomycosis
Cryptosporidiosis
Cyclosporiasis
Diphtheria
Ehrlichiosis/Anaplasmosis
Giardiasis
Gonorrhea
Haemophilus influenzae, invasive disease
Hansen disease (leprosy)
Hantavirus pulmonary syndrome
Hemolytic uremic syndrome, post-diarrheal
Hepatitis, viral, acute and chronic
HIV infection
Influenza-associated pediatric mortality
Legionellosis
Listeriosis
Lyme disease
Malaria
Measles
Meningococcal disease
Mumps
Novel influenza A virus infections
Pertussis
Plague
Poliomyelitis, paralytic
Poliovirus infection, nonparalytic

Psittacosis
Q Fever
Rabies
Rocky Mountain spotted fever
Rubella
Rubella, congenital syndrome
Salmonellosis
Severe Acute Respiratory Syndrome-
  associated Coronavirus (SARS-CoV) disease
Shiga toxin-producing *Escherichia coli* (STEC)
Shigellosis
Smallpox
Streptococcal disease, invasive, Group A
Streptococcal toxic-shock syndrome
Streptococcus pneumoniae, drug resistant,
  invasive disease
Streptococcus pneumoniae, invasive disease
  non-drug resistant, in children less than
  5 years of age
Syphilis
Syphilis, congenital
Tetanus
Toxic-shock syndrome (other than
  Streptococcal)
Trichinellosis (Trichinosis)
Tuberculosis
Tularemia
Typhoid fever
Vancomycin—intermediate
  Staphylococcus aureus (VISA)
Vancomycin—resistant
  Staphylococcus aureus (VRSA)
Varicella (morbidity)
Varicella (deaths only)
Vibriosis
Yellow fever

From National Notifiable Diseases Surveillance System, Centers for Disease Control and Prevention, 2008f. Retrieved on April 10, 2008, from http://www.cdc.gov/ncphi/disss/nndss/ndsshis.htm

Population Surveys

Health-related data are collected systematically in the United States through **population surveys**. One example of such a survey is the Behavioral Risk Factor Surveillance System (BRFSS). This survey tracks access to health care, presence of diseases and other conditions, and behaviors (preventive and risk) through a self-report telephone survey. Data collection is continuous in all of the states and approximately 350,000 U.S. adults are interviewed each year (CDC, 2008b).

The National Health Care Surveys are a set of surveys conducted among a representative sample of health care providers and health care settings. They provide data about resources for health care, types of procedures and disease management, and characteristics of patients and providers. The information collected can be invaluable for researchers, public health personnel, and policy makers (CDC, 2008e).

Censuses

Censuses originated in combination with the process of taxation in ancient Egypt and Rome. In the United States, the census occurs every 10 years in order to determine seats in the U.S. House of Representatives. Federal funding of some health and social services programs also depends on the number and distribution of people as measured by the U.S. census. As in all self-report surveys, caution is needed when using census data. For example, the ethnic and racial categories listed on the census survey have stirred controversy. There is such diversity in this country that many experts wonder if it is necessary or even possible to categorize ethnicity and race. Other data collected in censuses include gender, age, marital status, type of housing, ancestry, language spoken in the home, year the residence was built, place of birth, education level, employment status, plumbing and kitchen facilities, telephone and vehicle availability, and type of heating and cooling. Combining census data with data about disease helps health professionals gain a clearer picture of a community's health status.

Vital Statistics

In the United States vital life events are recorded and then counted. For example, each newborn receives a birth certificate, and death certificates are generated for each person who dies. The numbers of marriages and divorces also become vital statistics.

With censuses and other kinds of record keeping, there are inaccuracies. Sometimes diseases aren't diagnosed properly or the cause of death is inaccurately listed. As time progresses, diagnostic criteria may change, making comparisons of vital statistics between years less meaningful. Nevertheless, vital statistics provide a great deal of information that helps health professionals. Of course, the reason for collecting data, whether from primary or secondary sources, is to improve the health of individuals and communities. Although health is a great deal more than the prevention of disease, prevention remains one of the primary roles of the health educator.

Prevention

Helping people get the information they need to make healthy choices is one important aspect of prevention. You may even think that your involvement in prevention occurs only before an individual becomes ill. But two of the three categories of prevention take place after the onset of disease.

Primary Prevention

Efforts that occur before individuals become sick are called **primary prevention**. Programs that help people stop smoking before they develop heart disease or cancer reflect primary prevention tactics. Another example of primary prevention is vaccination of children against infectious diseases. Vaccinations trigger the production of antibodies, which in turn prevents future cases of the disease. These types of primary prevention impact the host. It is also possible to change the environment to bring about primary prevention. For example, mosquito control and water fluoridation programs are primary prevention efforts.

Secondary Prevention

Once a disease occurs in an individual, efforts to prevent its progression are called **secondary prevention**. Screening tools like mammography (breast x-rays that screen for cancer) are secondary in nature. They may identify a cancerous lesion at an early stage when it can be treated successfully, thereby preventing progression. Many women believe that if they have yearly mammograms they will not get breast cancer. In fact, mammograms do not prevent breast cancer. Regardless of the disease, any program that screens for disease is a secondary prevention program.

Tertiary Prevention

Tertiary prevention is concerned with the quality of life of individuals with disease. Regardless of a disease's effect on a person, tertiary prevention is practiced when efforts are made to improve the quality of life as much a possible. This may not seem like prevention at all, but the idea is to prevent situations from becoming worse. In other words, to help people with serious diseases live the best life possible. Home health care and hospice care are two examples of tertiary prevention programs.

Think of some actions that you could take to improve the quality of life for someone who has suffered major mobility issues due to the West Nile virus. Then work backward and consider how you would help prevent the individual from getting the virus in the first place. To do this, you will need information about the virus and how it spreads. It's wise to have some general information about disease transmission.

Infectious Disease

Infectious diseases spread from individual to individual or from insects, animals, or other carriers to humans. They are often caused by an easily identified single organism. Important aspects of infectious disease include causative organisms, modes of transmission, reservoirs, spectrum of disease, epidemic curve, immunity, and prevention.

Although many models have been used to illustrate the basic concepts of the epidemiology of infectious disease, the triangle is still relevant and easy to understand (Figure 3.4). The three apexes of the triangle represent the agent, host, and environment. The **agent** is the cause of the disease or causative organism. Another term used for agent in infectious diseases is **pathogen** (disease-causing microorganism). The **host** is the recipient of the disease. Anything internal within the host that influences the disease process should be considered part of the host. The **environment** consists of the external surroundings that influence the host.

Agent

The most common agents in infectious disease are viruses, bacteria, fungi, and worms. Viruses are the smallest agents and most difficult to treat. **Antibiotics**, which are substances that arrest the growth of or destroy pathogens, do not kill viruses. They do kill bacteria, which are also microscopic and come in shapes that range from rectangular to spiral. Although some bacteria are becoming antibiotic-resistant due to misuse among populations, most are still controllable with standard treatments. Some of the antibiotic-resistant strains can be controlled through the use of a combination of antibiotics or a "cocktail." Fungi, yeast, and molds cause many common conditions, such as vaginal

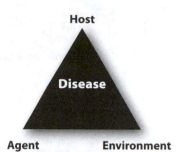

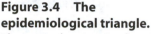

Figure 3.4   The epidemiological triangle.
There are three major factors that influence whether an individual gets an infectious disease. They are the agent, external environments, and host (individual or internal environment).

yeast infections and athlete's foot. Worms such as tapeworms, which can be many feet long, cause a variety of illnesses. See Figure 3.5 on the following page for common biological agents and examples of the diseases they cause.

The effects of agents on a host depend on many characteristics, such as their virulence, infectivity, pathogenicity, resistance, and the number of microorganisms that enter the host. For example, rabies is a very severe illness that almost always causes death in humans. The virus that causes it is **virulent**. An agent that can easily enter a body and multiply is **infective**. A highly infective agent causes measles. Measles is also a disease of high **pathogenicity**; once in the body, the measles agent almost always causes full-blown disease, not just a light case. HIV has low **resistance**, which means that outside of the body it is easy to kill.

You need to know the common biological agents because as a health educator you may be asked to teach people about the causes of their infectious diseases. Understanding terms like *virulence, infectivity, pathogenicity,* and *resistance* will allow you to help others communicate with their health care providers.

Host

The host is the individual who has the disease; *host* can be thought of as a person's internal environment. Think about the internal things that influence you. Did you come up with things like what you eat, how much you sleep, the presence of other diseases or disorders, genetics, and the ability to develop immunity? If so, you are absolutely right. Anything that influences the body internally has the potential to influence the outcome of a disease. Even factors like stress, exercise, and body temperature influence disease processes in the body. These factors don't cause the disease but rather determine, to some extent, how an individual will react to or fight a disease.

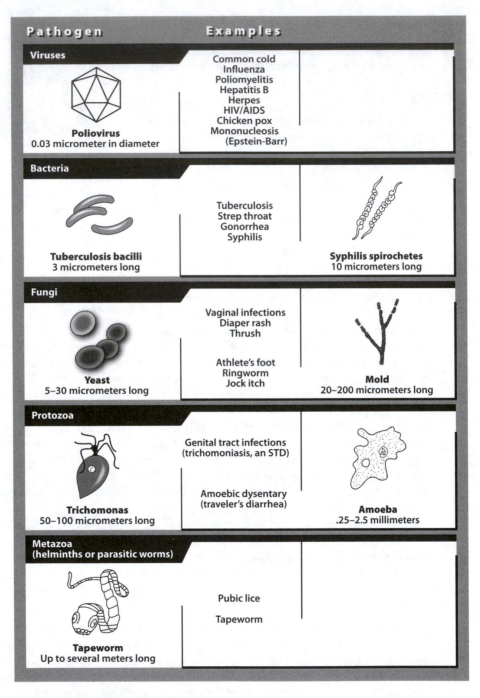

Figure 3.5   Common biological agents.

Infectious diseases are caused by a number of organisms. Some of the most common are shown in this illustration along with the types of diseases they cause. Adapted from *Environmental Health,* 2nd ed., by M.T. Morgan. © 1997 Brooks/Cole, a part of Cengage Learning, Inc. Used with permission.

The host's first line of defense is skin. What an amazing organ! It serves as a barrier to many agents. Tears and saliva do the same. The body's inflammatory response serves as the second line of defense. In an inflammatory response, the body sends fluids containing white blood cells and other substances to fight off the agent. The body's third line of defense is immunity.

Immunity

Immunity means that an individual is resistant or not susceptible to a specific disease. Immunity occurs when antibodies are produced in the body. **Antibodies** kill microorganisms or prevent them from multiplying and infecting the host. A person isn't immune to all diseases just because he or she is immune to one. In other words, immunity is disease-specific, and not all diseases stimulate antibody production. There are several ways in which immunity occurs. Individuals can produce it in their own body (**active immunity**) or receive the ingredients of immunity from outside the body (**passive immunity**). Both active and passive immunity occur either naturally or artificially. In **natural immunity**, individuals produce antibodies after having had a disease or received antibodies from their mother in utero. In **artificial immunity**, individuals become immune to a disease by producing antibodies after having had the weakened or killed agent responsible for the disease injected or by having actual antibodies injected. FYI 3.3 lists the types of immunity.

FYI 3.3   **Examples of Immunity**

Immunity can be acquired in two ways. Immunity is one of the human body's major lines of defense against disease.

Active Immunity	**Passive Immunity**
Artificially acquired active immunity (Vaccination)	Artificially acquired passive immunity (Antibodies injected)
Naturally acquired active immunity (Having had a disease)	Naturally acquired passive immunity (Antibodies passing from mother to baby)

Herd immunity occurs when a significant number of people in a population are immune to a disease. If many people in a community have a disease, it is much more likely that the disease-free people will get it; if few people have the disease, its spread to people who aren't immune will be less likely. Figures 3.6 and 3.7 will help you understand the concept of herd immunity. Imagine that the rain drops represent a disease agent and the umbrellas represent immunity. The first figure illustrates that most people in a group of 12 people will get wet (become infected with the agent) if there are only two umbrellas. The second figure illustrates an increase in the number of people in the group who stay dry (uninfected) if there are more umbrellas. If a large number of people become immune—by vaccine, for example—a protective barrier is created

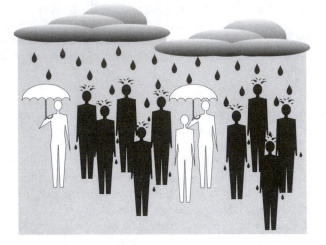

Figure 3.6   Herd immunity—low.
Low immunization levels fall short of protecting individuals within a group.

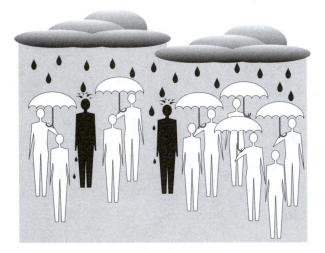

Figure 3.7   Herd immunity—high.
A high level of immunization within the group affords a good level of protection to most of the individuals within the group.

for those who are susceptible. People who don't have the disease, due to immunity or no contact, won't spread it. Almost the entire population or "herd" is protected.

As a health educator, you may help people gain the knowledge necessary to make good decisions about health. The range of information people might need concerning the internal environment of the host may vary from healthy food choices to reducing stress to the side effects of vaccines as well as their benefits. As we have mentioned before, it is important for you to be able to access information; in this case, you would need to research host issues. Consult Appendix A for Internet resources.

Environment

The external environment influences both the outcomes of disease and the very presence of the disease. The external environment has physical aspects (such as terrain, precipitation, and temperature) as well as social aspects (such as cultural characteristics). The numbers of people, plants, and animals influence the external environment. Insects or animals spread some diseases. If an insect carrier (vector) of a specific disease doesn't live in an environment, the disease is less likely to be present in the environment. If a disease is spread via tiny droplets in the air, a place crowded with people is going to have disease spread at a higher rate than will a location with very few people. Certain organisms live and spread best in places that are very hot and humid. The cultural environment influences everything from food choices to types of housing and stress-coping strategies. Although all cultural characteristics do not influence the external environment, all influence an individual's likelihood of contracting certain diseases. As a community health professional you will need to be prepared to answer questions about the environment and how it affects disease. If, for example, you live in a place where deer ticks, which carry Lyme disease, are common, your job may be to teach people that tick bites can be prevented by wearing long sleeves and tucking in loose clothing.

The interactions among agent, host, and environment produce the overall parameters of infectious disease. One example of the interaction occurs in the mode of transmission of disease. Characteristics of hosts, agents, and environments affect how the agent is transmitted from one person to another.

Mode of Transmission

The way in which an agent travels from one host to another is its **mode of transmission**. Some agents travel through the air, whereas others have to be picked up from a hard surface. As noted earlier, insects and animals also carry some agents from one host to another. Modes of transmission are direct or indirect. A *direct* mode of transmission means that an agent is passed directly from one person to another (person to person). *Indirect* modes involve a third element—an animal, insect, hard surface, or food. All modes of transmission fall within these two broad categories. Airborne transmission occurs when the agent is carried on small droplets of moisture or dust. Small droplets, forcefully expelled from someone's mouth or nose via a cough or a sneeze, can travel great distances if they aren't blocked. Vectorborne transmission occurs when an animal or insect serves as the agent's transportation. **Vectors** are living but nonhuman. **Fomites** are inanimate objects, such as cups, tables, doorknobs, and toys that can also serve as a means of transportation for some agents. Sometimes an agent remains in a **reservoir** and multiplies until it is transmitted to a host. Anything living or nonliving might serve as a reservoir, including the human body. Some humans or animals carry an agent and transmit it to others but do not get sick themselves. These *carriers* make prevention a challenge because their carrier status often goes undetected until many people around them get the disease. Typhoid Mary is the most famous example of the carrier phenomenon.

Mode of transmission involves the way agents get from person to person but do not determine how an agent enters the body (*portal of entry*) or exits the body (*portal of exit*). Portals of entry and exit and modes of transmission play important roles in the prevention as well as transmission of diseases.

Under the right conditions, once an agent enters a body the disease will progress through a fairly consistent set of stages. These phases are illustrated in Figure 3.8 on the following page. The *incubation period* is the time from the agent's entry in the body (*point of infection)* to the occurrence of signs or symptoms of disease. Signs and symptoms are actually different things. *Signs* are measurable changes in the body such as body temperature or number of white blood cells. *Symptoms* are subjective changes in the body such as pain or dizziness. Signs and symptoms begin to appear during the *prodromal period.* A disease is at its peak during the *fastigium period,* and signs and symptoms decline during the *defervescence period.* The individual recovers during *convalescence.*

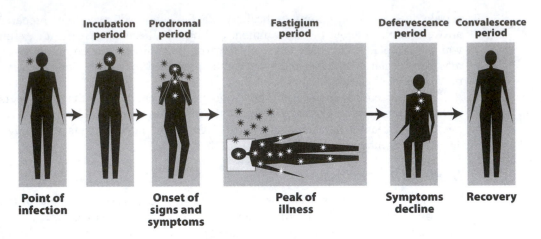

Figure 3.8   Progression of an infectious disease.
In this case, the disease affects the respiratory tract.

Noteworthy Infectious Diseases

Some infectious diseases are short term, or **acute**, and others are long term, or **chronic.** Although there are many acute and chronic diseases that we might discuss, we will discuss two that have been in the news in the recent past. Other significant infectious diseases and their modes of transmission are listed in Table 3.1.

Escherichia coli

Some forms of the bacterium *Escherichia coli* (E. coli) are virulent pathogens and many are carried by food products. You may have heard about recent outbreaks from contaminated foods. One such announcement was made on November 1, 2007. It

Table 3.1   Critical Biological Agents

Easy to Spread Agents	Moderately Easy to Spread Agents	Emerging Agents to Watch in Future

Anthrax
  Bacterium spread by contact with infected animals
	E. coli
	  Bacteria spread by eating undercooked food products that contain the E. coli toxin
		Hantavirus
		  Spread through exposure to infected rodent droppings

Botulism
  Spread by eating food containing botulism toxin
	Cryptosporidium
	  Parasite spread through contaminated water	

Smallpox
  Virus spread through air, person to person
	Mycobacterium Tuberculosis
	  Bacterium spread through air, person to person	

Source: "CDC's list of critical biological agents." *NSF Live Safer*. Retrieved January 25, 2009, from www.nsf.org/consumer/bioterrorism/bioterrorism_agents.asp#anthrax=

stated, "General Mills Operations, a Wellston, Ohio, establishment, is voluntarily recalling approximately 3.3 million pounds of frozen meat pizza products because they may be contaminated with E. coli O157:H7 and may be linked to an outbreak of E. coli O157:H7 illnesses, the U.S. Department of Agriculture's Food Safety and Inspection Service announced today" (USDA, 2007). Individuals who contract the illness caused by the 0157:H7 strain frequently have bloody diarrhea for short periods of time. Unfortunately, some individuals—especially very young children—die as a result. This illness is severe and acute in nature but can be prevented by adequate heating of the food reservoirs.

Avian Flu

As you may be aware, there are many types and subtypes of flu. One subtype of the Influenza A virus called H5N1 is highly pathogenic among birds. The CDC reports that there are two groups of H5N1; one of these two groups has also infected humans (CDC, 2007d). Although tracking these viruses can be tricky, the important thing to know is that human infections with H5N1 are rare. Even though rare, when human infection does occur the situation is grave. Infections in humans often cause death. The good news is that the majority of individuals who have been infected to date were in direct contact with infected birds; they did not get the virus from another person. The problem for public health officials, however, is that the H5N1 virus could change into a form that more easily infects humans and spreads from person to person. Think about our earlier discussion of immunity. If a new virus entered a population, what would happen? You are correct if you realized that there would be no immunity and the consequences would be devastating. Fortunately, many public health experts are working on this potentially serious circumstance with Influenza A H5N1.

Noninfectious Disease

The definition of noninfectious disease seems simple enough: diseases that are not transmitted from one person to another. However, there is nothing simple about most noninfectious diseases. These diseases are caused by chemical, metallic, electrical, psychosocial, genetic, or any number of other agents. The agent is not generally a pathogen, although it can be. In fact, noninfectious diseases are commonly caused by a combination of agents. A visual schematic of how agents work together to cause disease is found in Figure 3.9. The schematic, called a *web of causation*, demonstrates the relationship between agents. Finding the agents that cause a noninfectious disease or discovering how several agents work together to cause the disease is not simple. In the United States and most other developed countries, the burden of noninfectious chronic diseases is very heavy. If you refer back to Figure 3.1, you'll see that the four leading causes of death in 2004 were chronic diseases and were responsible for about 61% of all deaths in the United States that year (CDC, 2007d). The statistics were nearly the same for 2006, with diseases of the heart (26%), malignant neoplasms (23.1%), cerebrovascular diseases (5.7%), and chronic lower respiratory diseases (5.1%) accounting for 60% of all deaths (Heron et al., 2009). Diabetes, although not a leading cause of death, burdens many millions of people with serious consequences and in some cases death.

Heart Disease

In 2005, heart disease affected 37.1% of the U.S. population (American Heart Association, 2008). The category "heart disease" encompasses over 20 different conditions that make it difficult for the heart to function (CDC, 2007d). These disorders range from myocardial infarction, a heart attack, to congenital heart disease, something that occurred in the heart's development before birth. However, coronary artery disease is by far the most frequently occurring disorder.

Coronary artery disease is a condition in which the blood vessels on the heart get too narrow for blood to flow normally. You have probably heard of atherosclerosis, which is the collection of fatty plaque on the walls of arteries. The collection of plaque is what narrows the arteries, sometimes to the extent that no blood flows through them. When this happens in arteries on the heart, the result will be a heart attack.

The cause of diseases of the heart is multifaceted. Review the web of causation seen in Figure 3.9. You will see that food choices, body fat, use of tobacco, blood pressure, exercise, personality characteristics, other illnesses, and genetics can all play a role. While not all of these are under a person's control, many are. As a health professional, you may be asked to help individuals or groups understand their illness or change their negative health behaviors.

Cancer

All cancers combined account for the second leading cause of death in the United States. Lung cancer is the most common cancer among Americans; 213,380 new cases were diagnosed in 2007 (American Cancer Society [ACS], 2007). While not always easy to treat, lung cancer is the most preventable. Tobacco use, whether through cigarette, cigar, or pipe smoking, has the largest impact on the number of lung cancer cases. Eight out of 10 lung cancers result from the use of tobacco.

Cancer has become such a topic of concern that major newspapers like the *New York Times* run long articles on the subject. On July 29, 2007, the *Times* ran such an article entitled "Leading Causes of Cancer Deaths" in which they stated, "This year there will be 1.4 million new cases of cancer in the United States and 559,650 deaths." According to the National Cancer Institutes (2008), the five most common cancers by rank are lung, nonmelanoma skin, prostate, breast, and colorectal. The leading causes of cancer deaths include lung, colorectal, breast, pancreatic, and prostate cancers.

The diminished quality of life and death caused by cancer are tragic. However, those aren't the only issues that receive attention. "The cost of fighting cancer exceeds $171 billion annually in the United States; of this, over $12 billion is spent on sophisticated products to treat and support cancer patients" (MedTech Insight, 2003). The burden of cancer does not have to be so high! Many cancers can be prevented. As a health professional, you will want to have basic information about the leading cancers and how they can be prevented.

Diabetes

"The dramatic increase in the prevalence of childhood overweight and its resultant comorbidities are associated with significant health and financial burdens, war-

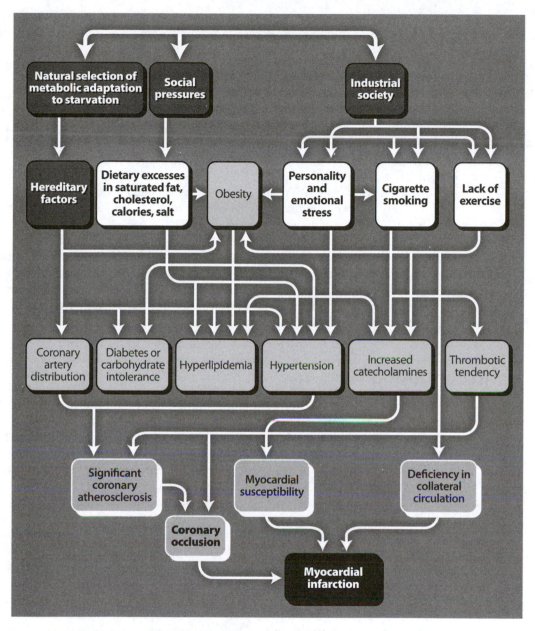

Figure 3.9   Web of causation for heart disease.

The cause of a myocardial infarction, or heart attack, is not simple to track. As you can see from this illustration, many things influence the onset of heart disease. In this illustration, the dark gray boxes are the factors outside the control of individuals, while the white boxes are behaviors or characteristics that people can change. The pale gray boxes are the first level of consequences, leading to the second level of consequences in the white-bordered boxes. The black box is the ultimate result. Adapted from *Primer of Epidemiology,* 4th ed., p. 4, by G. D. Friedman, 1994, New York: McGraw-Hill.

ranting strong and comprehensive prevention efforts" (American Academy of Pediatrics, 2003). Childhood obesity leads to obesity in adults, and 44 million Americans are considered obese as measured by body mass index. From 1991 to 2001 the number of obese adults increased by 74% (CDC, 2008h). Unfortunately, there is a strong correlation between obesity and diabetes.

Diabetes is actually a group of diseases in which insulin is not produced correctly or the action of insulin is not adequate. Consequences of uncontrolled diabetes include blindness, kidney damage, cardiovascular disease, and even death. Type I diabetes, which usually begins in childhood or young adulthood, occurs when an individual's immune system destroys the cells in the pancreas that regulate insulin. Insulin, in turn, controls blood sugar (CDC, 2007d). Most individuals with Type I diabetes require injections of insulin. Type II diabetes, which generally occurs in older individuals, is highly associated with obesity. The body does not use insulin well in this type of diabetes. Over 90% of diabetes cases are Type II.

As a health professional, you may have the task of helping an individual who is predisposed to Type II diabetes. You will need to let him or her know that the disease is influenced by many factors, including genetics, metabolism, behavior, environment, culture, and socioeconomic status. Because behavior and environment play such an important role, prevention may be possible. What an outstanding opportunity to implement the skills you will gain from this book and your other courses.

In Conclusion

Epidemiological studies provide much valuable information to health educators. Morbidity (incidence and prevalence) and mortality rates alone can assist health educators in helping individuals and communities obtain information about prevalent infectious or noninfectious diseases and plan appropriate education and prevention programs.

The epidemiological triangle is a guide to understanding how agent, host, and environment interact in the spread of disease. Understanding agents that are commonly found in a community will help determine the types of information that might be presented in an educational program. If highly infectious diseases are present, ill people may need to learn the importance of remaining at home or away from the uninfected population. On the other hand, if a disease that is highly resistant to normal treatments is present, people may need very specific information on what preventive measures to take.

Health educators play an important role in keeping the external environment healthy. You may be asked to help plan a recycling program or determine ways to solve overcrowding. Your largest role, however, may well be in helping people change their internal environments. You may have an opportunity to plan programs about food choices, exercise, or other lifestyle matters that affect the host.

You may be involved in determining what epidemiological information is needed to plan effective health programs. As a health educator you will need to know how to use the vast amount of epidemiological data available for the benefit of your community. Epidemiology is likely to be an important aspect of your job.

REVIEW QUESTIONS

1. Define incidence and prevalence.

2. Consider the question, "Can the incidence rate of any disease be higher than the prevalence rate for the same disease, at the same time and place, and with the same people?" Explain your answer.

3. Define morbidity and mortality.

4. Consider the question, "Can the mortality rates of two very different cities be compared to determine in which city there is more risk of death?" Explain your answer.

5. Define life expectancy.

6. Give possible reasons for disparities in life expectancies between ethnic groups in the United States.

7. Give examples of agents, host issues, and environmental issues that influence the spread of disease.

8. Briefly describe how the agent, host, and environment interact with one another in infectious diseases.

9. Give examples (other than those listed in the text) of each of the three types of prevention.

10. Describe the four types of epidemiological studies described in the chapter.

11. Identify and analyze a health issue that is currently in the news and the response of health officials.

FOR YOUR APPLICATION

You may have already selected or been assigned a partner community for a project. If not, just select a community. It's time to get to know the community by searching data sources for epidemiologic information about its members. You will want to find information such as life expectancy, leading causes of death, and leading causes of illness. Your search shouldn't stop with morbidity and mortality statistics but should also include health behavior information. As you know, behaviors such as tobacco use, drug and alcohol use, dietary intake, exercise, and other choices seriously impact health, so collect as much data as possible. If you will remember our discussion about the relationship between poverty and health, you'll realize that you also need information about average socioeconomic status, education levels, and common types of employment for your community members. (The entire needs assessment process is covered in chapter 6.) You should write a summary of the information you collected to add to your project report. Don't forget to use appropriate citations in the text of your summary and begin a reference list for the final report.

Special Populations

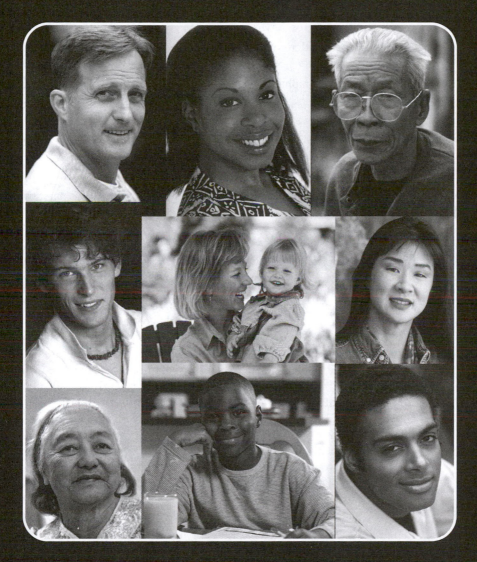

You've decided to work on gaining some community experience and building your résumé as you work through your degree program. Bravo! You choose to begin by volunteering at a local community center whose clientele is primarily ethnically diverse adults over the age of 65. The director asks you to develop a one-day workshop that focuses on preventing drug abuse. You enthusiastically agree. You particularly enjoyed learning about the prevention of adolescent drug abuse in the drug education course you completed. Addressing drug abuse among older adults couldn't be that different . . . could it?

CHAPTER OBJECTIVES

1. Explain the importance and challenges related to gaining information about the health status of Americans in age-, gender-, and ethnicity-specific groups.

2. Describe the underlying role of socioeconomic status and its effect on health status in the United States.

3. Describe demographic characteristics of age-specific groups in the United States.

4. Describe health issues and influencing factors for specific populations in the United States by age, gender, and ethnicity.

The Face of America

The face of America is changing. It is growing older and more diverse. Life expectancy in the United States increased from 47.3 years in 1900 to 77.7 years in 2006 (Heron et al., 2009). The total proportion of ethnic populations for all ages in the United States has also increased from 20.1% in 1980 to 33.5% in 2006. According to the National Center for Health Statistics, by 2050 nearly half of the total U.S. population is expected to identify with a specific ethnic group (NCHS, 2007a).

The overall picture of health in America is also changing, with notable declines in overall death rates. Of the 15 leading causes of death in the U.S. in 2006, the top five were heart disease, cancer, stroke (cerebrovascular diseases), chronic lower respiratory diseases (CLRD), and unintentional injuries (Heron et. al, 2008a). The overall age-adjusted death rate declined by 45% between 1950 and 2004 (see Figure 4.1), with particularly significant reductions in three of the five leading causes of death: heart disease (63% lower by 2004), stroke (72% lower), and unintentional injuries (53% lower). Though death rates for cancer and CLRD rose during part of that same time period, they have recently begun to decrease. In fact, between 2005 and 2006, statistically significant decreases in age-adjusted death rates occurred for 11 of the 15 leading causes of death and the decline was so significant for diabetes mellitus (originally number 6) that it switched places with Alzheimer's disease (originally number 7), which also declined somewhat (Heron et al., 2008b).

These trends in lower death rates for the total population are encouraging. But do these numbers tell the whole story about the health status of Americans? Despite increas-

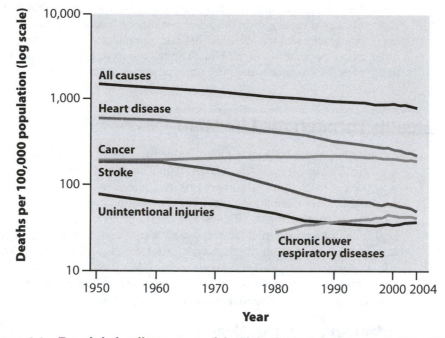

Figure 4.1   Trends in leading causes of death in the U.S. for all ages, 1950–2004.
From *Health, United States, 2007*, Figure 20, National Center for Health Statistics. Retrieved September 1, 2008, from http://www.cdc.gov/nchs/data/hus/hus07.pdf#032

ing longevity, Americans report an average of only 19 days per month during which they feel "healthy and full of energy" and "nearly one-third of Americans say they suffer from some mental or emotional problem every month" (CDC, 2007h, para. 1). This is partially due to the fact that longevity is often accompanied by an increased prevalence of chronic health conditions that can impact quality of life. And though death rates have been mostly declining for heart disease since 1980 and for cancer since the early 1990s, these two causes still accounted for 49% of all deaths in 2006 (Heron et al., 2008b).

The recent improvements in the overall U.S. health status "have not been equally distributed by income, race, ethnicity, education, and geography" (NCHS, 2007a, p. 3). The number of U.S. residents living in poverty, a strong health disparity factor, increased from 31.6 million (11.3% of total population) in 2000 to 37 million (12.5%) in 2007 (U.S. Census Bureau, 2008a). Some subgroups in the U.S. population (women, older adults, and some ethnic communities) are more vulnerable to the effects of poverty and face unique health challenges. That is why an understanding of health issues among **special populations** is so important. Measures of health and mortality for the total U.S. population can cloud the true picture of health and quality of life among Americans in different stages of the life span and from different walks of life.

In this chapter we highlight certain health and quality of life concerns of selected populations defined by age, gender, and ethnicity. As you would probably expect, we cannot include here all that you need to know to work effectively with these groups. And because each section must be brief, we risk inadvertently lumping together and making generalizations about members of these groups. We are certain that you are aware that each population or subgroup described consists of diverse and unique individuals. We encourage you to visit the Web sites listed in Appendix A to learn more about these and other special populations in the United States and to seek a better understanding of how to adapt health education and promotion processes to these unique groups.

Health Through the Life Span

In 2008, the CDC's **National Center for Health Statistics** integrated two Web sites, Health Data for All Ages (HDAA) and Trends in Health in Aging (THA), into a new site called Health Data Interactive (NCHS, 2008b). On that site you can access data and health information for the U.S. population broken down by age, gender, ethnicity, and state or region. Tables and charts provide statistics for causes of death, health conditions and risk factors, health status and disability, and access to health care, along with explanatory messages for selected health measures. You can also join a free Listserv to receive news about updates. We used information from this site and other reliable sources to provide a brief overview of demographic and health information throughout the life span and for special populations.

Infant and Maternal Health

Infant mortality and maternal health measures are critical indicators of a nation's health on a global scale. Though much has been accomplished in the United States to address the health of infants and mothers, more can be done to improve health and quality of life in this population. We will now explore some prominent health issues for this group.

Health and Demographics

According to the NCHS, an estimated 4.26 million babies were born in the United States in 2006 (Hamilton, Martin, & Ventura, 2007). This number represented "an increase of 3% from 2005, the largest single-year increase in the number of births since 1989" (p. 1). This increase in birthrates was evident among women in their 20s, 30s, and early 40s. But it was the rise in birthrates for teenagers that came as the biggest surprise. The teen birthrate had been on a steady 14-year decline since its peak in 1991 (61.8 births per 1,000 females) and had fallen 34% between 1991 and 2005 (see Figure 4.2). For that reason, the 3% increase in birthrates for those ages 15–17 (to 22 per 1,000) and 4% increase among those ages 18–19 (to 73 per 1,000) were noted as potentially significant by the NCHS. Also noted was the fact that 38.5% of babies were born to unmarried women in 2006 (a 20% increase since 2002).

A nation's **infant mortality** rate is considered a strong indicator of its health status. The United States made great strides in this area over a 40-year period, moving from an infant mortality rate of about 29 per 1,000 live births in 1950 to a rate of 7.6 in 1990 (NCHS, 1996). The rate further dropped to 6.8 per 1,000 in 2004, with improvements evident across all ethnic groups per 1,000 live births: Asian/Pacific Islander, 4.7; Hispanic, 5.5; non-Hispanic White, 5.7; American Indian/Alaska Native, 8.4; and non-Hispanic Black, 13.6 (USDHHS, 2007d, obj. 16-1c). The most

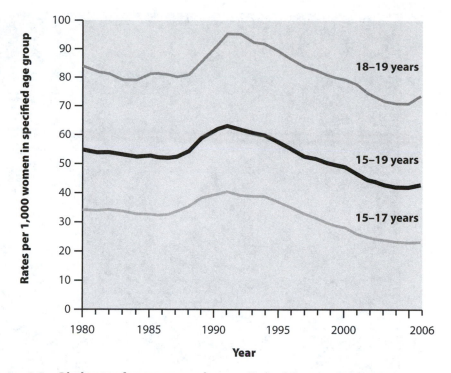

Figure 4.2   Birthrates for teenagers by age, United States, 1980–2006.
From "Births: Preliminary data for 2006," by B. E. Hamilton, J. S. Martin, and S. J. Ventura, 2007, *National Vital Statistics Report, 56*(7). Retrieved August 23, 2008 from http://www.cdc.gov/nchs/data/nvsr/nvsr56/nvsr56_07.pdf
*Note, 2006 data is preliminary.

significant decrease was evident for non-Hispanic Black women, with a 1940 rate of 70 per 1,000 compared to 13.6 in 2004. However, the decrease in the rate for this group has flattened over the past decade and, in fact, the total infant mortality rate was slightly higher in 2005 (6.9 per 1,000) than it was in 2004 (6.8).

Another important health measure is maternal deaths, which increased from a rate of 9.9 deaths per 100,000 live births in 1999 to 13.1 deaths per 100,000 in 2004 (USDHHS, 2007d, obj. 16-4). However, this increase is largely attributable to improvements in the reporting system. In 2004, the rates per 100,000 live births were 28.2 for mothers aged 35 years or older and 6.6 for mothers younger than 20 years. Of the four racial or ethnic populations for which reliable data were available, the maternal death rates in 2004 were 8.5 per 100,000 for Hispanic women; 9.6 for Asian/Pacific Islanders; 9.8 for non-Hispanic Whites; and 36.1 for non-Hispanic Blacks (obj. 16-4).

Factors That Influence Health

According to the March of Dimes Foundation (MOD, 2008), "Babies born too soon and too small" (para. 1) is the primary reason for infant mortality in the United States. Though the five leading causes of infant mortality in 2004 were categorized as congenital abnormalities (20% of deaths), short gestation or low birth weight (17%),

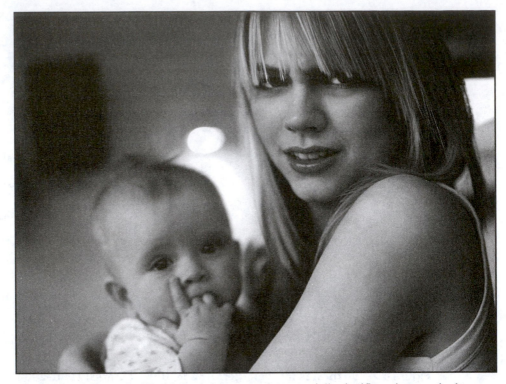

The National Center for Health Statistics reported a potentially significant increase in the teen birthrate in 2006.

sudden infant death syndrome (SIDS, 8%), maternal pregnancy complications (6%), and unintentional injuries (4%), a reanalysis indicated that 37% of those deaths were actually attributable to *preterm*-related causes (USDHHS, 2007d). "More than a half million babies are born prematurely (less than 37 weeks gestation) each year, and those who survive face the risk of lifelong health consequences, such as breathing and feeding problems, cerebral palsy, and learning problems. Mortality rates for infants born even a few weeks early, or *late preterm* (between 34–36 weeks of gestation), were three times the rates for full-term infants" (MOD, 2008, para. 5-6).

Low birth weight (LBW, less than 2500 grams or 5.5 pounds) and **very low birth weight** (VLBW, less than 1500 grams or 3.33 pounds) are highly associated with inadequate prenatal care; low socioeconomic status; ethnicity; the mother's age and marital status; environmental exposure to viruses, chemicals, and radiation; and a number of unhealthy behaviors—including smoking, inadequate diet, and alcohol and other drug abuse (Pan American Health Organization, 1998; Swartz, 1990). The mortality rate for VLBW infants is more than 100 times the rate of normal birth weight babies (MOD, 2008). According to the Federal Interagency Forum on Child and Family Statistics (FIFCFS, 2008), 14% of non-Hispanic Black infants were born in 2006 with LBW, a number that was higher than all other ethnic groups even when adjusted by maternal age (see Figure 4.3).

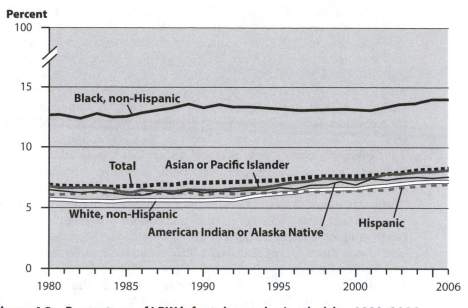

Percent

Figure 4.3   Percentage of LBW infants by mother's ethnicity, 1980–2006.
From *America's Children in Brief: Key National Indicators of Well-Being, 2008,* Federal Interagency Forum on Child and Family Statistics, 2008. Retrieved September 1, 2008, from http://childstats.gov/americaschildren/health.asp

Early and consistent prenatal care is important for the health of the infant and the mother. In 2004, 77% of non-Hispanic Black women and 89% of non-Hispanic White women received prenatal care beginning in the first trimester (USDHHS, 2007d). Among pregnant adolescents (less than age 15), only 49% received first-trimester care. These factors and the high rate of maternal mortality among low-income mothers are reasons why prenatal care and health promotion are important aspects of community health promotion.

Child Health

When the health of a nation suffers, its children are among those who suffer most. Conversely, when community partners work together to improve the lives of community members, children are among those most likely to gain. We encourage you to become familiar with the basic information provided here about child health in the United States and to consider how you can become part of the support system for America's children.

Health and Demographics

An estimated 73.9 million children under the age of 18 were living in the United States in 2007 (FIFCFS, 2008). This age group, representing 24.5% of the total U.S. population, consisted of approximately 57% non-Hispanic Whites, 21% Hispanics, 15% non-Hispanic Blacks, 4% Asian/Pacific Islanders. The remaining 3–4% were labeled as "all other races." Almost 69% lived with two-parent families, 23% lived with unmarried mothers, and 17.4% lived in poverty. Approximately 55% lived in counties with unhealthy levels of air pollution, 40% lived in inadequate housing, and 10% had no access to healthy drinking water.

According to 2003–2005 statistics for children ages 1 to 4 years (NCHS, 2008a), unintentional injuries (10.8 per 100,000) was the leading cause of death, followed by birth defects (3.5), cancer (2.5), homicide (2.4), and heart disease (1.1). For children aged 5 to 9 years, unintentional injuries (5.5 per 100,000) was followed by cancer (2.5), birth defects (1.1), homicide (.6), and heart disease (.5). Unintentional injuries account for more than 40% of all deaths of U.S. children, with close to half of those a result of motor vehicle crashes. Drownings, burns, suffocation, and firearms cause the rest.

Childhood obesity has increased to epidemic proportions over the past two decades (CDC, 2008c). The percentage of obese children 6 to 11 years of age has more than doubled over a 25-year period, increasing from 6.5% in 1980 to 17.6% in 2006. This heart disease risk factor is often linked with other risk factors such as high cholesterol and high blood pressure in adult populations. Because obese children are often likely to become obese adults, childhood obesity can serve as an early indicator of adult heart disease, type 2 diabetes, stroke, cancer, and osteoarthritis. Even during childhood, obesity can take its toll. Obese children are more likely than normal weight children to suffer from sleep apnea, bone and joint problems, and the social and psychological problems often associated with the stigma of being overweight.

Factors That Influence Health

The impact of poverty on health can be painfully obvious when discussing the health needs of U.S. children. According to a national survey conducted by the National Center for Health Statistics in 2006, the majority (54%) of U.S. children enjoyed excellent health and another 28% were in very good health (Bloom & Cohen, 2007). Yet, children in poor families were less likely to be in excellent health (just under 40%) than were children who were not poor (60%), and 6.9 million children (10%) had no health insurance coverage.

> Thirteen percent of children in families with an income less than $20,000 and 17% of children in families with an income of $20,000–$34,999 had no health insurance compared with 3% of children in families with an income of $75,000 or more. Children in poor or near-poor families were more likely to be uninsured, to have unmet medical needs, and to have delayed medical care than children in families that were not poor. About 1.8 million children (2%) were unable to get needed medical care because the family could not afford it, and medical care for 2.9 million children (4%) was delayed because of worry about the cost. (Bloom & Cohen, 2007, p. 6)

Children in poor families and those living in single-mother households were more than twice as likely to miss 11 or more days of school due to illness than children in two-parent families who were not poor. Poor children were also more likely to suffer from asthma than non-poor children (14% versus 9%), were twice as likely to have a learning disability than non-poor children (12% versus 6%), and were more likely to use a clinic or emergency room for health care (as opposed to a doctor's office) than children of non-poor families. The dental needs of 4.5 million children were unmet in 2006 because their families could not afford it, and 23% of uninsured children had no dental contact for more than 2 years (some had *never* had contact). These are but a few of the health disparities that exist for U.S. children that are driven by the socio-ecological factors we discussed in chapters 1 and 2.

Adolescent and Young Adult Health

The future of a nation is in many ways dependent on the health of its youth. You can impact the viability of the nation and influence tomorrow's health leaders through your efforts to promote health among today's adolescents. The following sections provide brief overviews of demographics, health issues, and the factors that influence them.

Health and Demographics

The **National Adolescent Health Information Center** (NAHIC) was established by the U.S. Maternal and Child Health Bureau in 1993 as a national clearinghouse for adolescent health information. Demographic information about adolescents and young adults released in 2008 included the following highlights:

- The adolescent and young adult population is more diverse than the adult population.
- Poverty rates among children and adolescents have decreased in the past decade.
- Family structure varies by racial/ethnic group.
- School enrollment rates have increased in the past few decades.
- The median age of first marriage has increased in the past few decades (NAHIC, 2008, p. 1).

The overall number of adolescents and young adults (ages 10–24) in the U.S. was 63.3 million in 2006. By the year 2020, that number is expected to increase to 64.1 million. This age group was already more ethnically diverse in 2006 than the adult population (25 years or more) and, by 2020, is expected to consist of 6.3% Asian/Pacific Islanders, 14.1% non-Hispanic Blacks, 22.2% Hispanics, and 57.4% non-Hispanic Whites. More than one in ten members of this age group was foreign born in 2006 (NAHIC, 2008).

Though the overall poverty rate for adolescents and children under the age of 18 decreased from 19.9% in 1996 to 17% in 2006, a disproportionate percentage of non-Hispanic Blacks (33%) and Hispanics (26.6%) in this age group were living in poverty in 2006. Differences in family structure were also evident in 2006 in that non-Hispanic Blacks aged 12–15 were most likely to live with only their mother (47.9%) and least likely to live in a two-parent household (35.4%, compared to the total percentage of 64.9%). Though school enrollment rates for youth 16–24 years old increased from 1980 to 2006, high school dropout rates were still higher in 2006 for Hispanics (22.5%) and non-Hispanic Blacks (10.8%) than for non-Hispanic Whites (6.0%). The median age for first marriage for males (27.5) and females (25.5) in 2006 was higher than it was in 1970, but the percentage of married young adults (20–24 years) varied widely from the Northeast (9.3%) to the South (41.6%). More than half of unmarried 20–24-year-old females who gave birth to an infant in 2006 were living with a male partner (NAHIC, 2008).

One of the more troubling statistics for this age group concerns the leading causes of death. According to the NAHIC (2006, p. 1), "71% of deaths among adolescents and young adults ages 10–24 were due to preventable causes of unintentional injury, homi-

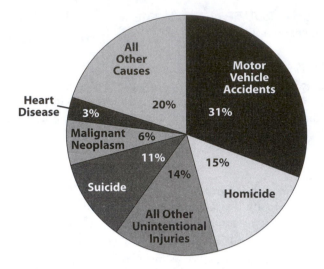

Figure 4.4   Leading causes of death, ages 10–24, 2003.

Source: *Fact Sheet on Mortality: Adolescents and Young Adults,* National Adolescent Health Information Center, 2006, San Francisco, CA: Author. Retrieved August 30, 2008, from http://nahic.ucsf.edu//downloads/Mortality.pdf

cide, and suicide" in 2003. Unintentional injuries accounted for 46% of those deaths, with motor vehicle accidents (31%) serving as the leading cause of death (see Figure 4.4). Death rates were higher in all categories for young adults (20–24 years) than they were for younger adolescents, and males were more likely than females to die from all causes of death as age increased. The gender difference was particularly significant for homicides: males were 5.7 times more likely than females to die from that cause.

Significant differences in death rates across ethnic groups were also evident in 2003. The highest death rates (per 100,000) were found among American Indian/Alaska Native (142.2) and non-Hispanic Black (124.4) males. Hispanic (82.3), non-Hispanic White (77.4), and Asian/Pacific Islander (44.4) males ranked significantly lower. The death rates of females in these groups were significantly lower, ranging from a high of 54.4 for American Indian/Alaska Native females to a low of 24.1 for Asian/Pacific Islander females. Non-Hispanic Black males die from homicide at rates that are as much as 12 times higher than some ethnic groups in the same age categories. American Indian/Alaska Native males were more likely to die from motor vehicle accidents and suicide. Though the death rates for 10–24-year-olds declined dramatically during the 1980s and early 1990s, these declines have largely leveled off in recent years (NAHIC, 2006).

Adolescents and young adults suffer from morbidity and social problems that are significantly impacted by behavioral choices. Approximately 757,000 pregnancies among women aged 15–19 years occurred in 2007 and a large proportion of those were unplanned and unwanted (CDC, 2008, June 6). Over 9 million cases of sexually transmitted diseases or infections, including 5,089 cases of human immunodeficiency virus/acquired immunodeficiency syndrome (HIV/AIDS), were recorded in 2007 among persons aged 15–24 years. Almost 16% of high school students were overweight and 13.0% were obese in 2007, and these percentages are expected to increase in ways that are already contributing to the chronic illnesses that plague American adults. The first step in reducing the incidence and prevalence of these health problems is to gain an understanding of the factors that contribute to them.

Factors That Influence Health

The Centers for Disease Control maintains a nationwide *Youth Risk Behavior Surveillance System* (YRBSS, see Appendix A) to monitor and address behaviors that place America's adolescents at health risk. According to a 2007 YRBSS survey report, the:

. . . leading causes of morbidity and mortality among youth and adults in the United States are related to six categories of priority health risk behaviors: behaviors that contribute to unintentional injuries and violence; tobacco use; alcohol and other drug use; sexual behaviors that contribute to unintended pregnancy and STDs, including HIV infection; unhealthy dietary behaviors; and physical inactivity. These behaviors frequently are interrelated and are established during childhood and adolescence and extend into adulthood. (CDC, 2008, June 6, p. 2)

Selected information on high school students from this report is highlighted in FYI 4.1.

FYI **4.1   High School Students: The Risks They Take**

Physical Activity—Over 65% did not engage in regular physical activity. Over 35% watched television and almost 25% played video and computer games for 3 or more hours on an average school day.

Eating—Almost 86% failed to consume enough milk and almost 79% bypassed needed daily levels of fruits and vegetable consumption. Yet, almost 34% drank at least one soda or pop per day.

Tobacco Use—Over 50% had ever tried smoking and 14.2% had done so by age 13; 25.7% had used a cigarette, smokeless tobacco, or cigar in the last 30 days.

Alcohol—Over 75% had ever tried drinking alcohol and 23.8% had done so by age 13. Almost 45% regularly used alcohol and 26% engaged in binge drinking.

Other Drugs—Over 38% had tried marijuana and 19.7% had used it within the last 30 days. Over 13% had ever used inhalants (glue, aerosol sprays, paints). Smaller percentages had tried hallucinogens (7.8%), cocaine (7.2%), ecstasy (5.8%), methamphetamines (4.4%), steroids (3.9%), or heroin (2.3%).

Sexual Activity—Almost 48% had engaged in sexual intercourse and 14.9% had done so with four or more partners. Of the 35% who were sexually active, 38.5% had not used a condom, 22.5% had drunk alcohol or used drugs, and only 16% had used birth control pills prior to their last intercourse.

Motor Vehicle Crashes—Over 29% had ridden in a vehicle driven by someone who had been drinking alcohol and 10.5% had driven while drinking. Over 11.1% had never or rarely worn a seat belt when riding in a car. Of those who had ridden a motorcycle (24.3%), only 33.9% used a helmet.

Violence—Over 35% had been in a physical fight in the past year, 18.0% (28.5% of males) had carried a weapon, and 5.5% had skipped school because they felt unsafe there or in route. Almost 10% had been physically hurt by a boyfriend/girlfriend and 7.8% (11.3% of females) had been forced to have sex.

Suicide—Over 28% reported having felt so sad or hopeless almost every day for 2 or more weeks in a row that they stopped doing some usual activities; 14.5% had seriously considered suicide, 11.3% had made a suicide plan, and 6.9% had attempted suicide in the past year.

Source: "Youth Risk Behavior Surveillance, United States, 2007," *Morbidity and Mortality Weekly Report*, *57* (No. SS-4), Centers for Disease Control and Prevention, 2008. Retrieved September 1, 2008, from http://www.cdc.gov/HealthyYouth/yrbs/pdf/yrbss07_mmwr.pdf

Many adolescents find themselves in a developmental stage of life in which their self-identity is forming, exploration of new ideas is common, and sensitivity to criticism and rejection is high. This stage renders many adolescents particularly vulnerable to peer pressure at a time when they also tend to live more in the present and are less concerned with long-term consequences. When these vulnerabilities are challenged by risk-promoting peer pressure, the results can be life threatening. Of the risk factors noted in FYI 4.1, we wish to highlight and discuss a few that are interrelated.

Alcohol use is a commonly accepted behavioral norm among adolescents and young adults (Komro, Perry, Veblen-Mortenson, Williams, & Roel, 1999) and has long been significantly related to the leading causes of death in that age group (Office of Disease Prevention and Health Promotion [ODPHP], 1988). In 1978, over 72% of 12th graders reported using alcohol within the past month (see Figure 4.5). That percentage significantly decreased to 48.6% by 1993 (Johnston, O'Malley, Bachman, & Schulenberg, 2008) largely because of effective peer leadership programs that changed normative perceptions about underage drinking (Komro et al., 1999; Perry et al., 1996). After a brief resurgence of use in 1996 (to 52.7%), reported alcohol use declined by 2007 to its lowest rate (44.4%) in over 30 years (Johnston et al., 2008). Between 1999 and 2006, the proportion of 12th graders who admitted initiating alcohol use by the end of 8th grade had decreased from 28.6% to 21.5%. In 2006, male and female adolescents ages 12–17 reported similar rates of alcohol use in the past month: 16.3% of males and 17% of females (NAHIC, 2007a).

These declines are extremely encouraging in light of the alarming alcohol-related death tolls of the 1970s. However, we urge you to be mindful of historical fluctuations

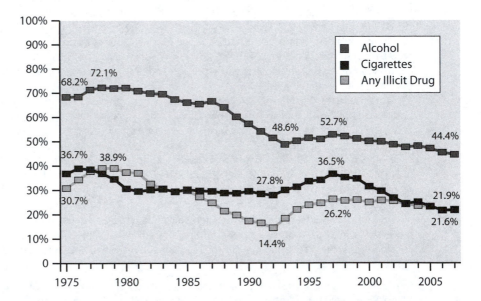

Figure 4.5   Trends in past-month substance use by type, 12th graders, 1975–2007.
From *Monitoring the Future National Results on Drug Use, 1975–2007. Volume I: Secondary School Students* by L. D. Johnston, P. M. O'Malley, J. G. Bachman, & J. E. Schulenberg, 2008, NIH Publication No. 08-6418A, Bethesda, MD: National Institute on Drug Abuse.

(as shown in Figure 4.5) in the use of alcohol and other substances among adolescents and the need for diligence to address these issues for each cohort that moves into this age group. In 2007, 33.4% of 10th graders and 44.4% of 12th graders reported using alcohol in the past month (Johnston et al., 2008) and one in four 12th graders reported **binge drinking behavior**, defined as drinking five or more drinks on one or more occasion over the past two weeks (NAHIC, 2007a). Alcohol use was particularly high among non-Hispanic Whites ages 18–25 (68.6%) compared to other same-age ethnic groups (47.4% to 51%) and was even higher among males (72.8%) in that age group.

Homicide is the second leading cause of death for the total population of adolescents and young adults and is the leading cause of death (accounting for 44.5% of all deaths) for non-Hispanic Black males (NAHIC, 2007b). The homicide rate for non-Hispanic Black males peaked at an alarming rate of 113.4 per 100,000 in 1993 (NAHIC, 2007b). That increase and an epidemic of students opening fire on school campuses generated widespread public concern for school safety, and the issue was designated a national public health and education priority (Hill & Drolet, 1999; Weiler, Dorman, & Pealer, 1999). By 1999, homicide rates had decreased to half the 1993 rates for non-Hispanic Black males (from 113.4 to 57.3) and Hispanic males (from 45.3 to 20.9).

Factors believed to contribute to violence among adolescents include increased exposure to violence involving weapons and escalating incidences of substance abuse, gang membership, victimization, hopelessness, and low academic performance (Powell, 1999). Poverty, a factor highly associated with violent behavior, has been said to rob young people of important deterrents such as positive role models, educational opportunities, and important social support systems. Attention to these factors and, particularly, to the fostering of adult social support and religious commitment, are recommended to promote nonviolent behavior among those at greatest risk (Powell, 1999).

Alcohol consumption also has negative effects on sexual activity (Dinger & Parsons, 1999). It increases the likelihood that young people will engage in sexual intercourse and decreases the chances that precautions will be taken to prevent unintended pregnancies and sexually transmitted diseases (STDs). Unintended pregnancies can lead to abortions or a host of other long-range problems for both mother and child. Among those STDs on the rise is AIDS. According to the CDC (2009b), by the end of 2006, an estimated 56,500 adolescents and young adults ages 13–24 were living with HIV infection or AIDS. Sex education for adolescents is a controversial issue in some political settings, but the consequences are grave when we fail to address this issue among sexually active teens.

Use of cigarettes and illicit drugs followed the same pattern of decline from the 1970s to the early 1990s (Figure 4.5), with a similar surge of use in the mid-1990s that tapered off again by 2006. Past-month use of these substances generally increases by grade level and continues to increase as 12th graders become college students. In 2006, 38.4% of young adults (18–25 years) reported past-month cigarette use and 19.8% in that age group reported past-month use of illicit drugs (primarily marijuana and nonmedical use of prescription-type drugs such as pain relievers) (NAHIC, 2007a). In that same year, over a fourth of young adult males reported dependence on or abuse of alcohol or illicit drugs with American Indian/Alaska Native (31.3%) and non-Hispanic White (24.6%) males reporting the highest rates of dependency (NAHIC, 2007a). The contribution of substance abuse to long-range health problems that emerge as primary causes of death (for instance, heart disease and cancer) and barriers to high quality of life are strong reasons for continued emphasis on substance abuse prevention for this age group.

The challenge of working with adolescents is sometimes tough, and the stakes can be very high. Yet fostering family and school connectedness and instilling in adolescents an optimistic sense of purpose about their future have been proven to positively affect risk-taking behavior (Fors, Crepaz, & Hayes, 1999). The more equipped you are with adolescent-specific knowledge and skills, the more likely you are to make a difference.

Adult Health in the Middle Years

The term *adult* can be misleading because it is commonly used to describe a wide range of age and experience. For instance, you can obtain adult mortality data from the NCHS's Health Data Interactive Web site. The data tables include, among other things, mortality rates for all adults age 18 and over (the total U.S. adult population) and for subgroups clustered by age ranges: 18–34, 35–44, 45–64, 65+, and 85+ years. These age ranges pose some challenges in interpreting the data. For example, the youngest adult age range (18–34) could include a single 18-year-old college student living in a dorm *and* a 34-year-old homeowner with a spouse, two children, and a mortgage. Differences in socioeconomic status, age, geographic location, education, ethnicity, and a wide variety of other factors exist among adults in these groups. However, despite these limitations, these data sets provide valuable information about the general health of U.S. adults in each age range and as a whole. This information can be used to compare the status of U.S. citizens to that of other countries, and it can be used by you to compare the status of local populations with which you work to national norms for specific age groups.

You can also access data through the NCHS National Vital Statistics System that are clustered in smaller and/or different age ranges. We have reported information in the following sections for two adult age groups, 25–44 and 45–64 years, because vital statistics are often reported for these two age ranges through the National Vital Statistics Reports that are periodically published by the NCHS. These reports are available online (see Appendix A).

Health and Demographics

In 2005, an estimated 154 million adults age 25–64 lived in the United States, which represented approximately 53% of all Americans (U.S. Census Bureau, 2008b). Of the total U.S. population, approximately 13% were 25–34, 15% were 35–44, 15% were 45–54, and 10% were 55–64 years of age (U.S. Census Bureau, 2008b). Of all U.S. adult women (18+ years), 12.9% were living in poverty compared to 8.9% of men and, when grouped by ethnicity, non-Hispanic Black (25.9%) and Hispanic (21%) women were more likely to be poor than non-Hispanic White women (9.3%) (Maternal and Child Health Bureau [MCHB], 2007).

In 2005, the five leading causes of death for U.S. adults ages 25–44 were, in rank order, unintentional injuries, cancer, heart disease, suicide, and homicide (NCHS, 2007a). For those 45–64 years old, the five leading causes were cancer, heart disease, unintentional injuries, diabetes, and chronic lower respiratory diseases (CLRD). As you can see, deaths caused by unintentional injuries are more prolific in the younger adult years but begin to be overshadowed by the onset of chronic health problems with age. (Also see the subsequent section in this chapter called *Health Factors in Ethnic Communities* for more information about adult health and leading causes of death.)

Perceptions of general health follow a similar pattern by age group. In 2006, the percentages of adults by age group who self-rated their health as only fair or poor were 6.3% (25–44 years old), 12.9% (45–54 years), and 18.8% (55–64 years) (NCHS, 2007a). The percentages of those who self-rated their health as fair/poor among impoverished non-Hispanic Blacks (23.0%), Hispanics (20.6%), and non-Hispanic Whites (19.5%) were much higher than ratings among higher-income adults in these ethnic groups (9.2%, 8.6%, and 5.5%, respectively) (NCHS, 2007a).

Factors That Influence Health

Three **controllable risk factors** that contribute significantly to heart disease and cancer are tobacco use, unhealthy dietary patterns, and physical inactivity. In 2005, 21% of U.S. adults were current cigarette smokers, 34% were overweight and another 34% were obese, and more than 40% were physically inactive (only 30% were *regularly* active) (NCHS, 2007a). Men (41.8%) were more likely than women (32%) to report engaging in vigorous physical activity.

Because these health-risk behaviors impact multiple body systems, it is common for some adults to develop more than one chronic health condition. **Multiple chronic conditions** are recorded as such for adults who have been diagnosed with three or more of the following: hypertension, heart disease, stroke, emphysema, diabetes, cancer, or arthritis (NCHS, 2007a). In 2005, 37% of adults aged 75 or older had multiple chronic conditions. That percentage was lower for adults aged 45–54 (7.3%) and 55–64 years (16.3%). However, the percentages were much higher for low-income adults in those two age groups (16% for those aged 45–54 and 30% for 55–64) (NCHS, 2007a).

Most adults know that regular exercise, proper diet, and abstinence from tobacco use are good for them. So, why don't they do "the right thing" when it comes to these three behaviors? To understand this, other influencing factors must be considered. Middle-aged adults (25–64 years of age) are a diverse group with a variety of needs and interests. Some common health-influencing factors for this age group include financial pressures at all levels of the socioeconomic scale, relationship and responsibility stressors at home and work, and low motivation to attend to personal health in light of these other pressures. The health professional who understands these needs will be better equipped to work in adult-based health promotion settings.

Older Adult Health

As longevity increases in the United States, health and quality of life among older Americans (aged 65 and older) has become a critical topic in discussions about national health. As the baby boomer generation moves into this span of life, some are already beginning to redefine what it means to be *older*. Some continue to work or pursue totally different interests long after the traditionally expected retirement age. Your contributions as a health professional to the well-being of older Americans has the potential to not only impact their quality of life but could, in some ways, positively impact your own experiences as an older adult.

Health and Demographics

There were approximately 34.8 million U.S. adults aged 65 and older in 2005, a number that represented 12% of the total population. This group is expected to grow to 72 million by 2030 and represent 20% of the population. By 2050, those 75 years of age and older will represent 12% of the total population, an increase from 6% in 2005. In all older age groups (65+ years), women outnumber men (6.9% of the population in 2005 versus 5.2%) (MCHB, 2007; NCHS, 2007a).

For adults aged 65 and older, the five leading causes of death were heart disease, cancer, cerebrovascular disease (stroke), CLRD, and Alzheimer's disease (NCHS, 2007a). Approximately 88% of these older adults have at least one chronic health condition and more than 20% have diabetes (CDC, 2007f). When diabetes, hypertension, and other conditions are not properly treated, they lead to conditions that impact one's ability to function and quality of life. Approximately 44% of adults age 75 or older report limitations to their usual activity due to a chronic condition. In addition to chronic diseases, this older population is also susceptible to vision and hearing difficulties, arthritis and joint pain, and compromised immune systems that make them vulnerable to infectious diseases (CDC, 2007f; NCHS, 2007a). In 2006, the percentages of older adults who self-rated their health as only fair or poor were 21.9% for those aged 65–74 and 28.1% for those 75 years or older (NCHS, 2007a).

Factors That Influence Health

As we have stated in previous sections, tobacco use, lack of physical activity, and poor eating habits are major contributors to chronic diseases. Older adults who replace these risk behaviors with healthy habits can significantly improve their health and quality of life even when chronic conditions are present. Yet, less than one-third of adults 65 years and older meet recommended fruit and vegetable intake standards. By age 75, one in three men and one in two women are physically inactive. Physical activity can reduce joint pain and stiffness, build strong muscles, and increase flexibility, all of which help to minimize the effects of arthritis and prevent falls and, in particular, hip fractures, a serious injury that impacts approximately 250,000 older adults each year (CDC, 2007f).

In 2005, 3.6 million older adults (10.1%) lived in poverty and an additional 9.5 million (26.7%) were near-poor (NCHS, 2007a). Though great strides have been made to help older adults gain access to needed health care, early detection and treatment of chronic conditions is not always realized. Ongoing health care and maintenance of positive self-esteem and independence are important goals for older adults interested in enjoying more of life.

Health Factors in Ethnic Communities

In 2006, 15% of the U.S. population was Hispanic, 12% was non-Hispanic Black, 4% was Asian, and about 1% was American Indian/Alaska Native or of more than one race (NCHS, 2007a). As you have learned through our descriptions of health issues throughout the life span of the U.S. population, some distinct health disparities exist between the predominantly White U.S. majority and some of these ethnic populations. For instance, the leading causes of death for adults (ages 18+ years) differ when broken down by ethnic group. As indicated in Table 4.1, heart disease and cancer were the leading causes of death for all groups in 2004. However, for American Indians/Alaska Natives, the third leading cause of death was unintentional injuries and stroke was ranked fifth. Diabetes was the fourth leading cause of death for all but non-Hispanic Whites, whose fourth leading cause of death was chronic lower respiratory disease (CLRD). For Asian American/Pacific Islanders, deaths due to influenza and pneumonia ranked fifth over unintentional injuries (their sixth leading cause at 21.4 deaths per 100,000). When causes of death are further differentiated by gender within each ethnic group (see Figure 4.6 on the following page), additional distinctions emerge (NCHS, 2007a).

Table 4.1   Five Leading Causes of Death among U.S. Adults (Age 18+) by Ethnicity, 2002–2004

Five Leading Causes of Death		Non-Hispanic White 66.5%*	Hispanic 14.7%	Non-Hispanic Black 12.3%	Asian American/ Pacific Islander 4.3%/0.1%	American Indian/Alaska Native 0.8%
	1	Heart disease 307.7**	Heart disease 229.9	Heart disease 404.0	Heart disease 169.8	Heart disease 208.5
	2	Cancer 258.0	Cancer 168.6	Cancer 318.4	Cancer 150.6	Cancer 165.5
	3	Stroke 69.3	Stroke 53.9	Stroke 100.5	Stroke 69.9	Unintentional injuries 66.7
	4	CLRD^ 62.2	Diabetes 46.2	Diabetes 66.9	Diabetes 23.0	Diabetes 46.6
	5	Unintentional injuries 48.2	Unintentional injuries 37.6	Unintentional injuries 45.5	Influenza & Pneumonia 22.5	Stroke 48.1

* Percentage of total U.S. population (Asian and Pacific Islander groups were separated in 2000 census. Some data/information still reported as one group).
** Deaths per 100,000 population.
^ Chronic lower respiratory disease; gray shading denotes a deviation from the majority of groups for that ranking.

Source: *Health Data for All Ages*, National Center for Health Statistics, 2008. Retrieved August 30, 2008, from http://www.cdc.gov/nchs/health_data_for_all_ages.htm

Even when mortality data and other health issues are ranked in the same order, the complications related to those health problems are often more pronounced among ethnic minorities. As we've emphasized in previous sections, a primary contributor to these health disparities across ethnic populations throughout the life span is poverty. In 2007, families living in poverty were disproportionately represented across these ethnic groups: 24.5% of non-Hispanic Blacks, 21.2% of American Indian/Alaska Natives, 21.5% of Hispanics, 16.1% of Native Hawaiian/Pacific Islanders, 10.2% of

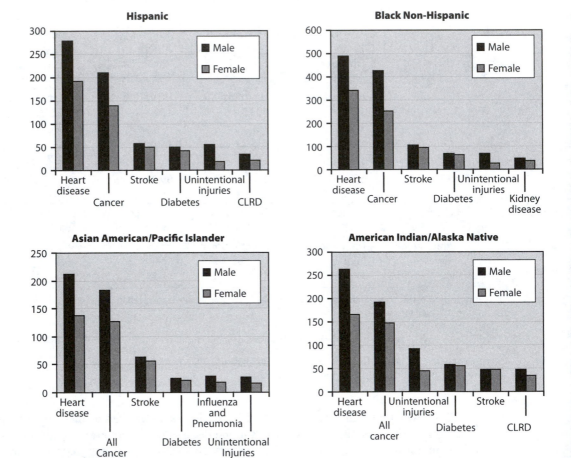

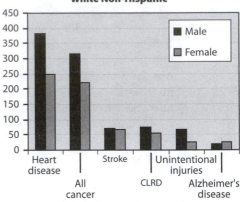

Figure 4.6   Leading causes of death for U.S. adults (age 18+) by gender and ethnicity, 2002–2004.

Source: *Health Data for All Ages*, National Center for Health Statistics, 2008. Retrieved August 30, 2008, from http://www.cdc.gov/nchs/health_data_for_all_ages.htm

Asian Americans, and 8.2% of non-Hispanic Whites. In contrast, the proportion of adults 25+ years of age who had completed a college degree was higher for Asian Americans (49.1%) and non-Hispanic Whites (30%) than for non-Hispanic Blacks (17.3%), Native Hawaiian/Pacific Islanders (15.4%), American Indian/Alaska Natives (13.6%), and Hispanics (12.2%) (U.S. Census Bureau, 2008a, b). These disparate education levels and financial opportunities across ethnic groups contribute in significant ways to differences in health status and access to health services.

Another major reason for health disparities across ethnic groups is that, according to a 2007 report on health in the United States from the NCHS (2007a), more traditional members often face barriers to health care access that include "ineligibility for many government-sponsored programs and difficulty in finding providers who speak their language and provide culturally sensitive care" (p. 4). Our chapter 2 discussion about developing cultural competence was meant as more than just a general suggestion. The lack of cultural competence in some pockets of the health professions is already seriously impacting the health and quality of life of many ethnic Americans. Quite simply, should you choose to neglect your personal growth in cultural competence, you will become part of the problem.

We offer the following overview of traditional health beliefs and communication styles with some hesitation; we are concerned that this information could be misconstrued or inadvertently applied in ways that perpetuate mislabeling and stereotyping. However, we trust that you will read the following material with a view toward understanding traditional norms and recognizing individual differences within any group.

We also encourage you to revisit this material after you've read the description in chapter 5 of the PEN-3 model (Airhihenbuwa, 1990). As explained there, cultural influences can be positive (health enhancing), negative, or *existential* (neutral). Most of what is described below is largely positive or existential. We hope you will learn to embrace and enjoy the diversity of traditional cultures in the United States. Even though health professionals might not agree with some practices, there is much that health educators can learn about life and total wellness from these traditional cultural perspectives.

Hispanic and Latino Americans

According to Dr. Rachel Spector (2004), a recognized authority on cultural aspects of health and illness, the terms *Hispanic* and *Latino* are sometimes used interchangeably to "refer to individuals who were born or whose predecessors came from Mexico, Puerto Rico, Cuba, Central and South America, Spain, and other Spanish-speaking communities and who now live in the United States" (p. 254). Think for a moment about the vast amount of geography, history, and diverse language and cultural nuances these original countries and continents represent, and you will likely more fully understand the diversity represented by those two terms and how easy it is to inadvertently stereotype Hispanics or Latino Americans.

Despite subgroup differences within the Hispanic umbrella, many of those groups share the traditional value of a family unit that extends beyond biological parents and children to include aunts and uncles, cousins, grandparents, godparents, and close friends (Purnell, 1998). These close relational ties contribute to a strong sense of community. Elderly family members usually move in with their children when they can no longer care for themselves. Sick relatives and friends are likely to receive hospital visits from many caring people. Health programs that promote nurturing family approaches can work well in these traditional settings.

The word *macho* may conjure up an image of a tough guy who believes himself superior to women. Its original meaning, however, was more positive; it referred to a man with "strength, valor, and self-confidence" (Purnell, 1998, p. 401). In patriarchal Hispanic tradition, male family members are the primary decision makers, while women monitor daily home and health care (Burk, Wieser, & Keegan, 1995; Purnell, 1998).

Traditional Communication Styles

Spanish is often the language of choice among traditional Hispanic families. Communication styles are rooted in views about *respeto, simpatía, personalismo,* and *confianza* (Paniagua, 2005; Purnell, 1998; Spector, 1996). *Respeto* (respect and courtesy to others) is often demonstrated by using titles (Señor or Señora) rather than first names and by avoiding direct eye contact, a sign of aggression. To uphold *simpatía* (avoiding conflict) and *respeto* for authority, traditional clients may not openly voice disagreement or dissatisfaction with your health promotion program. They may appear to agree in person and then simply not return. It helps to listen to what people *don't* say.

An overbooked health professional can suffer from a shortage of a critical commodity: time. In an ideal world, there would be enough hours in the day to embrace a more leisurely, caring approach when working with our clients. We sometimes forget that rushing through client visits can result in having more time on our hands than we'd like when those clients quit coming back. To counter this, *personalismo* (personalizing interaction) can be established with traditional Hispanic clients by first asking about the well-being and recent activities of the family. This approach often puts clients at ease and helps them feel as though you truly care about them. If you can recall interacting with a person who always took time to ask about your life, you can likely understand the significance of doing so with your clients.

Adapting your health promotion style to the traditional Hispanic views of *respeto, simpatía,* and *personalismo* will enhance the degree to which community members trust and accept you and your program. But don't expect to win their *confianza* (trust) overnight. You probably regard newcomers in your life with a bit of preliminary caution. Expect the same from your new clients. Be as consistent as possible in your efforts, openly admit when you make mistakes, and keep working at it. Patience pays.

Traditional Health Beliefs and Practices

Traditional health beliefs and practices vary and sometimes differ widely across Hispanic subgroups. Most of the examples provided below are based in Mexican or Puerto Rican traditions but can also be found in some form among traditional members of other subgroups (Spector, 2004).

Hot and cold theory.   Some traditional Hispanics believe illness is caused by improper balances of "hot" and "cold" foods (based on healing properties, not temperature) (Purnell, 1998; Spector, 2004). There is much disagreement about specific foods and illnesses that are classified as "hot" or "cold." For that reason, it is best to simply ask a client who adheres to this theory about his or her beliefs. In general, the treatment goal within this theory is to bring the body back to a state of balance (Spector, 2004). Thus, if a disease is considered a "hot" illness (for example, some view infections, fever, and diarrhea as "hot"), then "cold" foods (for some this means fresh fruits, milk, and fish) should be eaten. "Cold" diseases (some view arthritis, pneumonia, and cancer as "cold") are treated with "hot" foods (for some, eggs, beef, pork, cheeses, liquor, and spicy dishes) (Purnell, 1998).

Mal de ojo.   Some people associate *mal de ojo* or "evil eye" with what they've seen in movies about witches casting spells with wicked looks. But in Hispanic traditions, *mal de ojo* is an illness (such as fever, vomiting, irritability) that can be passed on to another person through well-meaning but excessive admiration and direct eye contact; an example is an adult making a great fuss over a cute baby (Spector, 2004). The spell can be broken, however, if the admirer touches the child as she looks. You may notice a child wearing a seed bracelet or a bag of seeds pinned to her clothing to prevent *mal de ojo* (Purnell, 1998).

Susto.   The condition called *susto* (fright or soul loss) is believed to result from a traumatic event that causes the soul to leave the body. Spector (2004) reported three common symptoms: restless sleep; listlessness, anorexia, or lack of interest in personal appearance and hygiene; and malaise, depression, and introversion. Treatment often involves a *curandero* (a traditional healer) and herbs to coax the soul back into the body (Purnell, 1998; Spector, 2004).

Black Americans

The first Blacks to arrive on the North American continent were not slaves. According to historians (Bullough & Bullough, 1972), Blacks arrived on the continent prior to the Pilgrims' arrival and also traveled to the Americas with Columbus in the fifteenth century. However, between 1619 and 1860, more than 4 million individuals were transported to the Americas as slaves from their homes on the African continent (Spector, 2004).

Though not all Black Americans are of African descent, some traditional African norms can be found in some Black American families. For example, the traditional **Afrocentric worldview** embraces the seven principles of *nguzo sabo* as a guide to appropriate living (Campinha-Bacote, 1998). The principles include "*umjo* (unity), *kujichagula* (self-determination), *ujima* (collective work and responsibility), *nia* (purpose), *imani* (faith), *ujamaa* (cooperative economics), and *kuumba* (creativity)" (p. 57). These seven principles contribute to a traditional culture that values hard work, self-discipline, and a cooperative community spirit.

Traditional Communication Styles

As is true for most White Americans, English is the dominant language spoken among Black Americans. And, as is true for some White Americans and others, Blacks employ ways of speaking English that do not necessarily match the standard rules of English grammar. However, according to the California Center for Applied Linguistics (CCAL, 2008), there exists a specific dialect (a regular, systematic language) used in some traditional Black American families that is currently referred to as *African American English* (AAE).

AAE is a systematic language variety, with patterns of pronunciation, grammar, vocabulary, and usage that extend far beyond slang. Because it has a set of rules that is distinct from those of Standard American English, characterizations of the variety as bad English are incorrect; speakers of AAE do not fail to speak Standard American English, but succeed in speaking African American English with all its systematicity. Linguists are less concerned with whether or not AAE is a language or a dialect (terms that are more important socially and politically than linguistically) than with recognizing the systematic nature of AAE. (CCAL, 2008, para. 4)

Examples of AAE-based speaking styles can include the use of the verb *be* in a nonstandard way, as in "He be going there," or following a noun in a sentence with a repetitive pronoun, as in "My mother, she lives in New York" (Campinha-Bacote, 1998; Landrum-Brown, 2000). However, note that the CCAL description of AAE is not presented as an insulting statement about bad grammar but, rather, as a systematic language. As a health professional, your goal should be to understand and respectfully work through any communication barriers that may arise when serving a traditional Black American whose primary dialect is AAE, just as you would with a traditional Hispanic American whose primary language is Spanish.

Regarding other aspects of communication styles, traditional Black American communication is dynamic and expressive, with feelings openly expressed among trusted friends and family. A louder voice volume doesn't necessarily correlate with anger or aggression and may, instead, be used with wit and humor among friends (Campinha-Bacote, 1998).

Traditional Black Americans are reportedly more comfortable with closer personal space than are Whites. However, touch is personal and reserved for close family members, while eye contact with an authority figure can be viewed as aggressive behavior (Campinha-Bacote, 1998). As with Hispanic Americans, we suggest that you call older Black American clients by their title (such as Dr., Mr., Mrs.) unless invited to do otherwise.

Traditional Health Beliefs and Practices

Black American communities can be as diverse as Hispanic American communities with regard to the spectrum of religions and spiritual beliefs as well as traditional health practices. We provide below a few of the more commonly identified traditional beliefs and practices.

Spirituality.   Christian teachings have historically played a strong role in the Black American community (Campinha-Bacote, 1998; Spector, 1996). The Black church is often an integral part of community function regardless of the degree of religious commitment among individual community members (Campinha-Bacote, 1998). In some traditional circles, illness is believed to be caused by evil spirits or sinful deeds. Healing comes from God through the power of prayer and "the laying on of hands" (Spector, 1996, p. 66). Belief in Satan-induced illness may lead some to a fatalistic view about sickness prevention (Campinha-Bacote, 1998), but belief in a spiritual source of strength and healing can also have positive health-enhancing results. We invite you to develop a healthy respect for the spiritual beliefs of traditional Black Americans and infuse positive spiritual components into your health education programs.

Voodoo. A very small portion of Black American communities reportedly practices voodoo, which derives its name from a West Indies god, *Vodu* (Spector, 2004). Over time, traditional voodoo rites and ceremonies merged with Catholic beliefs so that some ceremonies became a mixture of tribal dance, sacrifice and blood drinking, and the attribution of special powers to Catholic saints and relics. Health-related voodoo treatments include the use of good and bad *gris-gris* (spirit-powered oils and powders) and lighting candles of various colors for positive or negative hexes and spells (Spector, 2004).

Rooting. In the practice of rooting, derived from voodoo, a folk healer or root doctor may prescribe a variety of treatments. Many of these home remedies involve herbs or household products, such as an herbal tea made from goldenrod root used to treat pain and fever, or a potato poultice used to fight infection and inflammation (Spector, 2004).

Asian Americans

Like the word *Hispanic*, the term *Asian* represents a rich array of origins that include "the Far East, Southeast Asia, and the Indian subcontinent; for example, Cambodia, China, India, Japan, Korea, Malaysia, Pakistan, the Philippine Islands, Thailand, and Vietnam" (Spector, 2004, p. 210). Though the U.S. Census Bureau designated *Pacific Islanders* as a separate category in 2000, health data are still commonly reported as representing *Asian American/Pacific Islander.*

You have probably noticed the importance of family in most traditional ethnic cultures. In Asian traditions, individual success is most valuable in light of the honor it brings to the family (Paniagua, 2005; Spector, 2004). Obedience and respect, particularly in relation to age and status ranks, are very important. Relatives are expected to use their connections to support each other (*guan xi* in Chinese), and adult children are obligated to care for their aging parents (Matocha, 1998). Traditional family leaders and decision makers are usually the oldest male in the family. Traditional women are considered family nurturers and caregivers (Matocha, 1998).

As in most cultures, religion provides a rich context for health beliefs and practices among traditional Asian Americans (Spector, 2004). The four traditional religions of Buddhism, Confucianism, Taoism, and shamanism share a central theme of harmony and balance (Spector, 1996). Buddhism teaches respect for life, moderation in behavior, self-discipline, and selflessness. Confucianism emphasizes harmonious relationships, a behavioral code, respect for superiors, and the pursuit of learning. Harmony with nature and between humans is a primary principle of Taoism, and shamanism supports the belief that everything in nature possesses a spirit.

The yin-yang philosophy originated in ancient China, where it was commonly believed that all life is regulated by two forces that constantly work in opposition to each other (Spector, 1996). *Yang* is the positive and dynamic energy force (light, hot or warm, full) and *yin* is the negative and static energy force (dark, cold, empty). Traditional belief says that if one is to function in harmony with self and the world, an appropriate balance of this yin-yang life force must be maintained (Matocha, 1998).

Traditional Communication Styles

The diversity of languages represented within the Asian American population is as vast as the number of countries of origin and subcultures. Among Filipinos, the fastest growing Asian group in North America, more than 100 languages are spoken (Miranda, McBride, & Spangler, 1998). Because modesty is considered a virtue, some Asian Americans may closely guard against public embarrassment over health-related issues that imply personal failure, for example marital difficulties and mental disorders (Jack, Harrison, & Airhihenbuwa, 1994). To maintain "face," a traditional client may pretend to understand and agree with your instructions or suggestions. When working with traditional Asian American clients, you may need to maintain a respectful distance (arrange chair choices at varying distances), minimize direct eye contact (try sitting side by side) and touch (explain why and when touch is necessary), and ask for ample communication feedback (use short, simple sentences and list directions) (Matocha, 1998).

Traditional Health Beliefs and Practices

There is often confusion in mainstream American culture about some traditional Asian American health practices and beliefs. For example, the practice of t'ai chi is viewed by some as simply a physical exercise or art, but is viewed by others as a practice that is steeped in mysticism. In truth, neither view is accurate. We provide below a brief explanation of qi and t'ai chi along with some additional traditional practices.

Qi and t'ai chi.   Some traditional Asian Americans believe the human body contains an invisible system of channels or meridians through which energy (*qi*) flows (Matocha, 1998). Traditional healers are trained to know the precise points along these meridians at which an acupuncture needle, physical pressure or massage, or moxibustion (heat application) can be applied to induce healing.

T'ai chi is an ancient practice in which individuals attempt to achieve a healthy balance in energy flow (called *chi)* through a variety of movements or exercises. Some seek chi through the martial arts. Others prefer less definitive movement patterns that are dictated by one's inner sense of the yin-yang balance. T'ai chi has been found to reduce stress levels and benefit the circulatory system (Matocha, 1998).

Coining and cupping.   Some traditional Asian American healers may provide spiritual cleansing through *coining* (lightly scraping the skin with a coin) or *cupping* (creating suction through heat on the skin with a "cup") to rid the body of illness-causing spirits (Matocha, 1998). Demonstrated respect for these existential practices can foster community acceptance of your health promotion programs.

Traditional remedies.   Some Asian American cultures have long employed herbal roots, plants, and other products, which are ground and boiled in water for the patient to ingest or use as a poultice (Spector, 1996). Examples include eating snake flesh for clear vision; applying rhinoceros horn to boils; and taking ginseng tablets or tea for anemia, digestive problems, impotence, and depression. Because it can be dangerous to combine these treatments with physician-prescribed medicines, you should be aware of home remedies used by your clients.

American Indians and Alaska Natives

The U.S. government has officially recognized more than 560 tribes (Office of Minority Health, 2009). The five largest American Indian Nations include the Cherokee, Navajo, Latin American Indian, Choctaw, and Sioux (Spector, 2004). The vast diversity across and within these groups can complicate attempts to provide generalized information about traditional American Indian cultures. However, knowledge about some recognized commonalities (Paniagua, 2005; Spector, 2004; Still & Hodgins, 1998; Waldram, 2004) can enhance your competence as a health professional.

In many traditional American Indian cultures, the family unit is important and elderly members are highly respected (Paniagua, 2005; Still & Hodgins, 1998). Competition is often discouraged (Paniagua, 2005; Waldram, 2004) and, in some tribes (such as the Navajo), families with more wealth are expected to provide for those with less (Still & Hodgins, 1998). Family leadership roles differ across American Indian subgroups, but many tribes are matriarchal, meaning that mothers and grandmothers are the center of society and commonly are health-related decision makers (Still & Hodgins, 1998).

Health-related beliefs vary across cultures and individuals. However, common tradition embraces the concept of *Mother Earth* (Paniagua, 2005; Spector, 1996), the idea that the earth is a living organism with which one must seek harmony to be well and happy. Caring for one's body and the land on which one lives creates a harmonious environment in which a person can fulfill one's spiritual destiny. Disharmony results in illness.

Traditional Communication Styles

Language and dialect differences across more than 560 tribes sometimes serve as communication barriers between tribes (Still & Hodgins, 1998). Like some Asian-oriented languages, American Indian languages often rely heavily on differing voice inflections to convey different meanings. Talking loudly or using the wrong voice inflection when trying to pronounce an Indian word can be insulting. For that reason, using an interpreter in professional settings is often a good idea (Still & Hodgins, 1998).

When working with a traditional American Indian client, don't be alarmed if you are met with a deadpan expression or if direct eye contact is avoided. Some individuals may seem aloof until they know you better, and those who interpret eye contact as a sign of aggression may avoid it (Paniagua, 2005; Waldram, 2004). Although touch is usually reserved for intimate friends, a handshake is often the appropriate greeting.

Traditional medical healers are expected to know the cause of illness without asking the patient. In a clinical setting, physicians may be considered incompetent if they have to ask many questions. With traditional clients, it may help to begin with observational statements (such as "You appear to have a chest cold") rather than questions.

Traditional Health Beliefs and Practices

As with the cultural traditions of other ethnic populations, the nature and scope of healing beliefs and practices among 560 American Indian nations are diverse. We provide a few examples of these beliefs and practices below.

Divination.   Traditional American Indian healing is rooted in beliefs about the mind-body-spirit connection and the place of plants, animals, and humans in the spirit world (Spector, 2004). Medicine men and women are often believed to possess a spiritual gift that allows them to first diagnose the cause of an illness without asking the patient (called *divination*). Hopi medicine men and women often use *meditation* to determine the cause of an illness. They sometimes use a crystal ball or chew on trance-inducing jimsonweed to identify the evil that caused the disease. A Navajo medicine man or woman may be gifted with the *motion of the hand* in which sand or pollen is ceremonially sprinkled around the patient while the diviner chants and waves a hand to determine the cause of illness. Sand art is sometimes created in these ceremonies or incorporated into *stargazing* (determining the cause by noting the colors of light shafts) or *listening* (interpreting various sounds) (Spector, 1996).

The singer.   The diviner often meets with the family to discuss the discovered diagnosis, discuss treatment, and recommend a healer or *singer* if the diviner does not have the healing gift or training. A singer may be called on to treat the condition through "the laying on of hands" or by drawing disease-causing elements out of the body while singing.

Purification.   *Purification* (cleansing the body and spirit) is brought about by total water immersion and the use of sweat lodges and herbal remedies in special rituals. Remedies differ across groups. For example, the Micmac Indians of Canada use milk-weed plant to cure warts and juniper berries to treat rheumatism. The Oneida Indians treat colds with witch hazel and ear infections with skunk oil. The Hopi Indians use sunflowers to treat spider bites and the ground stem of the yucca plant as a laxative.

White Americans

Because White European Americans represent a large portion of the U.S. population, the natural tendency is to think of this group as the majority rather than an ethnic population. However, there are special populations within this group who also adhere to traditional cultural norms that differ from that of mainstream society. The historical origins of White Americans are as diverse as that of other ethnic populations we have described. Most traditional White American ethnic groups identify themselves with German, Irish, English, Italian, and French heritages. In some large U.S. cities such as New York, Los Angeles, Chicago, Houston, and Philadelphia, Whites represent a minority of the city population (Spector, 2004).

At the risk of sounding repetitive, we note that the family unit is an important component of most traditional White American populations. This was particularly true for original immigrant families who established neighborhood enclaves for solidarity and support. Some multiple-generation families still live in these social enclaves and, because of that, are more likely to practice high heritage consistency (see chapter 2) than are those who have moved from these neighborhoods and live within more culturally diverse segments of U.S. society.

Traditional Communication Styles

As with other ethnic groups, communication styles across traditional White American populations can vary widely. They can represent various languages (for example, English, Italian, German, and French) and dialects within those languages. We encourage you to explore resources (CCAL, 2008) about languages and dialects (such as *Southern English*) used among traditional White Americans.

Traditional Health Beliefs and Practices

Health beliefs and practices among traditional White American groups can be as diverse as the original countries and global regions they represent. We provide below some examples that derive predominantly from Italian and German traditions.

Malocchio and castiga.   Some traditional Italian Americans believe that certain illnesses can be caused by *malocchio* (evil eye), the Italian equivalent to the Hispanic term *mal de ojo*, or to *castiga* (curses sent by God as punishment for sins or by evil people). *Malocchio* is commonly thought to cause less severe illnesses such as headaches, but illnesses caused by *castiga* can be fatal. One treatment for *malocchio* is the practice of using eggs, olive oil, and water in a religious ritual combined with prayer. The belief that illness can be a punishment from God for wrongdoing is common among traditional Italian, German, and Polish Americans (Spector, 2004).

Germ and stress theories.   The belief that stress and germs cause illness is common in many ethnic cultures and is particularly dominant in some traditional White American cultures. For example, one traditional Italian belief is that suppressed emotions can make one ill, a belief that may contribute to strong emotional approaches to communication observed in some traditional Italian American families. Traditional German Americans also believe in stress-related theories and also strongly adhere to cleanliness and fresh air approaches to ridding the environment of disease-causing germs.

Home remedies.   Home remedies are commonly used across all traditional ethnic communities. These remedies vary widely from family to family. Examples of remedies used among some traditional White American groups include the use of herbs and teas; pendulums or wire bracelets (to ward off illness-causing curses); and topical salves or poultices that contain spices/herbs, aloes, or fats. Honey with lemon, chicken soup, and gargling with salt water are common remedies for a cold or sore throat. The periodic use of laxatives (including Black draught and Castor oil) to clean or purge the system of unclean, illness-causing elements is also common (Spector, 2004).

In Conclusion

In this chapter we highlight some health issues relevant to selected age, gender, and ethnic groups in the U.S. population. We also briefly touch upon some traditionally ethnic communication styles and health-related beliefs and practices. Though the information provided lacks the depth and breadth that you will need to fully understand, appreciate, and effectively work with each group, it can be a useful starting place for learning more about these and other special populations. We encourage you to consider the information in this chapter as you explore the application of processes described in subsequent chapters. Keep in mind what we said in chapters 1 and 2, that becoming an effective, culturally competent health professional is an ongoing developmental process. You are not expected to be fully proficient in all special populations today. Your goal should be to identify where you are in this developmental process, establish some personal development goals, and take the next step.

REVIEW QUESTIONS

1. Explain the importance of learning about the health status of Americans in terms of age-specific and ethnic groups.

2. Discuss strengths and weaknesses of health-status data sources in the United States.

3. Describe the underlying role of socioeconomic status and its effect on health status in the United States.

4. Describe some general demographic characteristics for each age-specific group in the United States.

5. Name some leading causes of death and prominent health issues for specific age groups, genders, and ethnic populations in the United States.

6. Describe some traditional communication styles and health beliefs and practices of at least four ethnic communities in the United States.

7. Explain the utility as well as potential risks of attempting to apply general information about traditional ethnic groups to local communities and individual members of those ethnic groups.

FOR YOUR APPLICATION

Tracking Health Issues throughout the Life Span

Select a health problem (such as alcohol abuse) that can be tracked through the life span. Create a three-column table and label those columns *Age-Specific Group*, *Potential Risks,* and *Potential Solutions.* Add a row to the table for each of the age-specific groups addressed in this chapter (for example, infants, children, adolescents). Place those group labels in the *Age-Specific Group* column of each row. At the top of the paper, give your table an appropriate title (such as *Alcohol Abuse Throughout the Life Span*). Then, in the *Potential Risks* column, list what a person in each age group could face if exposed to the health problem. For example, if exposed to alcohol abuse, an infant might be born with fetal alcohol syndrome; a child might be abused/neglected by alcoholic parents; an adolescent might be in an alcohol-related traffic accident; a middle-aged adult could develop chronic liver disease; and an older adult could suffer from other illnesses known to be intensified by life-long alcohol misuse (such as diabetes and heart disease). For the *Potential Solutions* column, list capacities and resources available to individuals in each age group that could reduce potential alcohol-related problems or reduce exposure to alcohol misuse. Note differences across the life span.

CHAPTER
five

Theory-Based Approaches

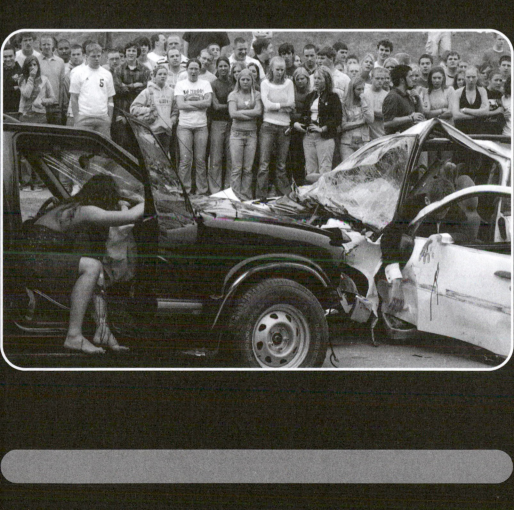

You realize that understanding theories is important. But you've seen an illustration of a theory and it seemed like a jumbled collection of boxes, circles, and lines. And then, when you tried to review more than one, it became just plain overwhelming. How can theories and models be so helpful if they don't even make sense?

CHAPTER OBJECTIVES

1. Describe the primary components of individual behavioral theories such as the health belief model, transtheoretical model, theory of planned behavior, and the precaution adoption process theory.

2. Explain how the interpersonal behavioral theory—social cognitive theory—differs from individual behavioral theories.

3. Discuss how the PEN-3 model can be used to distinguish between positive, existential, and negative cultural influences on health.

4. Detail how PRECEDE/PROCEED would be a useful model for identifying factors that influence community health problems.

5. Analyze how behavioral theory relates to public health.

Importance of Theory to Health Education

Having to memorize theories and models for a college course can be a nuisance. You may suspect that some professors include them in required materials just to keep you busy or to satisfy some egotistical "ivory tower" personality quirk. We don't deny that in some cases you could be correct. However, theories and models can be useful in the real world when they serve as a framework for accuracy and efficiency. Used appropriately, they enable you to competently evaluate large, complex issues. To illustrate the value of using a model in needs assessment, program planning, or evaluation, we invite you to consider a fictitious story we lovingly refer to as "The Elephant Story."

Our story is derived from a well-known poem called "The Blind Men and the Elephant" written by John Godfrey Saxe in the 1800s (Bornstein, 1996). The poem was fashioned after a portion of the Udana, canonical Hindu scripture (Ireland, 1999). Both are about blind men who believed they understood all there was to know about an elephant but, in reality, understood only certain parts. Our elephant story helps make the point about needing to see the whole picture. We hope it will help you in your quest to unscramble the meaning behind behavioral theories and their use.

The Story

Once upon a time, there were a number of different research groups who were all attempting to assess a certain health phenomenon called "The Elephant." Part of the problem inherent in seeing the full picture of this elephant phenomenon was that the research groups were not cooperating with each other. Members of each group feared that sharing information with others would threaten their access to limited resources. The result was that each group had only a partial picture of the whole elephant issue. This, of course, distorted the truth about the elephant phenomenon and crippled any effective attempts to address the issue as a whole.

One day, a student who had recently joined one of the research teams voiced the unspeakable. She suggested that all of the teams be invited to a conference to share what they'd learned about the elephant phenomenon. She even launched an awareness campaign to help each team realize the advantages of being able to see the whole elephant picture. She then booked the conference in the Bahamas to add to the appeal. Miraculously, it worked. The teams came.

On the first day of the conference, all of the big names in "elephant phenomenon" research entered the conference hall, and the excitement (not to mention the competitive tension) was high. The first research team representative walked to the podium and the crowd expectantly hushed. He started speaking: "Ladies and gentlemen, I am honored to be the first to speak on this momentous occasion about the phenomenon we all know to be the elephant. As you know, our research team has been tirelessly working for a number of years to carefully assess the elephant and we have clearly identified some interesting physical characteristics and movement patterns. We now know that the elephant is shaped much like a tree trunk, is flat on the bottom, and often appears in clusters of four" (Figure 5.1). With a self-satisfied look on his face, the researcher returned to his seat.

A representative of another research group then came to the podium with a slight frown on her face. She leaned into the microphone and stated, "Ladies and gentlemen, I respectfully submit that the previous speaker may think he's been researching the elephant. However, I can only surmise that he must be mistaken." The first speaker gasped from his seat, and his face turned red. But she continued, "My team has been researching the elephant phenomenon for over a decade and we've found our data to accurately reflect its characteristics." She paused for effect. "The elephant is not at all shaped like a tree trunk, nor does it move in clusters of four." The first speaker angrily grasped the arms of his chair. "To the contrary, elephants almost always move in

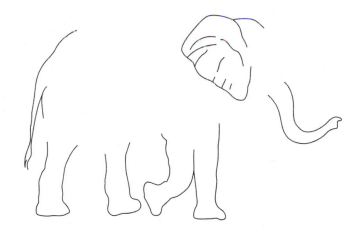

Figure 5.1   The elephant story.
The "elephant story" illustrates how a model can be used to create a more complete picture of a community health issue from previously isolated pieces of information.

pairs. (We believe they mate for life.) They are shaped much like a huge, flat fan and, under certain conditions, may move in wavelike motions." She shot a pointed look at the first speaker and returned to her seat.

The tension mounted as a representative of yet a third research group approached the microphone. He solemnly eyed his audience and, with a thoughtful expression, said: "Distinguished colleagues, I am perplexed by what we have heard today. There is nothing in my 20-year experience of elephant phenomenon research to validate the previous two speakers' descriptions. In our assessments, we have never encountered elephants in close proximity to each other. Each elephant is shaped like a garden hose and often behaves like one with an occasional spray of water coming out the end." He sat down amidst the hubbub of agitated whispers and angry looks between research teams.

Just as total crowd chaos was about to break forth, a tall, white-haired, distinguished-looking gentleman suddenly stood from the back of the room and shouted above the noise "Enough!" Heads turned toward his voice and in the ensuing hush you could have heard a pin drop. This man was recognized by all as a long-time researcher and scholar in the field. Though he, too, had selfishly guarded his findings over the years, he remained a recognized authority in elephant research, predominantly because he'd been researching the longest. All eyes were on him as he purposefully made his way to the front of the room. He turned his intense gaze onto the hushed audience and said, "I've heard enough! I am appalled at your lack of understanding and true knowledge about a phenomenon that affects the lives of so many people. This elephant phenomenon is no joking matter!" Fixing his fiery gaze on each of the three speakers, he virtually shouted, "You have embarrassed our profession with your misguided attempts to describe the elephant! The elephant is like . . . it's small . . ."

The crowd leaned toward him, sensing that what he was about to say would change forever how they saw the elephant. But the intensity of the moment became too much and, before he could finish his sentence, the gentleman fell to the floor in a dead faint. The crowd rushed to his aid, almost smothering him in the process. Some were shouting instructions to unbutton his collar, get him some water, call 911. Others shouted for the crowd to back up and give him some breathing space. In a moment, the gentleman came to and instantly grabbed the collar of the researcher who kneeled beside him. Pulling him close, the gentleman urgently whispered in a hoarse, strained voice, "The elephant is like a very large, stiff worm with no eyes." Those close enough to hear him looked at each other in surprise. "A worm?" someone asked incredulously. "Yes," he hissed. "A worm that grows out of the rump of a hill." He paused to catch his breath and then moaned, "But, to this day, I can't for the life of me determine the source of that awful smell."

The Meaning

Okay, so it's a silly story. It's difficult to imagine any thinking human having difficulty seeing the full picture of an elephant. After all, we all know what an elephant looks like, right? But what if we were talking about a real community health issue that was a little more difficult to define and assess? What if it were something that affects the well-being of a large array of community members, such as violence in schools? Imagine that some teenagers walk into a high school and open fire on students with automatic weapons. The aftermath is devastating, and the whole country gets in on the act of trying to assess what happened and why.

The discussion could sound a lot like the comments of those researchers who saw only parts of the elephant. Some might blame the school system for loose security and call for metal detectors at all doors or specialized training for school personnel. Others might point to violent media sources and demand that they be banned. The parents would certainly be scrutinized, and some would argue for more counseling programs for troubled families or for stricter laws holding parents accountable. Most assuredly, a large array of resources and potential solutions would be suggested, some of which might actually work within the context of the whole picture. However, without broad understanding of all potential influences and solutions, some parts of the "elephant" might be overlooked.

That's how theories and models help. They provide a framework through which we can accurately assess large, complex health issues and their potential solutions. They remind us to look for common relationships between factors and help us ask the right questions. A number of theories and models are used in the health education field. We will address only a portion of them in this textbook. Most are useful in a number of ways, including needs assessment; program planning, implementation, and evaluation; and program marketing. The theories you use will depend on your unique work situation, the participants, and the target behaviors. For that reason, we encourage you to learn enough about the commonly used theories and models to gain some idea of where to start when selecting a theoretical foundation for your work.

Commonly Used Theories in Health Education

Words abound when discussing theories and models so let's start by considering a few definitions. Some individuals use the word *theory* to mean simply an idea about how something works. However, most fields that are grounded in science use the word *theory* only when that idea has been studied through research and determined to be true in at least one circumstance. When we talk about behavioral theory, especially behaviors related to health, we are talking about the scientific use of the word *theory*. Because human behavior is complex, behavioral theories are generally multifaceted; that is, they contain several concepts and/or constructs that work together to explain a behavior. **Construct** is a term for a theoretical concept that was created for a specific theory (Glanz, Rimer, & Viswanath, 2008). As a theory is studied, relationships between concepts are clarified and put together to explain why a behavior occurs.

According to Glanz, Rimer, and Lewis (2002), a model uses concepts or constructs from several theories to explain a phenomenon or behavior. In a sense, it's like melding several theories into a new theory. When a theory is studied through research, concepts and constructs are called **variables**. Of course, it would be easier if the same words were used, but research and evaluation carries a set of specific terms that have meaning to researchers, so it is important for you to understand how those terms relate to your work. You will learn more about research and evaluation in an upcoming chapter.

One of the reasons that studying behavioral theories becomes frustrating is the sheer number of them. There are theories that work best with individuals, while others were created for use with entire communities. Some theories focus on attitudes and beliefs while others regard consequences of actions as most important. An appropriate first step is to become familiar with some of the commonly used behavioral theories in health education. The following sections will assist you in this endeavor.

Health Belief Model

The **health belief model** (Hochbaum, 1958) was initially created to explore people's willingness to participate in screening x-rays for tuberculosis and to evaluate that willingness in relationship to their perceptions of susceptibility to the disease and perceptions of disease severity. It is a model that helps explain the behaviors of individuals. Although the theory originated out of a study of individuals in a screening program, it can be applied to other behaviors.

Did you ever watch a film or video in school that was designed to deter you from drinking and driving? If so, you may still remember some of the more graphic scenes of automobiles ripped in half and human blood everywhere. Did the scare tactics work? If so, for how long did the message influence your behavior?

What if you had been the person hired to make that video? Would you have done it any differently? You might have, if you understood the average adolescent mind-set. Adolescents who take risks rarely believe that behavioral consequences affect them. They may fully accept statistical evidence that shows a high correlation between fatal accidents and drinking while driving. But they may not fully believe themselves to be at risk, even though they drink and drive. Their attitude may be, "I know it can happen to the other guy—that doesn't mean it's going to happen to me." In some cases, showing a dozen graphic videos about the severity of the consequences may do little to change that perception.

As illustrated in Figure 5.2, an individual's perception of the severity of a behavioral consequence plus the perception of their personal susceptibility to the consequence will determine their perception of threat from the behavior. In other words, risk-taking adolescents are more likely to refrain from drinking when they drive if they truly feel threatened or at risk of experiencing the potentially awful consequences. So, how would you convince them they are at risk? How would you increase their levels of perceived threat? The graphic video might not work if it addresses only one of the two types of individual perceptions that often influence perceived threat. An adolescent can truly believe bad stuff can happen when a person drinks and drives (high perceived severity) but still think "It won't happen to me!"

According to the health belief model, adequate levels of both perceived severity and perceived susceptibility must be present for perceived threat to be a behavioral motivating factor. Even with both those elements in place, other modifying factors

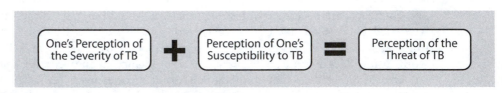

Figure 5.2   Perceived threat in the health belief model.

sometimes come into play (Strecher & Rosenstock, 1997), as illustrated in Figure 5.3. Of course, we already know that differences in age, personality, culture, experience, and so forth can influence perceptions about threat. For example, an adolescent who has been in a car hit by an intoxicated driver will certainly have different perceptions of threat than other adolescents.

Perceived benefits and barriers (pros and cons) to engaging in healthy behavior also increase the likelihood of behavior change if the benefits outweigh the barriers (Nardi & Petr, 2003). Adolescents may believe that their friends want them to drink, which may serve as a powerful momentary barrier that may outweigh the benefit of keeping mom and dad happy. So, the key is that perceptions of barriers must be decreased while the perceptions of benefits increased.

Even with all those health-enhancing components in place, individuals may still need a little nudge to help them get started on changing behavior for the better. In the health belief model, that little nudge is referred to as a cue to action, usually a single event that serves to jump start behavior change. In our example, a cue to action among adolescents might be the death of an admired celebrity in an alcohol-related accident. Any event that brings the threat closer to home can serve as a cue to action.

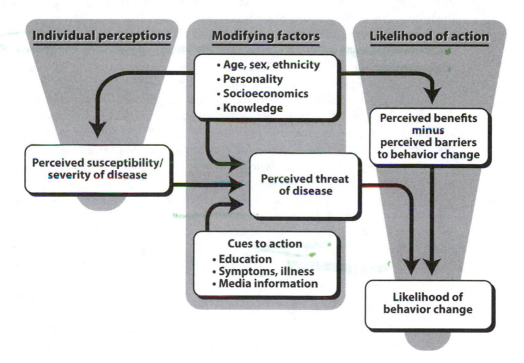

Figure 5.3   Health belief model.
According to the health belief model, adequate levels of perceived severity and perceived susceptibility must both be present for perceived threat to be a behavior-motivating factor.
From "Health Belief Model," by V. J. Strecher and I. M. Rosenstock, in *Health Behavior and Health Education: Theory, Research, and Practice* (p. 48), edited by K. Glanz, F. M. Lewis, and B. K. Rimer, © 1997 by John Wiley and Sons. Used with permission.

The construct of self-efficacy was added to the health belief model (Rosenstock, Strecher, & Becker, 1988) when the model started being used for more complex behaviors. Self-efficacy is a perception about how well one can perform a specific task. If adolescents don't believe they can say no to alcohol being offered by peers, they have low self-efficacy regarding this behavior. We will learn more about self-efficacy in the discussion about social cognitive theory, the theory for which it was created.

Now that you've learned about the health belief model, how would you increase the likelihood that adolescents would choose to refrain from drinking and driving? Even with your new knowledge, it won't be an easy task and other theories and/or models might better fit the adolescents in your community.

Theory of Planned Behavior

Have you ever done something you knew was risky? Though you may have had a number of reasons, none may have been related to your perceptions about the severity of the consequences or your susceptibility to them. That's why the health belief model doesn't work in every situation. There are times when people know all about severity and susceptibility and still forge ahead. So we encourage you to consider some of the influencing factors in Figure 5.4, which illustrates another individual behavior change theory, the **theory of planned behavior** (Ajzen, 1991).

Like the health belief model, the theory of planned behavior includes an attitude component that reminds us to think about behavior-related perceptions, beliefs, and expected outcomes. An individual's belief about a behavior (what will happen if a behavior is performed) plus his/her judgment about that outcome (positive or negative) make up the attitude toward the behavior which, in turn, impacts the intention to perform a behavior. The behavioral intention, then, influences the actual behavior. For example, a woman who believes that quitting smoking will improve health but does not value her health or believes that quitting will be physically and emotionally difficult will have a negative attitude toward the quitting behavior. That negative attitude will lessen the intention to quit.

The theory also prompts us to think about another common influencing factor we've not yet discussed. It's called **subjective norm** (see Figure 5.4). A person's subjective norm is made up of his or her perceptions about whether others approve or disapprove of the behavior (normative belief) plus the degree to which he or she values their opinions (motivation to comply). In our smoking example, the woman may believe that her doctor wants her to quit, but there would also have to be a motivation to comply with the doctor for the behavioral intention to be increased. A more likely scenario is that friends of the smoker, who also smoke, don't want her to quit. There may be stronger motivation to comply with friends, which would lessen the behavioral intention.

Perceptions of behavioral control, made up of control beliefs and perceived power, will influence both the behavioral intention and the actual behavior. The perception that there are factors that facilitate or prevent a behavior are *control* beliefs, while the weight that an individual gives each of those factors determines whether there is a negative or positive perception of behavioral control. Our smoker will have a positive perception of behavioral control if she believes there are useful factors that will help her quit.

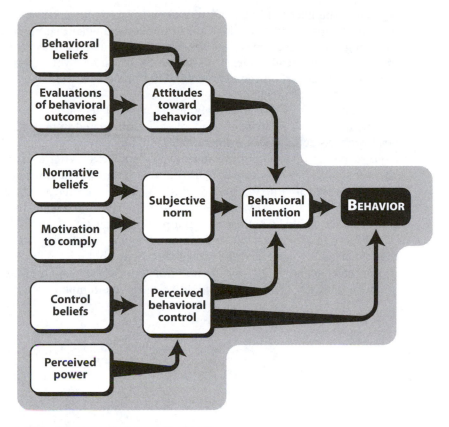

Figure 5.4   Theory of planned behavior.
In the theory of planned behavior, subjective norm is measured as a person's perceptions about and motivation to comply with the opinions of others. From "The Theory of Reasoned Action and the Theory of Planned Behavior," by D. E. Montano, D. Kasprzyk, and S. H. Taplin, in *Health Behavior and Health Education: Theory, Research, and Practice* (p. 92), edited by K. Glanz, F. M. Lewis, and B. K. Rimer, © 1997 by John Wiley and Sons. Used with permission.

If all of the people in your community of interest acted like clones, if they all had the same perceptions and moved at the same pace in their decision-making processes, we could end our discussion of theory here. After all, we've already discussed different types of behavior-related attitudes and beliefs (health belief model) and the powerful influence of peers (theory of planned behavior). What we haven't covered, however, is how the behavior-change process can evolve over time. We think that's important because we don't want you to become impatient or discouraged if you don't witness immediate results with your health education efforts.

Transtheoretical Model

The process of educating a community about health and observing positive changes is sometimes like planting a seed and watching it slowly grow into a flowering plant. You have to be patient and willing to "feed and water" the behavior-change process along the way. You also have to understand what that process needs at each stage of growth. That's one of the benefits of referring to the **stages of change** portion of the **transtheoretical model** (see Figure 5.5). It will help you determine where community members are in the decision-making process as well as ways to adapt your health education strategies.

In our previous discussions about behavior-related attitudes and beliefs, we've assumed that our participants had already formulated some opinions about the health-related behaviors of drinking and smoking. However, some of those participants, even the ones who drink and drive or smoke, may have never really thought about it at all. They may have been too busy with the ups and downs of life to contemplate the risks of drinking and driving. According to the transtheoretical model (Prochaska, Redding, & Evers, 1997), those who haven't given any thought to a particular behavior would be in the **precontemplation** stage.

What if most of the adolescents in our drinking and driving example had already thought about it a great deal due to some recent alcohol-related deaths in their school? In that case, spending all your limited time and money on an awareness campaign might be a waste. The majority would be in the **contemplation** stage, meaning that

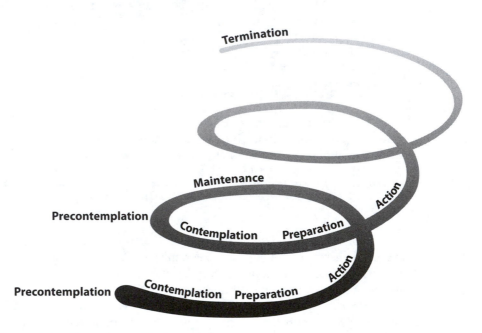

Figure 5.5   Transtheoretical model.
The transtheoretical model (stages of change) illustrates how a person can progress through a series of stages, from not even considering a behavior change to actually infusing the behavior change into one's lifestyle. Loops and repeated stages depict potential relapse and repeated change cycles. From "The Transtheoretical Model of Change and HIV Prevention: A Review," by J. O. Prochaska, C. A. Redding, L. L. Harlow, J. S. Rossi, and W. F. Velicer, *Health Education and Health Behavior 21*(4), pp. 471–486. © 1994 by Sage Publications. Used with permission.

they have been thinking about the need to change their drinking and driving habits but are, perhaps, hesitating because of what they'd have to give up.

As you have probably guessed, each stage of change has its own characteristics and information needs. Individuals in the **preparation** stage have already decided to make a change and are planning to do something about it in the very near future. They are the ones who need more information about how to avoid drunk driving situations in the face of peer pressure. On the other hand, it would be a waste to start with this "how to" information if individuals are in the precontemplation stage and haven't even decided yet that they need such information.

Those in the **action** and **maintenance** stages have already been practicing the desired behavior at different levels of success. Different health education strategies are required to promote consistency in practicing the newly acquired behavior change and prevent relapse. Strong support groups can help individuals who have reached these last stages to continue making good choices.

Other aspects of the transtheoretical model demonstrate, once again, how important beliefs, perceptions, and attitudes are in making behavior changes. Decisional balance and self-efficacy are core constructs of the transtheoretical model. Decisional balance describes concepts we discussed earlier; simply, the pros and cons of making a behavioral change. And as you know already, self-efficacy is one's belief that he/she can perform a task.

The transtheoretical model goes beyond theoretical concepts and offers actual strategies for helping individuals move through the stages of change. These strategies are termed **processes of change** and include the actions listed in Table 5.1 on the following page.

Precaution Adoption Process Model

We want to give you a very brief introduction to the precaution adoption process model (PAPM). This model has seven stages that document an assumption that behavior change is dynamic and occurs over time (Elliott, Seals, & Jacobson, 2007). The stages include the following: unaware, unengaged, deciding about action, deciding not to act, deciding to act, acting, and maintenance. Do you see the similarities to the stages of change in the transtheoretical model? The stages are much the same in both processes but we include PAPM because it addresses individuals who choose not to act.

In the stages of change, people who have no knowledge of a new healthy behavior and those who know about the healthy behavior but choose not to act are placed together in the precontemplation stage. In reality, a different strategy may be needed to motivate people who have decided not to act compared to those who just don't know about the healthy behavior. We believe this issue is important because you will be working with many people who choose not to act. For example, how many people do you know who smoke and have no idea that the behavior is unhealthy?

Weinstein and Sandman (1992), who developed the model for the precaution adoption process, believe that concepts and constructs from other theories such as perceptions of susceptibility and severity (health belief model), self-efficacy (social cognitive theory) and social norms (theory of planned behavior) can be used to help individuals move from the stage of "deciding to act" to the stage of "acting." If an

Table 5.1   Processes of Change

Process	Goal	Interventions
Consciousness Raising	Increase awareness	Feedback, education, confrontation, and media campaigns
Dramatic Relief	Increase emotional experience	Psychodrama, role-playing, grieving, personal testimonies, and media campaigns
Environmental Reevaluation	Assess thoughts and feelings	Empathy training, documentaries, and family interventions
Social Liberation	Increase social opportunities	Advocacy, empowerment procedures, and appropriate policies
Self-reevaluation	Assess one's self image	Value clarification, healthy role models, and imagery
Stimulus Control	Decrease negative cues to action and add positive cues to action	Avoidance, environmental re-engineering, and self-help groups
Helping Relationships	Increase social support	Rapport building, a therapeutic alliance, counselor calls, and buddy systems
Counter Conditioning	Learn healthy behavior	Examples—relaxation can counter stress; assertion can counter peer pressure; nicotine replacement can substitute for cigarettes, and fat free foods can be safer substitutes
Reinforcement Management	Add consequences and rewards for specific behaviors	Examples—a day off after 6 days of exercise; a special low-calorie food treat after several days of very low-calorie meals
Self-liberation	Increase belief that one can change and stick with it	New Year's resolutions, public testimonies, and multiple rather than single choices can enhance self-liberation

Source: "How Do We Do It: Health Behaviors," Center for Health Communication Research, 2008. Retrieved June 1, 2008, from http://chcr.umich.edu/how_we_do_it/health_theories/healththeories5/chcr_document_view

individual does not know anything about an unhealthy behavior, providing base knowledge about the consequences of that behavior may be enough to facilitate the transition. However, if a person has chosen not to act, it may be more useful to address his or her perceptions of susceptibility and severity. This might entail a combination of strategies including providing knowledge, introducing well-known and respected individuals who support a behavior change, and guided practice with a behavior for the purpose of increasing self-efficacy.

Social Cognitive Theory

An interpersonal theory, **social cognitive theory** (Bandura, 1977) provides an understanding of how the social environment influences behavior. Figure 5.6 illustrates our conceptualization of social cognitive theory (SCT); the relationships depicted in the illustration have not been verified through research but they might help you clarify the theory's components.

An underlying assumption of the theory is that a dynamic relationship between a behavior, an individual, and the environment occurs. The three continuously interact with one another; as one changes, so do the others. It's fairly easy to see how the physical environment, thunderstorms for example, impacts the exercise behavior of a man who has started a new exercise regime of walking 30 minutes every day. What's more difficult to understand is how the emotional consequences of not walking for a few

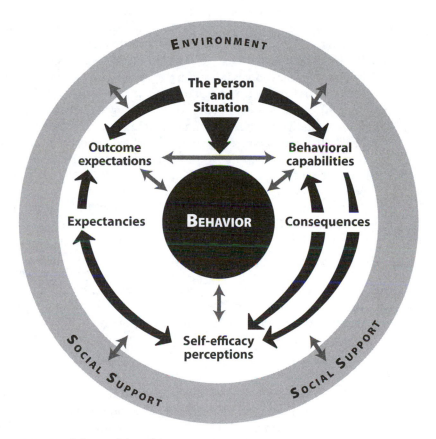

Figure 5.6   Social cognitive theory.
Social cognitive theory helps to explain why people choose behaviors. Among other things, it suggests that a person's belief about an outcome of a behavior and confidence in his or her ability to perform it will influence the frequency of the behavior. It also suggests that the environment influences a person and the behavior, which, in turn influence the environment.

days will impact the new exercise behavior and how that will change aspects of his environment. For example, he may not feel comfortable exercising outside again. You can see how that would make a difference in the program.

According to the SCT, the (a) environment and situation, (b) outcome expectations and behavioral capabilities, and (c) self-efficacy perceptions and expectancies will influence an individual's behavior. *Environment*, as we stated in chapter 3, includes anything external to the individual, including social, cultural, and physical aspects of the person's life. The situation is an individual's perception of the environment. As you know from personal experience, perceptions are not always 100% accurate. Accurate or not, the situation influences both the environment and behaviors.

Outcome expectations are an individual's beliefs about potential outcomes of a behavior. When individuals state that they believe they will lose weight as a result of exercise, they are expressing outcome expectations. **Behavioral capabilities** are the skills and knowledge necessary to make a behavior change. According to SCT, outcome expectations and behavioral capabilities influence behavior directly. For example, a person who wants to lose weight, believes that exercise will result in weight loss, and knows a little about exercise is more likely to choose exercise as a means of weight loss than individuals who don't have the same knowledge and beliefs. However, individuals who place importance on weight loss and believe they will be successful at exercise are more likely to follow through. The belief in success is powerful. The value an individual places on an outcome is called **expectancy**, and **self-efficacy** is the belief that one can perform a specific behavior. So, an individual must value losing weight, have some knowledge and skills, and believe he or she can do it in order to have the most success.

Bandura (1977) believes that values (expectancies), beliefs (self-efficacy), and skills (capabilities) can be influenced through **observational** or **vicarious learning**. Observational or vicarious learning occurs when individuals watch someone else perform the behavior successfully. The next step would be actual practice with small elements of the final behavior until each is performed successfully.

Once a behavior is performed, consequences of the behavior will influence expectancies, self-efficacy, and capabilities. These, in turn, influence future behavior and the environment. This interactive influence is called reciprocal determinism. Social support from individuals in the environment can also influence the individual and behavior in a powerful way.

PEN-3

An important dimension of the health education picture is how you view your professional role in relation to it. It would be a sad mistake for you to see yourself as a "knight in shining armor" who arrives at a community's doorstep with all the answers and resources in hand. That isn't how effective community health education works. Most individuals and communities prefer to fight their own battles and shape their own futures. Ideally, your role will be to serve as a catalyst and support person rather than a bearer of all the right answers. This difference in perspective may seem slight, but making that shift can greatly influence the results of your efforts, particularly as you strive to become a culturally competent health educator.

PEN-3 (Figure 5.7) is a conceptual model designed by Collins Airhihenbuwa (1990), a leader in multicultural health education, as a guide for culturally appropriate health education. Each of the three model dimensions contains components health educators should consider when working with a particular ethnic community. In each dimension, the first letter of each component composes the acronym PEN. In the dimension labeled "Health Education," we are encouraged to consider whether our health education program is designed to reach only an individual **per**son or the broader scope of that person's **e**xtended family or **n**eighborhood (school, community). In most instances, efforts that encompass the entire community result in more effective and long-lasting results.

In the dimension labeled "Educational Diagnosis of Health Behavior," we are encouraged to assess community

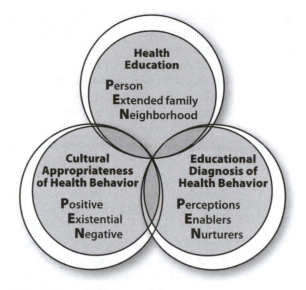

Figure 5.7   PEN-3 model.
The PEN-3 model encourages us to consider the health-related influences of an individual person's extended family or neighborhood (health education); community perceptions, enablers, and nurturers (educational diagnosis); and positive, existential (exotic but harmless), and negative cultural norms (cultural appropriateness). From "A Conceptual Model for Culturally Appropriate Health Education Programs in Developing Countries," by C. O. Airhihenbuwa, 1990, *International Quarterly of Community Health Education, 11,* pp. 53–62. Used with permission from the author.

perceptions (such as attitudes, knowledge, beliefs), **e**nablers (that is, available and accessible resources), and **n**urturers (such as family, peers, religious leaders, health professionals) that influence health behaviors and health status within the community. This dimension was derived from a well-known needs-assessment model called PRE-CEDE/PROCEED that you will read about in the next section. Its primary precept is that few people live in a vacuum with no need for human or resource support. Most are dependent to some extent on the influence of others and the accessibility of health services. Thus, to bring about health-related improvements, our health education programs should address attitudes, beliefs, and behaviors not only of the individuals we serve but also of the people who influence them. And, of course, enhancing health service availability and accessibility is another important component of health promotion efforts.

The third PEN-3 dimension, "Cultural Appropriateness of Health Behavior," calls on us to carefully examine cultural characteristics in light of how they truly affect the health status of the community. Airhihenbuwa (1990) pointed out that culture-based knowledge, attitudes, beliefs, and practices of a group can exert **p**ositive, existential, or negative influences on the community's health. (*Existential* means "affirming existence"; existential effects are neutral or harmless, though they might seem exotic to someone from another culture.) Unfortunately, negative influences are sometimes the only characteristics of a culture that receive attention in health promotion. Although minimizing negative influences is an important aspect of promoting wellness, problems arise when all cultural influences are assumed to be negative and when positive cultural aspects are ignored.

Many cultures foster health-enhancing beliefs and practices that, when used as motivators in your health promotion program, can make your job easier. For example, traditional Chinese respect for older family members (Matocha, 1998) can foster support for health promotion programs designed for the elderly. The traditional African American belief that personal choices and behaviors affect one's destiny (Spector, 1996) can be useful when health-related behavior change is needed. The positive cultural influences of a traditional community can and should be integrated into your health education program to enhance program acceptance and participation.

Airhihenbuwa (1990) maintains that some health beliefs and practices may be existential; they may seem exotic or strange to the Western medical perspective but, in truth, are harmless. One example is the practice of "coining" in some traditional Asian communities where illness is believed to be caused by evil spirits who gain control of one's body (L. Rasbridge, personal communication, December 15, 1999). A traditional healer scrapes the skin with a coin to release illness-bearing spirits. The resulting red marks are usually harmless but can alarm an untrained school or health official, particularly when they appear on a child. Recognizing this practice as an existential influence could prevent you from reacting inappropriately and help you avoid jeopardizing community trust.

PRECEDE/PROCEED Model

One of the most widely used health assessment, planning, and evaluation models, developed by Green and Kreuter (2005), is called **PRECEDE/PROCEED**. Although not specifically a theory, the model has components that provide a theoretical perspective. We will discuss these shortly, but for now, take a look at Figure 5.8. As you can see in the figure, this model is complex and can seem a bit overwhelming at first, until you realize that its purpose is not to belabor the process with needless attention to detail. Instead, it is designed to help us develop a full picture of our community of interest—its health needs and the factors that influence them. It isn't the only existing needs-assessment and program-planning model, but it is a good place to begin your exploration of needs because it offers a broad community-assessment perspective and provides a framework in which community members can participate in the process.

The model originally focused on the assessed health problems of communities and the ability of a central agency or organization to develop programs as solutions. It has been adapted, however, to promote community involvement in the needs-assessment and program-planning process and to incorporate a more positive approach through assets mapping, capacity building, and resource and policy development (Green & Kreuter, 2005). With a lot of teamwork and careful attention to a variety of contributing components, you can help a community develop a full picture of the

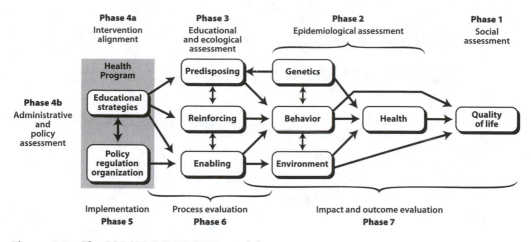

Figure 5.8   The PRECEDE /PROCEED model.
This model can be used to identify factors that contribute to health and quality of life within a community. The arrows depict lines of causation and how health promotion efforts can produce positive impacts and outcomes. From *Health Program Planning: An Educational and Ecological Approach* (4th ed., p. 11), by L. W. Green and M. W. Kreuter, © 2005 by McGraw-Hill. Used with permission of the McGraw-Hill Companies.

quality of life and health status of its members and develop a plan of action to enhance them.

The first four phases comprise the PRECEDE components and are implemented phase by phase, from right to left in the model. Phase 1, on the far right, entails the **social assessment** of the community's quality of life. This is the ideal place to start because the ultimate goal of health education is to foster life satisfaction and total well-being among community members. Starting here enables you to involve the community in subjectively defining the social issues of greatest import and determining how they can be addressed for the common good (Green & Kreuter, 2005).

In the social assessment, community members are encouraged to identify **social indicators** that reflect the community's levels of satisfaction with their quality of life. These indicators vary depending on the community members' unique perspectives. FYI 5.1 (on the following page) provides examples of social indicators that may be identified during Phase 1 of the assessment. Assets mapping is also conducted during this phase to identify available resources and the individuals and organizations that control them (Green & Kreuter, 2005).

In the **epidemiological assessment** (Phase 2), data are collected to determine the incidence and prevalence of community health problems that affect the community's quality of life (see FYI 5.1 for indicators). These can include communicable diseases (such as measles and hepatitis), chronic diseases (such as cancer and heart disease), health-related risk factors (such as malnutrition, anemia, and hypertension), and other recognized health problems (such as domestic violence and adolescent pregnancy). **Behavioral indicators** may include compliance, consumption patterns, self-utilization, or care. The environment also impacts behavior as well as health status. **Environmental indicators** include such things as hazard sites, community resources such

FYI 5.1   **Examples of Social Indicators**

Community Level Indicators	Organization Level Indicators
Aesthetics	Absenteeism
Civil Unrest	Productivity
Comfort	Achievement
Crime	Employee Morale
Crowding	Attention
Discrimination	Property Damage

Source: *Health Program Planning: An Educational and Ecological Approach* (4th ed.), by L. W. Green and M. W. Kreuter, 2005, New York: McGraw-Hill.

as hospitals or clinics, conditions of the physical environment such as public transportation, safe walkways, and clean air. Environmental factors may be beyond the individual's control, such as the lack of low-fat selections in fast-food restaurants. If so, you may need to include long-range environmental change efforts in your action plan.

Genetic indicators were recently added to the PRECEDE/PROCEED model to acknowledge what years of scientific research have proven: that one's inherited biological code can render a predisposition to certain health conditions. For example, much has been written about the breast cancer gene and how women who have a family history of the disease may determine their course of prevention by taking a genetic test. The interactions between genetics, behavior, and environment are represented by arrows in Figure 5.8. Green and Kreuter (2005) explain these interactions by stating that "most controls on the gene-environment interactions depend on the behavior of individuals and populations in their exposure to environmental risks, so we place behavior between genetics and environment" (p. 15). By the end of Phase 2, community health professionals and stakeholders should prioritize the identified issues in terms of their degree of importance to and changeability within the community.

We stated earlier that beginning with Phase 1 of the model is the ideal. We should point out, however, that Phase 2 may be where you actually begin. Why? Because most health education jobs have a predefined focus. For example, if you were hired by the American Heart Association, you would know during job interviews that the "health problem" focus (Phase 2) is heart disease. Under those circumstances, you would first devote attention to how the community of interest perceives heart disease and its effects on community members' quality of life. Thus, in this instance, you would move from Phase 2 to Phase 1 and then back to Phase 3 (Green & Kreuter, 2005).

Phase 3, the **educational and ecological assessment**, is composed of predisposing, reinforcing, and enabling factors. Distinguishing among these three categories can be a challenge when you are first learning the model, but recognizing their different but related influences will be critical for your health education program. These factors provide the theoretical perspective to the model. You will be collecting information on the factors with the assumption that they impact health-related behaviors. **Predisposing**

factors (attitudes, values, beliefs, knowledge) involve those thought processes that motivate the targeted behaviors. For example, predisposing factors that sometimes influence adolescents to smoke include the belief that smoking is cool, the desire (value) to be accepted by peers, and an attitude of rebellion against authority figures who say they shouldn't. On a more positive note, adolescents may exercise regularly if they know about and value its benefits and are motivated by a desire to stay fit and trim.

Reinforcing factors are rewards or encouraging feedback (positive or negative) that community members receive from other people. In our example, smoking adolescents may receive encouragement from smoking peers, but can be positively influenced by nonsmoking role models (such as popular athletes) willing to help in your health education program. Individuals who are providing negative reinforcement may also be educated or trained through your program to shift to a more positive influence, as in the case of physical education teachers being trained to tailor their classes to the abilities and interests of their students so that adolescents develop positive attitudes about exercise.

Enabling factors include resources and skills needed for behavior change to occur or barriers that may prevent it from happening—or both. Regular exercise will be easier to maintain if exercise resources, such as a safe and convenient place to jog or engage in recreational sports, are available and accessible. Because improper exercise can cause needless muscle soreness and injury, adolescents also need training in appropriate exercise skills. Enabling factors that contribute to negative health behaviors may also need to be targeted, as in the case of cigarette accessibility for minors.

Now that you have collected information for Phases 1–4a, you are ready to transition into more of the planning phases, which comprise the beginning of the PROCEED portion of the model. Realize that this is the portion that comes after you have identified and prioritized needs. In Phases 4b and 5, you must determine what program components, strategies, and services are necessary to bring about the intended change. Does the program have the resources and the administrative infrastructure to make it happen? This is where assets mapping comes into play. Resources such as time, personnel, and budget are three primary considerations that can be matched at this point with identified community assets and capacities. In Phase 5, you can begin to assess barriers to implementation such as staff commitment and attitudes or community concerns. In the policy assessment, local politics and organizational systems that may influence program implementation are also considered. This is a good place to begin emphasizing your community of interest's resources and develop community coalitions to develop solutions. Another important aspect of the PRECEDE/PROCEED model is that it emphasizes evaluation (the PROCEED portion). We will discuss evaluation in chapter 9, but Green and Kreuter make an important statement when they include evaluation as a component of program planning. Evaluation cannot be an afterthought; it should be an integral part of the entire planning process.

As valuable as the PRECEDE/PROCEED model is for broad-based community assessment and program planning, it does not address every aspect of what health professionals should know about human nature and the factors that often influence the way people think. For example, the model includes "attitudes" among the predisposing factors that often influence health behavior, but it doesn't provide detailed descriptions of the types of attitudes or perceptions that influence health most often.

Other theories and models can help you further explore these psychological influences. Understanding such influences can help you be more specific in your chosen health education strategies.

Selecting the Appropriate Theory

Selecting the right theory takes some time and effort on your part. The first thing to consider is the specific use for the theory. Are you preparing to conduct a needs assessment or are you ready to develop the actual prevention program? Perhaps you will be evaluating an existing program. Take time to think through what has been done and what needs to be done. You will not want to use the PRECEDE portion of the PRECEDE/PROCEED model if you are evaluating an existing program. You will not want to plan a program based on the social cognitive theory if the needs assessment was based on the health belief model. So, first be very clear on what tasks need to be completed and which theories have been used in other aspects of the program.

As you may know, all programs *should* be developed with the use of data collected in a needs assessment, if at all possible. You will learn more about needs assessment in chapter 6 but for now, keep in mind that using a theory or model as a framework for your assessment can be the best decision you make. If your needs assessment is grounded in theory, you will have a direction for your program development and evaluation.

So, how do you choose the right theory? You will first need a good working knowledge of behavioral theory gained from the professional literature. Yes, you will need to read professional journals, seek new information, and keep up with the field. You must know how to access professional literature, so if you have some confusion about that, we urge you to get some help! The selection of a theory will depend on three aspects: (a) the behavior being changed, (b) the characteristics of the participants, and (c) the environment. Each aspect must be considered and some of the best information will come from the professional literature. In studying professional literature, you will note that some models such as PRECEDE/PROCEED include assessments on the three aspects (behavior, participants, and environment) as part of the model.

Health-Related Behaviors

The fact that there are so many behavioral theories tells us that behaviors are not all equal. Some are deeply rooted in culture while others have a biological foundation and still others result as a reaction to another behavior. And, of course, cognition plays a powerful role in most behaviors. So, what does all this mean?

You will need to know a little about the behavior being changed in order to select the appropriate theory. If, for example, the target behavior involves a physical addiction, success is unlikely if your program is based solely on a theory that addresses only attitudes and beliefs. In fact, there may be a need to combine theoretically and medically-based program components in order to fully address the behavior. For example, some smoking-cessation programs might include strategies to change perceptions, attitudes, and skills as well as the use of a medical treatment such as the nicotine patch.

On the other hand, some theories and their relationship with specific behaviors have been extensively studied. Adolescent sexuality and social cognitive theory is an example. Studies have shown that interpersonal relationships are powerful influences on teens (Hogben, 1998). Therefore, social cognitive theory may be an excellent choice for programs working with adolescents and sexuality.

Some behaviors will require more emphasis on the process of change—taking small steps before getting to the final objective. In these cases a theory that involves change over time, such as the transtheoretical theory, might be a good choice.

How do you learn more about the behavior? As we've mentioned, reviewing what others have found through research and reported in professional literature is a good place to start. But don't hesitate to talk with other professionals and consider what you have learned through experience. Use many sources of information (unlike our elephant researchers) so you can see the whole picture. Don't forget that you also need to know something about the participant to make a good decision.

The Participant

We've already mentioned that some theories work best with individuals. These may focus on perceptions, beliefs, and attitudes. Other theories work best with behaviors highly influenced by interpersonal relationships and focus on how they interact. Still others work with community or organizational cultures and focus on belief structures of the entire community (large or small). So it will be important to understand with which you are working. Are you working with a group of individuals who, even though attending a program with others, will be working on their own beliefs, attitudes, and skills in order to make a behavior change? Or are you working with a community to help members change behaviors within their cultural beliefs? You will need to know in order to select a theory.

There are characteristics of groups that may also help guide your choice of theory. We've already discussed the mind-set of many adolescents. They often feel invulnerable to risk and are learning new things about themselves and others at every moment. Early elementary children are concrete thinkers, which means they may not understand abstract concepts about health. Individuals may have religious beliefs that preclude participation in certain activities while others have cultural beliefs that don't match some prevention plans.

Understanding the internal environments of your participants may also aid you in choosing a theory. For example, locus of control—whether an individual believes that he or she is personally in control of an outcome—could heavily influence program outcomes. For example, if individuals in your group believe incorrectly that an outside source has caused a health problem, they are not likely to change their own behaviors to make it better. Locus of control has been found to be an important predictor of healthy behaviors (Steptoe & Wardle, 2001). If control beliefs are a strong influencing factor in behavior, you will want to select a theory that addresses this issue.

How do you learn about the participants? First, you must know who they are. There is no way to plan a generic prevention program. Will it be adolescents, new mothers, or men from a senior living center? Your needs assessment, agency, funding source, or even personal interests will all play a role in determining the participants. Just be certain that you know with whom you will be working. It may sound silly, but many programs have gone wrong because they were planned for different people than those who eventually attended the program.

You will also, as always, want to refer to the professional literature to learn more about your participants. But most importantly, learn about the participants *through* the participants. Learn by talking and asking questions. Your participants are the ones who know the most about themselves.

As you consider your participants and the target behavior changes, you will also want to fully understand the environment in which you are working. Again, all three aspects are important in your decision making.

The Environment

There are many things to consider in regard to external environment besides the evident physical aspects. These include time, money, social and political influences, and others, some of which were discussed in chapter 2. Nieuwenhuijsen, Zemper, Miner, and Epstein (2006) discuss the impact of environment on an exercise program for a student using an electric wheelchair. "If the student is attending a university that offers accessible sport and recreation for wheelchair users, with personal assistants and/or supportive faculty members, her chances of successfully engaging in regular physical activity will be much better than if she is attending a university with no wheelchair-accessible sport or recreation facilities; her chances grow even fewer with no accessible transportation or support from staff or faculty." So, choosing a theory that involves only changing attitudes and perceptions will not work in this situation. An appropriate theory would also involve the removal of actual barriers.

It's pretty clear how money, time, and other resources impact the success of a program. If you choose a theoretical foundation that will require costly strategies and you don't have the resources, the program will not succeed, even if you understand the behavior and participants well. If you are planning a sex education program in a political environment that will not support it, you will not get far, even if you select the perfect theoretical base. Knowing the environment will help!

Sometimes, extensive reviews of literature, communication with other professionals, and talking with participants doesn't point you in a definite direction for choosing a theory. Combining theoretical components may be the best choice if a behavior is complex or a good match to an intact theory can't be found. Christine Jackson (1997) developed eight principles that might assist you in combining theories. In summary, the principles describe behavior change as a process that is powerfully influenced by attitudes, beliefs, and values. They remind us that a rewarding experience is more likely to be repeated and that the experience will influence future values, beliefs, attitudes, and behaviors. Jackson's principles suggest that participants should drive the behavior change and that health educators should understand the magnitude of influence wielded by important others in the lives of those participants. It's also important to understand the concept of reciprocal determinism, in which changes in values and beliefs change behavior, which, in turn, changes values and beliefs. The final principle returns to the idea that programs should be based in research and evaluated for effectiveness.

We know that studying theories and models for the first time can be frustrating and overwhelming. However, if you think about it, you are already using theories on a daily basis. After all, why do you do the things you do? Talk to other practitioners, practice using the theories, and read the literature. Before long it will all make more sense than you can imagine.

In Conclusion

Theories help us analyze why people behave the way they do and provide models or frameworks for action. Keep in mind that some theories are best used with individuals, others with small groups, and still others with entire communities. The basic tenets of theories vary also. For example, some theories use attitudes and beliefs as the foundation for behavioral change and others include time and practice as important elements. Some theories are fear-based while others involve cues to action. As a community health professional, you will need a firm understanding of a variety of behavioral theories and planning models. You will also need to know how to assess the individuals and groups with whom you will work. This knowledge will help you build successful health education and behavior change programs.

 REVIEW QUESTIONS

1. Describe the primary components of the health belief model, theory of planned behavior, and transtheoretical model.
2. Discuss how the precaution adoption model differs from the transtheoretical model.
3. Explain how the PEN-3 model can be used to distinguish between positive, existential, and negative cultural influences on health.
4. Diagram the PRECEDE portion of the PRECEDE/PROCEED model and explain how its components can influence community health.
5. Analyze how theories and models influence public health.

☞ **FOR YOUR APPLICATION**

Draw a figure that illustrates how constructs, concepts, theories, and models relate to one another. To give you an idea of what we mean, let's say that the assignment asked you to *build* a structure that showed how constructs, concepts, theories, and models related to one another. You might use tinker toys and indicate that theory is represented by the base of the structure and the model is the structure as a whole. We are asking you to put your ideas on paper. Be sure to include constructs and concepts too.

PART II

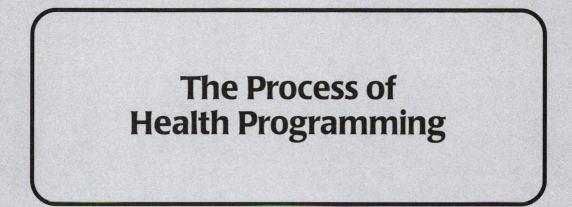

The Process of
Health Programming

Needs and Capacity Assessment

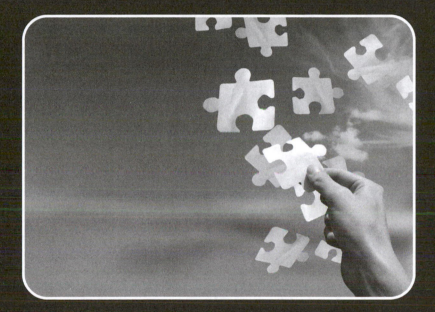

It's your first week in your role as a health educator at a county health department in Rural, USA. You've been given the directive from your supervisor to develop a culturally competent HIV/AIDS prevention curriculum for adolescents that can be implemented in the area's middle and senior high schools. Your supervisor informs you that the school district's superintendent is supportive of the initiative but has asked that you meet with members of the district's Health Advisory Committee before developing the curriculum. Although the county epidemiological reports show a surge in HIV/AIDS cases within the last five years, the committee is quick to inform you that there isn't really a problem with HIV/AIDS in "their schools" and what the kids really need is a "healthy eating program." You sense some tension in the room and realize that there may be a discrepancy between the perceived and actual needs among the community members. Now what do you do?

CHAPTER OBJECTIVES

1. Define needs assessment.
2. Discuss the difference between actual and perceived needs.
3. Explain why it is useful to assess both actual and perceived needs and establish common ground.
4. Review the four phases of needs assessment and the steps involved with each phase.
5. Compare and contrast individual vs. group strategies for data collection.
6. Identify community assets.
7. Use the PRECEDE portion of the PRECEDE/PROCEED model to identify factors that influence an identified health need.
8. Conduct a needs assessment within your own community.

Needs-Assessment Concepts and Definitions

Now that you have a general picture of America's health problems, it is time to consider the process through which those problems were identified and the methods you should use to develop a broader view of America's subgroups. In chapter 1 we introduced the concept of quality of life and highlighted the importance of assessing community health needs, a primary competency for health educators. Our goal here is to expand your understanding of the purpose and character of needs assessment, how it is evolving, and how it relates to other assessment and community organization terms and principles.

We know our health education programs are on target when we base them on accurate needs-assessment data and a careful interpretation of their meaning. The goal of **needs assessment** is to identify gaps between what exists and *what ought to exist* so that you can design a program to reduce those gaps (Gilmore & Campbell, 2005).

Actual and Perceived Needs

Gilmore and Campbell (2005) define needs assessment as "a planned process that identifies the reported needs of an individual or a group" (p. 7). They explain that two important groups of people are expected to provide input in needs identification: (a) health professionals and (b) community members. Ideally, both groups will be involved in planning and implementing the proposed community health program. The needs identified by these groups may be **actual needs** (true needs often based on incidence and prevalence data) or **perceived needs** (what individuals report based on their subjective views). These two types of needs sometimes differ, but they are both important pieces of assessment information.

Why Both Are Important

Why would perceived needs be as important as actual needs? The answer can be readily understood if you picture, like the introductory example, a community in which a high rate of HIV infection has been documented, although most community members deny that the problem exists. Health professionals would likely suggest you implement an HIV/AIDS education program to address this actual need, but community members might be less than cooperative. The community might be more concerned about a recent, single, well-publicized incident of school violence and prefer a violence prevention program rather than an HIV/AIDS education program. The more information you have about actual and perceived needs in the community you serve, the more equipped you will be to educate the community and work with others to prioritize program goals.

A slightly different scenario could exist if the community actually wished to address both health concerns but was still more concerned about violence (perceived need) than HIV/AIDS (actual need). Finding the common ground where data-based evidence and community concerns match is an ideal place to begin community health promotion efforts, but it doesn't always exist. When this convergence doesn't occur, it helps to respectfully acknowledge perceived needs, promote community awareness about real needs, and work within a partnership format to build and maintain a collaborative effort.

What Type of Information Should You Collect?

When conducting a needs assessment, it is important to understand the different types of data available about your community, county, state, or country and how to collect this information in order to prioritize health needs. Archival documents, county or country reports, testimonials, pictures, registration logs, attendance records, budget spreadsheets—all of these are examples of data. As mentioned in chapter 3, **primary data** refers to information that stems from its original source, such as a first-hand account in a diary or a taped interview. Other examples of primary sources are letters, autobiographies, focus groups, blogs, speeches, stories, photographs, and survey responses. **Secondary data** refers to information that is not first-hand; in other words, it is information drawn from an unoriginal source. Examples of secondary data include county health reports, hospital discharge data, and national databases such as the National Primary Care database and DATA 2010, a database relating to *Healthy People 2010*. Both primary and secondary data are instrumental in assessing a community's perceived and actual needs.

Collecting Secondary Data

National and international databases and sources are valuable because they can help you determine how the nature and extent of needs identified in your community compare to those of other communities. You can learn from those sources which approaches were effective or ineffective in other locales and you may gain insights you would otherwise have missed. You can then consider the specific characteristics and needs of your community and adapt what you learned from those secondary sources.

Other important secondary sources are organizations and groups that have worked or are presently working in your community of interest. Although leaders of some organizations may view you as competition and respond in a territorial fashion, others will likely welcome your efforts and be willing to share what they know. Tapping into these local secondary sources before you begin any primary data-collection efforts can save you time and resources by avoiding needless duplication. It can also be a useful way to learn from the experience of other professionals about the culture, history, and characteristics of your community—who the real leaders and gatekeepers are, and how to best establish trust and mutual respect between you and community members. These secondary source connections can develop into future collaborative relations that will broaden and strengthen your efforts.

Collecting Primary Data

Primary data collection is a critical component of the needs-assessment process because it helps accomplish two things: First, it can provide accurate, community-specific data about problems, influences, and potential solutions to health issues. Second, if conducted appropriately, collecting primary data can help you establish important relationships with community members. Involving them in the early stages of your work helps develop community ownership. From this joint effort you can gain an insider's perspective on community culture and characteristics and the degree to which members will respond positively to your work. Their input will help you incorporate perceived needs into your program planning. It will also help you determine the best methods to collect primary data and the types of questions to ask. Primary data-collection methods are usually categorized as individual or group assessments; these will be discussed later in the chapter.

The Four Phases of Community Needs Assessment

Conducting a community needs assessment is a lot like working a jigsaw puzzle: there are myriad pieces of information scattered around your community that, when put together, help form a vivid picture of the quality of life that exists in that corner of the world. As you begin the process of collecting these "pieces," you will continue through four stages of needs assessment: (a) gathering preliminary data and generating assessment questions, (b) collecting community data, (c) analyzing the data and interpreting results, and (d) prioritizing needs, identifying assets, and providing recommendations. You will move through the phases of needs assessment by completing 13 steps. These phases and steps are illustrated in Figure 6.1.

Phase I: Gather Preliminary Data and Generate Assessment Questions

You are ready to begin the vital first step in planning an effective, evidence-based program that will improve the health and/or quality of life of members of your targeted community.

Step 1: Gather Basic Community Information

Start by collecting some basic resources such as maps of the area, phone books, and Chamber of Commerce information (such as brochures or welcome packets). Keep in mind that the Chamber of Commerce materials will read like a travel brochure, so be sure to read past the propaganda and focus on the facts. You may want to check Web sites, visit the local library and health department, and speak to individuals within the community to gather the following information:

- What are your community's demographics (i.e., characteristics of a population such as mean age, average family size, ethnic group composition, median yearly salary, etc.)?
- How many schools and universities are within the area?
- What is the average level of education?
- What local churches are in the area?
- What are property values like?
- Are there parks, trails, and places for recreation and exercise?
- How many fast food restaurants are in business?
- What kinds of medical services are available?
- What is public transportation like?
- Are there supportive services for the elderly or those without housing or medical insurance?
- What is the history of the community? What are the current issues impacting the community?
- What types of local media exist, and who reports the news in your community? What types of stories are covered by this media?
- Is there a community Web site? If so, what can you learn from it?
- Who appear to be the "gatekeepers"?

Examining the "pieces" of community information listed above may provide clues about the health status of your community and lead you to explore factors that impact its overall health picture.

Step 2: Observe and Take Notes

While gathering secondary data is important, you will learn best through first-hand experience in the field. Take a drive through the community. If your community is defined by geographical boundaries, then you will be able to easily determine its parameters. However, some "communities" are not always defined by geography. For example, if you're working with a refugee Hmong group in your region of the state, find out where people within this ethnic community gather, such as refugee centers, neighborhood gardens, grocery stores, churches, community clinics, restaurants, and so forth. Talk to the people within the community to decide which sites are most relevant.

In addition, pay attention to environmental cues. For example, what areas might be potential hazards? Is there a lack of pedestrian walkways? Is there graffiti on build-

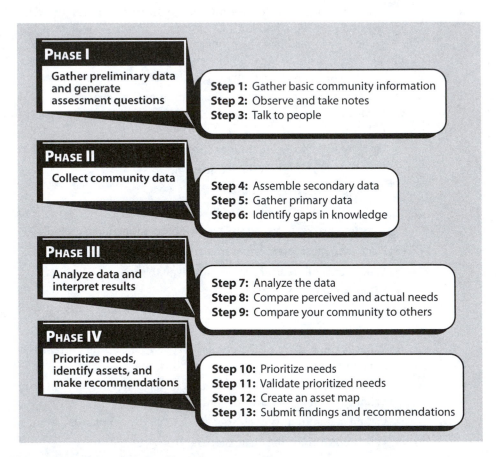

Figure 6.1   Four phases of needs assessment.

ings, and if so, what does it say? Are lawns well kept? What types of stores and advertising surround the community? Is alcohol sold in the area? You may want to write your observations in a notebook or record audio notes on an MP3 or audio voice recorder. Taking photos of various public places will reinforce your memory and enhance your field notes. Your observation notes offer yet more pieces of the community "puzzle" you are assembling.

Step 3: Talk to People

After you've taken the time to collect your own field notes, it's time to talk to members of the community to gain their perspectives. You will want to talk to an array of individuals, from those who hold powerful leadership positions to those who vote for the leaders (and of course those who do not vote at all). **Gatekeepers** are members of the community who hold some position of influence. Examples of gatekeepers are listed in FYI 6.1. It's also important to converse with individuals who live within the community and who are served by some of the services and individuals mentioned below. Community perspectives differ according to the roles people play within the community, so listening to multiple voices is essential to gaining a broader perspective.

When you contact gatekeepers and members of the community, what should you say? You might start with some general questions, such as "How long have you been a

---

FYI **6.1   Examples of Community Gatekeepers**

- The mayor and city officials
- School officials and PTA leaders
- Ministers and religious leaders
- Realtors and other business people
- People who work in social service agencies
- Representatives from nonprofit organizations and grant-funded programs
- Community activists
- Physicians and health professionals
- Local health educators and epidemiologists
- Rotary or Kiwanis Club presidents
- University professors or school teachers
- Presidents of neighborhood associations
- Members of Congress
- Local journalists and members of the news media
- Law enforcement officials
- Town historian
- People who are well-respected and lead informally

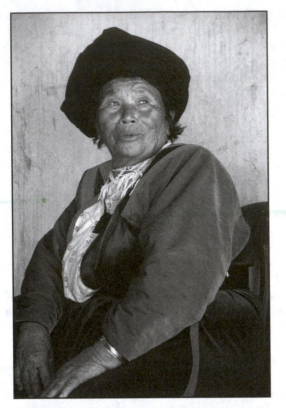

This grandmother is a well-respected member of her community and thus serves as an informal gatekeeper. (© Teoman Alemdar)

member of the community?" and "How do you feel about the community overall?" If the individual is a long-standing resident of the area or a member of a target group, you might ask about some historical events that have impacted the community. You might then transition into more health-related questions, not giving any probes (such as facts or statistics), but allowing the individuals to voice their own perceptions about quality of life. You might ask, "What health issues are most pressing?" and "Why do these health issues exist?" You can follow up with questions about issues that are not health related (chances are, these are related to health anyway). Keep in mind that everyone will have their own interpretation of what is "pressing," another reminder of why it is important to gain multiple perspectives from people in a variety of community roles.

After you've interviewed these members of the community, be sure to thank them for their time and insight. Be sure to follow up with a thank-you note or a token of appreciation. It leaves a good impression and speaks to your level of professionalism. Remember, too, that networking within the community is key to developing "buy in" and to building support for future health education or public health initiatives.

Phase II: Collect Community Data

Now that you've gained some subjective viewpoints from local community members and leaders, it's time to seek out facts and figures that will add to the store of puzzle pieces you've already collected.

Step 4: Assemble Secondary Data

There are myriad resources at your disposal. The Community Toolbox, an online resource that promotes community health and development (http://ctb.ku.edu), offers the following examples:

- The state or county health department can help you determine health indicators on a variety of issues.

- The state human services department should be able to tell you the number of Medicaid recipients and food stamp program participants.

- Hospital admission and exit records can give you information on issues such as teen births, causes of deaths, etc. Depending on the community, some of the data may not be part of the public record, but it may be possible to purchase or arrange to use it in some form.

- Census data and demographic information are available for your community and the United States as a whole. This information is found in the *Statistical Abstract of the United States* on the Census Bureau Web site at http://www.census.gov. Many states have similar information on their own Web sites, and state departments of health may also have links to the census on their sites. One note of caution about using census data, however. It has not always proven reliable. For example, lack of documentation of nonnative immigrants, homeless persons, or those who simply refuse to participate in the census survey can influence the accuracy of census data.

- Police records can give you crime rates and the incidence of problems such as domestic violence or motor vehicle accidents.

- Chamber of Commerce data include statistics on job growth, unemployment rates, and property values.

- Nonprofit service agencies, such as the United Way or Planned Parenthood, generally have records on a variety of different issues. These agencies may have already conducted surveys and found the information you need.

- School district reports may indicate graduation rates, test scores, rates of school violence, and truancy rates for local schools. For comparative figures across school districts, check with your community's state department of education.

- Centers for Disease Control reports national information on rates of many diseases, such as HIV/AIDS and diabetes. Access this at http://www.cdc.gov

- Healthy People.gov can provide progress reports about areas of priority for U.S. health initiatives.

- The Bureau of Health Statistics and Research of the Pennsylvania Department of Health provides you with the capability of compiling reports on a number of health issues from adolescent health to yellow fever. Visit the site at http://dsf.health.state.pa.us

- A reference librarian at a public or university library can point you to valuable local resources.

- Specialized local, statewide, or national organizations may help. For example, if you were interested in substance abuse or diabetes, you would want to track down and consult an organization specializing in that topic. You may want to look in *Gale's Encyclopedia of Associations* as a resource. In addition, most organizations have their own Web sites with abundant topic-specific information.

Step 5: Gather Primary Data

In addition to the informal interviews you conducted in step 3, you may want to gain more detailed information about community members' knowledge, attitudes, behaviors, and perceptions of various health issues. You may need to use a survey to collect this type of data. As you will learn later in this chapter, this type of data is only as good as the survey you use to collect it. Therefore, search out existing community health surveys for sample questions and formats. You might also check the Internet, your health texts, and professional journals (are there specific survey titles listed in articles related to your subject matter?). Chat with the local health department staff, or contact representatives from professional organizations related to your topic. Be sure that the survey is culturally relevant as well as conducive to the reading level of your community members. If you cannot find an existing survey that "fits," it might be necessary for you to prepare your own. The important steps in this process are detailed in chapter 10.

Other strategies for collecting primary data from your community include facilitating focus groups, conducting interviews, moderating town meetings, and using **Photovoice** (a process that allows community members to take pictures reflecting their unique perceptions of community needs and assets). FYI 6.2 provides a more complete list and description of these data-collection strategies.

Individual Assessments

FYI 6.2 provides an overview of the four types of individual survey methods. The information provided there is described in great detail by Gilmore and Campbell (2005), well-respected authorities in needs assessment. They define a **survey** as "a structured process for gathering information directly from individuals by asking questions" (p. 46). The type of survey you choose will depend on a number of factors, including who and how many people you are trying to reach and how much time and money you have to put toward the effort.

Mailed surveys.   Mailed surveys have the potential to reach large numbers of individuals and may generate thoughtful replies (since participants have time to complete the survey at their leisure). The expense involved varies, depending on postage and the cost of the survey itself. If you are using an existing survey, there may be a fee associated with its use. You may also have to pay for the mailing list. Mailed surveys can reduce the bias and influence that interviewers may exert in telephone or face-to-face surveys; however, you cannot always verify if the person completing the mailed survey is the individual intended to receive it. Gilmore and Campbell (2005) suggest using a mailed survey if the type of information you need could be considered private and more personal contact would seem threatening to survey participants.

Telephone surveys.   Telephone and face-to-face surveys usually result in higher response rates than do mail-outs; and face-to-face surveys in particular can be more effective among those with low literacy or minimal English. Telephone surveys can be conducted more quickly, but face-to-face interviews are best for open-ended questions.

Face-to-face surveys.   A face-to-face survey is the best way to distribute a lengthy questionnaire (Fowler, 2002, p. 71). More complex questions are best handled with face-to-face surveys because follow-up questions are more easily asked. Also, those without access to a phone or the Internet would be better reached through a written, face-to-face survey. However, there are several drawbacks to this format. First, anonymity may be sacrificed. Second, participants may answer a certain way because you

FYI **6.2   Overview of Individual and Group Data-Collection Strategies for Needs Assessment**

Individual Surveys	Advantages	Disadvantages
Mail surveys	Low cost, wide distribution possible, valid information (allows time for thinking before answering)	Lengthy process, low response rate, limited questions, no control over answers (no clarification possible), mailing list required
Telephone surveys	Shorter process than mailing, better response rate, more/different questions possible, better control over answers (can ask for clarification)	More costly than mailing, less valid information (may receive socially desirable answers)
Face-to-face surveys	Best opportunity for questioning, most control over answers (can read nonverbal expressions), effective for low-literacy individuals	Most costly (time and travel expense), least valid information (socially desirable answers), access to participants may be difficult (privacy and security issues)
Online surveys	Potential to collect a large amount of data in a short period of time; flexibility; convenience for participants; ability to garner participation across the globe; ability to reach unique populations; has equal or better response rate than mailed surveys if incentive is provided; allows for anonymity; may be less expensive than paper format	May not reach individuals from older or lower socio-economic groups; technological errors can occur while individuals are completing the survey; hard to verify whether individuals from intended sample are actually the ones completing the survey or are only completing it once
Group Participation		
Community forum	Allows a large number of people to assemble in one setting (one-time effort vs. repeated attempts); encourages a diversity of perspectives; may allow for community "buy in" and support from community members and leaders	Requires time to plan and advertise; facilitation skills are essential in order for forum to remain orderly and effective; may result in backlash
Nominal group	Direct involvement, planned interactivity, allows for diverse opinions, full participation of all group members, creative atmosphere, recognition of common ground fostered	Time commitment, competing issues may slow process, participant bias can emerge, segmented planning involvement
Focus group	Low cost, convenient, creative atmosphere, ease of clarification, high flexibility potential	Qualitative information only, limited representativeness, dependence on moderator skill, preliminary insights only, some group members dominate
Photovoice	Imbues community members with ownership in the process; uses photography to reflect community members' perspectives of community barriers and assets; initiates discussion for community members; creates awareness	Can be time intensive; participants must be trained; may be expensive depending on type of equipment used; qualitative information only; may require a translator

are present. Third, face-to-face surveys can be expensive because those distributing and collecting the surveys must travel. Fourth, the interviewee may talk longer in person than by mail, e-mail, or telephone, and large projects could require several interviewers. Fifth, interviewers may need to be trained beyond the scope of those who survey by e-mail or phone because the interviewers may have to make decisions in the field without the benefit of consulting with a supervisor. Finally, as modern living has gotten busier and concerns with security and privacy are increasing, it may be harder to reach participants through face-to-face methods than by other delivery modes.

Online surveys.   Online surveys are gaining momentum as a popular survey mode because they allow for a larger participant sample, convenience, and anonymity (Wright, 2005). However, technological errors can occur, and this mode is not appropriate for those without access to computers. Also, there is a risk that those completing the survey are not really part of the intended sample or that people will complete the online survey more than once. It is important to carefully consider all of these factors—type of information, audience, money, time, and personnel—in order to choose a method that will work well for your purposes (Wright, 2005).

Another individual assessment method that bears mentioning is the **Delphi technique**; it is used when objective information is not available from other sources and generates "a consensus through a series of questionnaires" (Gilmore & Campbell, 2005, p. 68). It is often used to identify goals and establish priorities, brainstorm possible alternatives, or gather information about group values and perspectives. The process usually involves three to five rounds of mailed questionnaires in which participants are first asked to respond to a few broad questions; from those responses, more specific questionnaires are developed to further clarify and specify the information. Although this approach can be useful in clarifying important issues, it is more likely that you will be involved in various local survey methods when you first enter the profession.

Group Assessments

Advantages and disadvantages of the nominal group, focus group, and community forum are also outlined in FYI 6.2.

Nominal group.   As can be deduced from the description there, the nominal group process is more structured than the focus group process. In the nominal group process, five to seven individuals who are knowledgeable about community issues meet to address a particular issue. In the beginning, each member is asked to write down, without discussion, personal responses to a single question (such as, "What do you think are the most pressing health concerns in our community?"). Each written response is shared with the group in round-robin fashion, until every response is recorded. The group then discusses and clarifies items on the list and ranks them according to what is considered most important. The process continues until a prioritized list is agreed on, through a vote if needed. This high-structure approach is designed to foster equal input for every member.

Focus group.   The focus group process is a much more relaxed approach in which 6 to 12 fairly homogenous group members answer questions asked by a trained moderator. The moderator's role is to help the group stay focused, stimulate interaction, and encourage clarification and expansion of ideas without biasing the results. These sessions are usually taped so that ideas expressed in this free format will not be lost or forgotten. This format is designed to encourage spontaneity in generating ideas through the process of free expression. It is particularly useful in collecting qualitative information for a preliminary assessment of community opinions and goals. It does, however, require a well-trained, experienced moderator who will remain impartial and focused on the assigned group task.

Community forum.   Of all the individual and group strategies mentioned here, the community forum is the least structured and can involve the greatest number of participants. Community forums, or public meetings, are often used to distribute information but can also be helpful in gaining initial feedback from any community member who wishes to voice an opinion about a particular health issue. Although it is not considered the most rigorous approach to community assessments, it does allow all community subgroups or segments to voice their views and can be a positive communication channel when carefully planned and implemented. The key is to maintain a positive, objective tone during the meeting and avoid possible degeneration into a gripe session.

Photovoice.   This method employs a participatory action technique that allows individuals to photograph their everyday realities and highlight factors that may enhance or diminish their individual health status or that of the community. As Baker and Wang (2006) explain, "It [Photovoice] is also structured as a mechanism to engage participants in group discussions about their images and to present these images in public forums" (p. 1408). Photovoice is gaining momentum as an empowering strategy in public health. The technique has been used to "capture" health issues among diverse and unique populations. Some of these examples include a clinical and nonclinical sample of older adults in Michigan who chronicled their daily pain levels; factors impacting inner-city adolescents' health and well-being (Strack, Magill, & McDonagh, 2003); health and community issues of rural Chinese women in the Yunnan province (Wang & Burris, 1997); quality of life among rural African American breast cancer survivors (Lopez, Eng, Randall-David, & Robinson, 2005); men's experiences with prostate cancer (Oliffe & Bottorff, 2007); perceptions of safety among battered women (Frohmann, 2005); barriers to orphan care-giving in Sierra Leone (Walker, 2008); and the cultural and social context of physical activity and dietary intake among U.S. Hispanic women (Keller, Fleury, Perez, Ainsworth, & Vaughan, 2008). The main goals of Photovoice are to engage people in active listening and dialogue, create a safe environment for introspection and critical reflection, and move people toward action (Baker & Wang, 2006). There is a specific protocol when using Photovoice, and these steps are listed in FYI 6.3.

When choosing data-collection methods for assessing community needs, remember that each alternative has pros and cons. We suggest you consider using multiple strategies, depending on your available time and resources. The nominal or focus group can be a good way to get started because each provides insight into community values and concerns in a relatively short amount of time. We recommend, however, that information gleaned from small-group processes be used to develop surveys or questionnaires for implementation among larger representative groups within the community. An appropriately balanced collection of group and individual assessment data can help you develop a truer picture of your whole community.

FYI **6.3   Using Photovoice to Assess Community Needs**

Photovoice is a component of participatory research that uses photography to create and encourage social change. Caroline Wang (2006) and Mary Burris (Wang & Burris, 1997) present a nine-step methodology to successfully carry out the goals of Photovoice.

1. *Recruit Photovoice participants.* Wang and Burris recommend that a Photovoice group should include six to ten people. This provides efficiency in collecting data and adequate discussion.

2. *Select a target audience of policy makers or community leaders.* The participants select this group based on the target audience's ability to make decisions that will improve the problems identified through Photovoice activities.

3. *Introduce Photovoice to the participants.* The researcher must conduct a workshop or training session to explain Photovoice and to demonstrate proper use of the cameras. This session is also used to educate the participants about obtaining consent when photographing others.

4. *Obtain informed consent.* The researcher must obtain informed consent from each participant. This is typically completed during the training session.

5. *Brainstorm with participants.* A brainstorming activity is highly recommended to familiarize the participants with initial themes for taking photographs. This helps facilitate the Photovoice activity because participants will gain a clearer focus to guide their picture taking. Brainstorming can be done at the training session.

6. *Distribute cameras.* This is done at the training session. Each participant will need a camera to complete the Photovoice activity. The facilitator (researcher) will decide which type of camera to distribute to participants.

7. *Provide time for participants to take pictures.* The most commonly allotted time frame for picture taking is seven days. This provides each participant enough time to take a sufficient quantity of pictures related to the research project.

8. *Meet to discuss the photographs.* After the seven days, the participants are asked to return with the cameras and their images to discuss the photographs taken. This can be done as a group or individually. Each participant will review his or her photographs with the facilitator and select the photographs that best tell the story. The facilitator will then work with participants to contextualize their photographs using the SHOWeD Method. Common themes are identified and discussed with participants.

9. *Plan with participants a format to share photographs and stories.* The facilitator and participants will choose the best medium to present the photographs and descriptions to the target audience. Formats used in the past include Web sites, slide shows, and exhibits.

Sources: Adapted from "Photovoice: Concept, methodology, and use for participatory needs assessment," by C. C. Wang and M. Burris, 1997, *Health Education and Behavior, 24*(3), 369–387; "Youth participation in Photovoice as a strategy for community change," by C. C. Wang, 2006, *Journal of Community Practice, 14*(1/2), 147–161.

Keep in mind that you need to set limits to how much information you will collect. Too much information will be just as much of a problem as not enough. You can easily become overwhelmed. Consider what is feasible—given your time frame—and then establish your limits.

Step 6: Identify Gaps in Your Knowledge

This is where you begin to put the puzzle together. Go back to the questions you generated in Step 1 and use the data you've collected to answer them. What pieces are missing? What information might help you form a complete picture? You may need to extend the data collection at this point or decide it's time to stop gathering information. Try to fill in the knowledge gaps as best you can with solid information—remember what happens when we assume anything. It sometimes helps to invite others who have not been involved in the process to join you at this point to view the overall set of information you have gathered so far. The fresh perspective of people who have not been closely involved in the process can help you identify what's missing. They may also help you discover new ways to use the data you have collected to more fully answer your assessment questions.

Phase III: Analyze Data and Interpret Results

Collecting community data can be hard work that takes both time and patience. However, once the information is collected, knowing how to interpret this data can also be a challenge.

Step 7: Analyze the Data

Data analysis, the process of examining and interpreting data, can be either formal (as in using computerized statistical analysis) or informal ("eyeballing" the data in search of obvious differences between what is and what should be). If your community's perceived needs match obvious gaps in health education or services, the less formal approach will suffice. For example, during a town meeting you may learn that community members are concerned about alcohol-related traffic accidents in the area. Local police and hospital emergency room records confirm that alcohol-related accidents are a frequent problem, with often tragic results. Further, a review of community settings in which the much-needed education could occur reveals inadequate efforts. All of this information combined points to an obvious need; therefore, more rigorous data collection and analysis may not be necessary because the prioritized need is obvious.

Step 8: Compare Perceived and Actual Needs

What if data about the community members' perceived needs, local secondary data, and available services or education don't match? Or, what if several needs from each of these sources are evident and the results are mixed? There are no foolproof solutions to this common dilemma, but there are some steps you can take to help clarify the issue. The first is that you may need to collect more data. If local records indicate a high incidence or prevalence of a health risk, you may need to go back to community members for more primary data about their perspectives and experiences with that specific issue. If a particular health issue is evident in the primary data but is not showing up in secondary data, you may need to consult local health professionals and community members to determine why the issue is not evident in local records. These decisions about "what is" should be driven by input from all stakeholders, with the desired end result being a list of identified problems, their nature, and their extent.

To further illustrate what we mean by working with both perceived and actual needs, consider the following story about an international public health group that decided to build a hospital in a very remote region of a developing country. The group decided to build the hospital because of the high rate of maternal and infant deaths in childbirth in that region, a problem attributed to the scarcity of trained physicians and appropriate medical facilities. So the group diligently raised the money needed, built an amazingly modern facility in view of the surrounding conditions, and flew in well-trained professionals to do the work. But after some time, childbirth death rates remained high and few local people had even visited the new facility. Someone decided to ask "Why?" and learned from the people who lived there that they trusted the local midwives and preferred to remain in their familiar home surroundings to give birth rather than move to a new and unfamiliar building to be cared for by strangers. The public health group realized it had failed to accurately assess the situation. It decided to try again, this time armed with needed information about the local community, its interests, and perceived needs. With time, the health group was able to reach out to the locals by inviting their midwives to train in the facility and work in the birthing room along with the "imported" professionals. Had someone fully understood the need to assess the whole picture before the plan was implemented, things might have progressed quite differently.

Step 9: Compare Your Community to Others

It is important to put the information you have collected into a context, either positive or negative. For example, pinpointing that the rate of HIV/AIDS in your area is ten times higher than the national rate could have a significant impact on whether grant-funding organizations decide to fund your proposed HIV/AIDS awareness program.

Phase IV: Prioritize Needs, Identify Assets, and Make Recommendations

Now comes the hard part, deciding which needs to address first. This important step determines the direction your health education program will take. Often, there are several important needs on the list and people disagree about which should receive immediate attention. Yet limited resources and time rarely allow you to address them all at once. You have to start somewhere.

Step 10: Prioritize Needs

McKenzie, Neiger, and Smeltzer (2005) suggest that you evaluate each listed need in light of four questions:

1. What is the most pressing need?
2. Are resources adequate to deal with the problem?
3. Can the problem best be solved by a health promotion intervention, or could it be better handled through administration, politics, or changes in the economy?
4. Can the problem be solved in a reasonable amount of time?

Reality dictates that you have to consider questions 2 through 4 due to time and resource constraints imposed by your employer or by funding sources who have agreed to support your efforts. Green and Kreuter (2005) would likely categorize these four questions under the heading of how "changeable" the health situation is. They suggest you assign each of the identified needs to one of four areas (FYI 6.4). These categories weigh levels of pressing need (importance) with the potential for change (changeability) as a result of health education efforts. Any decision-making process should also consider the degree to which other community agencies and organizations are providing similar programs. This can help you avoid duplication of existing services and minimize potential territorial issues with leaders of other organizations.

FYI **6.4**   **Prioritizing Health Needs**

A community's health needs should be prioritized according to their importance and changeability as determined by community members and the health professionals who serve them.

	More important	**Less important**
More changeable	Needs that are highly *changeable* and *important*	Needs that are highly *changeable* but are less important
Less changeable	Needs that are highly *important* but are less changeable	Needs that are neither changeable nor important

Source: Adapted from Green & Kreuter (2005).

Step 11: Validate Prioritized Needs

After putting all of the puzzle pieces together, an image of your community will emerge. How do you know, however, that your picture is accurate? Validating needs may seem unnecessary because it calls for a return to previous steps, such as conducting focus groups to determine the community's reaction to the prioritized needs or gaining second opinions from other health professionals. If careful groundwork has been laid, this step may be less important. However, because so many people have likely provided input to the process, some may have lost sight of the final goal along the way. If the needs are not properly validated, you could possibly proceed with costly programs that are less effective than expected. For that reason, we suggest you consider this step as an important reminder to constantly validate your prioritized needs as you proceed. You can confirm your decisions through careful, consistent communication with community members and collaborating health professionals as you move from the assessment to the program-planning stages.

Even if you arrive in a new employment situation where much of the data collection and prioritizing groundwork has been completed, we encourage you to at least spend time establishing personal relationships with primary and secondary data contacts to foster your awareness of the situation.

Step 12: Create a Community Asset Inventory or Map

After prioritizing needs, it is important to identify existing community resources that may help address those needs. For example, if the data you've collected and the responses you've received from community members indicate that obesity is the health priority for this community, you should next determine what services, organizations, and resources relating to obesity already exist in the community and may be included as part of the solution. For example, is there an obesity task force already in place in a local school district? Identifying existing resources allows for greater community involvement, prevents replication of services, and allows for more efficient allocation of funding.

Health programs and services that are built upon **community assets,** or existing resources, are more effective because they already have roots in the community. The process of identifying community assets is also known as **community capacity building** because it encourages program planners to build upon community strengths, not deficits. Specifically, **capacity-focused assessment** identifies capacities, skills, assets, or contributions that can be provided by community individuals, associations, and institutions (Gilmore & Campbell, 2005). FYI 6.5 provides examples of community assets. The information collected in capacity assessment (or assets mapping) can be used later to form community coalitions and advisory panels for program planning and implementation (see chapter 7). All of this can lead to community empowerment, which is the ideal. As we explained in chapter 2, community health professions have moved toward a community empowerment approach that involves community members in the health education process.

As defined in chapter 2, community empowerment is a social-action process by which individuals, communities, and organizations gain mastery over their lives, change their surroundings, and improve their overall quality of life. In other words, community empowerment is about helping people help themselves in a way that encourages them to take ownership of their health problems and use their abilities and resources to develop solutions. By having a stake in assessing, planning, and implementing health programs, community members are more likely to accept, participate, and adopt health interventions and behaviors that support a healthier community overall.

FYI 6.5   Types of Community Assets

Individual Assets

Individuals and their
- Skills
- Talents
- Experiences

Consider:
- Professional
- Personal
- Resources
- Leadership

Institutional Assets

Churches
Colleges and universities
Elderly care facilities
Fire department
Hospitals and clinics
Mental health facilities
Libraries
Police department
Schools
Utilities

Organizational Assets

Community centers
Radio/TV stations
Small businesses
Large businesses
Home-based enterprises
Religious organizations
Nonprofit organizations
Clubs
Citizen groups
Business associations
Transportation networks
Cable and phone companies

Governmental (State and Federal) Assets

City government
State capital
Bureau of Land Management
Economic development
    departments
Forest service
Military facilities
School service center
Small business administration
State education agency
Telecommunications agency

Physical and Land Assets

Agriculture
Emergency resources
Forest
Industrial areas
Lakes, ponds, streams
Mining
Natural resources/landmarks
Parks/recreation areas
Vacant land
Waste resources

Cultural Assets

Historic/arts groups
Ethnic/racial diversity
Heritage
Crafts, skills
Cultural traditions

Step 13: Report Findings and Make Recommendations

As you've noted from the prior 12 steps, completing a thorough community needs assessment takes time and diligence. After you've validated your findings and have included community members in the prioritization process, it's time to compile a report and provide suggestions for addressing these needs. When writing the formal needs assessment report, be sure to include the following components: (a) introduction and community description, (b) methods for data collection, (c) data analysis, (d) findings, (e) implications for health education and program development, and (f) conclusion. FYI 6.6 provides a detailed description of each component.

FYI 6.6   Components of a Formal Community Needs Assessment Report

Title Page	Title of your assessment project, name of author/s, and date.
Executive Summary or Abstract	A brief (250 words or less) summary of the purpose of the assessment, methods used, and findings.
Table of Contents	List all of the paper content sections with appropriate first page number.
Introduction & Community Description	Overview of the community (history, demographics, geographic boundaries, etc.). Provide facts collected through secondary data.
Data-Collection Methods	Discuss the data collection strategy used along with the step-by-step protocol.
Data Analysis	Explain how the collected data was analyzed.
Findings	Illustrate and discuss results from the data analyses. Include graphs and charts to display your findings.
Community Assets	Identify community assets that would be helpful in program development, coordination, implementation, evaluation, and maintenance.
Implications for Health Education and Program Development	Discuss the implications of what you found, explain emergent health priorities, segment health needs by group, provide suggestions for health education and health interventions, and suggest guiding theoretical frameworks.
Conclusion	Provide a few summary statements and offer some of the limitations of the needs assessment. Explain how the results of the study will help plan or assist programs within the community.
References	Be sure to list all references in a format such as APA and provide parenthetical reference citations throughout.
Appendixes	You may want to include copies of the surveys or questions you used for data collection; articles or handouts relating to the community and any miscellaneous documents you feel enrich the community assessment.

Using a Theoretical Lens to Assess Community Needs

So far, we have discussed how needs-assessment data are collected and how that information is combined with a capacity assessment to develop a health education program plan. What we haven't addressed is what to look for in those assessments or how to use a theoretical lens. As we discussed in chapter 5, applying a theoretical basis to program development is necessary if you want the program to be relevant to the community and have a significant impact.

How can we approach the assessment process with any assurance of knowing what to look for? This is rarely a simple process because each community has its own unique characteristics and a variety of influences that have shaped it (see chapter 2). However, some helpful guidelines and models used in the health education profession can increase our chances of identifying a full assessment picture. One of the models we find most helpful for community needs assessment is the PRECEDE portion of the PRECEDE/PROCEED model described in chapter 5. An explanation of how to use the constructs of this model for community assessment and asset mapping follows.

You may recall from chapter 5 that the PRECEDE/PROCEED model can seem a bit overwhelming at first, until you realize that its purpose is not to belabor the process with needless attention to detail. Instead, it is designed to help you develop a full picture of your community of interest—its health needs and the factors that influence them. It isn't the only needs-assessment and program-planning model, but it is quite useful for your exploration of needs because it offers a broad community-assessment perspective and provides a framework in which community members can participate in the process.

Applying PRECEDE to Community Needs Assessment

In chapter 5, we presented the history and purpose of the PRECEDE/PRO-CEED model and discussed the various phases that comprised its framework. Now it's time to apply it! Figure 6.2 (on the following page) presents a sample PRECEDE assessment of adolescent smoking. The words or phrases in each PRECEDE box represent factors we might identify and target if we were conducting a needs assessment among adolescents in a local school system. We invite you to use this visual as a guideline to create your own PRECEDE assessment of a similar adolescent health issue, such as drug abuse. FYI 6.7 (on p. 149) lists needs-assessment strategies you might employ as you move through the four phases of the PRECEDE model.

To begin, draw a small "quality of life" box on the far right side of a sheet of paper. Record in it social indicators you think would emerge from a needs assessment about high school drug abuse. Draw a "health" box to the immediate left of the quality-of-life box and list in it some possible health indicators of drug abuse. Add behavioral, environmental, genetic, predisposing, reinforcing, and enabling boxes to your drug abuse model and insert relevant examples in each.

Suppose there have been a number of incidents related to drug abuse in a local high school; various students have been involved in alcohol-related traffic accidents, drug overdoses, and the like. School authorities and parents are alarmed about drugs pervading the school system, and the issue is a primary discussion topic among students. You've been asked to develop a school-based drug education program and you wish to apply the PRECEDE /PROCEED model to assess influencing factors. What quality-of-life factors would you expect to emerge in the social assessment? In other words, what social indicators might be detected as evidence that drugs are a problem in the school? Any number of indices could emerge, including drug-influenced domestic problems, school absenteeism and dropouts, and even arrests.

How would you know whether drug abuse is actually prevalent in the school and should be a health education priority? You would look for incidence and prevalence rates of specific drug-related health problems. Examples of indicators you could name

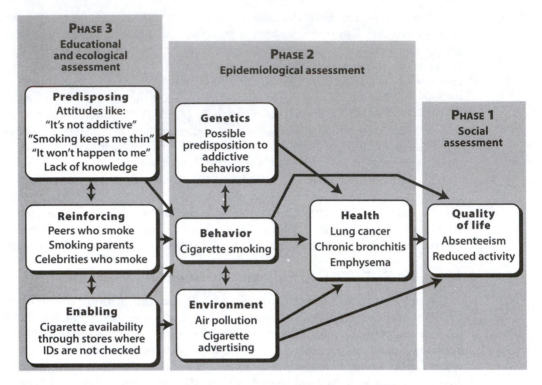

Figure 6.2   A sample PRECEDE assessment of adolescent smoking.
Based on Green and Kreuter's (2005) PRECEDE model, this example shows selected factors known to influence smoking behavior and its long-range effects as outlined using the first three phases of PRECEDE.

include the frequency of alcohol-related traffic accidents, drug overdoses, and diagnosed drug addictions recorded over the past year. These statistics could be compared to other possible health problems such as injuries or sexually transmitted diseases to validate drug problems as an important priority.

With drug problems confirmed as an important target, what behavioral and environmental factors might you find to be contributing to the drug problems? In an educational and ecological assessment, what predisposing, reinforcing, and enabling factors might emerge? Individual surveys and group assessments could reveal important answers, such as the need to address social drinking and drug experimentation (behaviors) commonly practiced at parties and sporting events (a social environment factor). Common adolescent attitudes, values, misconceptions, and beliefs about drug and alcohol use (predisposing factors) might be similar to those associated with cigarette smoking, and just as damaging. Your needs assessment might reveal that a well-designed health education campaign could counter the usual negative peer pressure if it involved recognized role models and school heroes (reinforcing factors). The assessment could also help you understand drug accessibility issues and identify the skills needed to refuse drugs in a social setting (enabling factors).

FYI **6.7**   **Needs Assessment Strategies Using Phases 1–4 of PRECEDE**

Phases	Strategies
1. Social Assessment (Quality of Life)	Observe and take field notes, use photos or facilitate Photovoice, interview community gatekeepers and residents, conduct public forums and/or focus groups.
2. Epidemiological Assessment (Health, Genetics, Behavior & Environment)	Collect secondary data such as reports from the state health department, county health department, and hospital data. Other sources include police records; school district reports; CDC data, reports, and publications; Center for National Health Statistics data; nonprofit organization data, reports, and publications. Use Photovoice; conduct geographic information system mapping (GIS); review or distribute community surveys to collect primary data.
3. Educational and Ecological Assessment	Review existing research from credible sources; develop and/or implement community surveys; conduct interviews, focus groups, or public forums to assess the predisposing, enabling, and reinforcing factors that impact the health issue; observe ecological factors that impact health and use field notes; take photos.
4. Administrative and Policy Assessment & Intervention Alignment	Map community assets; use Delphi group, nominal and/or focus groups, and/or public forums to discuss and prioritize community needs; review media and public policies; select theory or theories to guide program; list appropriate program strategies.

The PRECEDE assessment results we just described could serve as a visual framework for a needs-specific drug abuse prevention program. Specific aspects of program development, including goals, objectives, and implementation, will be addressed in chapter 7. Then, in chapter 8, we will revisit the model to discuss program evaluation plans and strategies.

In Conclusion

As mentioned throughout this chapter, assessing community needs and assets is a vital first step for those planning health-related programs or services. It is important for health educators and other health professionals to understand the unique characteristics and health needs of each community in order to provide effective and relevant health education and services. In this chapter we present needs assessment and community-capacity-building concepts that will serve you well in the future. We outline steps in the assessment processes and highlight a way to map community assets. Planning models are helpful when developing programs and the PRECEDE/PROCEED model is one of the most comprehensive tools of this kind. In chapter 7 you will have the opportunity to learn how to use the model to move from needs assessment to program development.

REVIEW QUESTIONS

1. What is a needs assessment and why is it important?
2. Discuss the difference between actual and perceived needs and explain the value of assessing both.
3. Explain the benefits and drawbacks of using various types of data-collection methods in community needs assessment.
4. Explain how models and theories can be useful in the needs-assessment process.
5. Draw the PRECEDE portion of the PRECEDE/PROCEED model and explain how its components can influence a community's health.
6. Discuss why community asset mapping and community empowerment are important for program development.

FOR YOUR APPLICATION

Develop a PRECEDE Assessment

1. Choose a specific health problem in an age- or ethnicity-specific community and use the PRECEDE/PROCEED model to identify factors contributing to the health problem and subsequent quality-of-life issues.

   A. Draw the same PRECEDE boxes you see in Figure 6.2 on a sheet of notebook paper. Write the PRECEDE labels (quality of life, health, behavior, and so forth) at the top of each box.

   B. Write your chosen health problem inside the "health" box. (If it's a behavior, such as smoking, enter it in the "behavior" box instead.)

   C. Move to the right and enter some quality-of-life issues that might arise in your chosen community as a result of this health problem. (If you began with a health behavior, complete both the health and quality-of-life boxes.)

   D. Now move back toward the left. Fill in each box with factors you think contribute to the problem. Try to be specific to your chosen community.

   E. Make a list of potential community resources, capacities, and solutions.

2. Apply the four phases (and 13 steps) of community needs assessment to your chosen community. Practice using some of the data-collection strategies outlined in this chapter, analyze the results, and create a formal report to submit to your instructor and peers.

Using Photovoice in Your Community

Purchase a few disposable cameras and ask some community members (i.e., members of a local community group) to take pictures of what they perceive to be community barriers or assets that impact quality of life and overall health within the area. Use the steps of Photovoice (FYI 6.3) and analyze the results. Prepare a presentation of your findings to share with your classmates and members of the community.

Creating Assessment Opportunities

Contact a local health department or health agency that provides health education programs. Ask about health issues and programs the agency is planning to address in the future. Volunteer to conduct a literature search to (a) clearly define the health issue, (b) identify factors that could potentially influence the targeted health problem, and (c) locate existing needs-assessment survey instruments that could be used by the agency. Use the PRECEDE model as a guide, and create a brief report of your findings. Give one copy to the agency and place one in your portfolio. Create a folder in your portfolio labeled "Needs Assessment (Responsibility I)." Ask an agency representative to write a brief evaluation of your efforts to include in that portfolio folder.

Planning Processes for Evidence-Based Programs

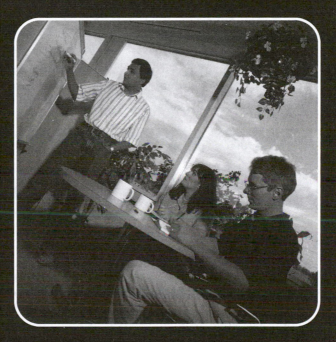

You are invited to serve on a planning team to develop a wellness promotion program for students on your university campus. The task seems easy enough until your planning team discovers that students are too busy with course work, jobs, and personal lives to squeeze in time for regular exercise. Conversations with coordinators of student health services, the campus wellness center, and the academic department that offers wellness courses reveal that students don't effectively use these resources to their full advantage. You discover that a number of students struggle with health-related issues that are seriously impacting their quality of life and placing their futures at risk. Where do you begin in your attempt to make a difference?

CHAPTER OBJECTIVES

1. Describe benefits and general characteristics of the planning process.
2. Describe the use of the PRECEDE/PROCEED model in the planning process.
3. Describe the phases of the MAPP model.
4. Name and describe the general components of a grant proposal or program plan.
5. List steps commonly used in the planning process.
6. Explain the purpose and characteristics of a vision, mission, goal, and objective.
7. Explain the utility of process, impact, and outcome goals.
8. Develop a measurable objective.
9. Conduct a SWOT analysis for program planning.
10. Describe common budget categories.

Planning Concepts and Strategies

"So, what's the plan?" This is a common question in everyday life. Whether it is asked among friends putting together a last-minute social event or among coworkers responding to an emergency, the general assumption is that a good plan can be useful. Our goal in this chapter is to equip you with basic planning concepts and strategies that can help you develop good planning skills. We begin with a general description of planning concepts.

Planning Benefits and Characteristics

Success in community-based health promotion can be thwarted by complex health issues, conflicting opinions, and shifting community dynamics. Trying to overcome these challenges to achieve long-range goals can feel like aiming at a moving target from a rocking rowboat. The precious commodities of time, momentum, funds, and other resources can be wasted when no clear sense of direction is in place. A well-designed plan can serve as:

- A communication tool to help partners focus on established goals, minimize unrealistic expectations, understand roles, and build trust.

- An action guide to streamline efforts, use resources effectively, and foster productivity.

- An evaluation guide for measuring progress and success.

Effective planning calls for patience, diligence, flexibility, and the realization that few plans are ever perfect or finished. Planning is an ongoing process.

Planning partners from different backgrounds sometimes struggle to find a common language to use in the process. Some groups stall over confusion about whether they are planning a "program" or an "intervention." Green and Kreuter (2005) define a **health program** as "a set of planned and organized activities carried out over time to accomplish specific health-related goals and objectives" (p. 1). McKenzie, Neiger, and Thackeray (2009) define an **intervention** as a "theory-based strategy or experience to which those in the priority population will be exposed, or in which they will take part" (p. 201).

Though these terms are often used interchangeably, when used together, "the term *intervention* will usually refer to a specific component of a more comprehensive *program*" (Green & Kreuter, 2005, p. 192). We have included in this chapter a sequence of planning steps that you can use to design an intervention. This intervention could be the only program component or could serve as one of several components of a large program.

A Model-Based Approach to Planning

Planning models can be useful planning guides. McKenzie, Neiger, and Thackeray (2009) identified more than a dozen program planning models, most of which contain five common elements: "assessing needs, setting goals and objectives, developing an intervention, implementing the intervention, and evaluating the results" (p. 17). The PRECEDE/PROCEED model (Green & Kreuter, 2005) described in chapter 5 is one of the most widely used planning models in public health and health education. As illustrated in Figure 7.1 (on the following page), needs assessment data collected in Phases 1–4 can be used by a planning group to set priorities, develop a vision, create goals and objectives, and align the planned intervention with available resources and administrative support. Phases 5–8 can be used to plan implementation and evaluation strategies.

An online strategic planning guide called the MAPP Tool may serve as a useful resource as you develop your planning skills. The tool is based on the Mobilizing for Action through Planning and Partnerships (MAPP) model created by the National Association of County and City Health Officials (NACCHO, 2008) to help "communities apply strategic thinking to prioritize public health issues and identify resources to address them" (para. 1). In Phase 1 of MAPP, Organize for Success, collaborative groups discuss partnership benefits and barriers, identify and organize participants, design the planning process, assess resource needs, secure commitments, assess readiness for planning, and develop needed tools for a successful planning process. In Phase 2, Visioning, the group discusses current and past community visions and develops a shared vision for the next 5 to 10 years. In Phase 3, Assessments, the group

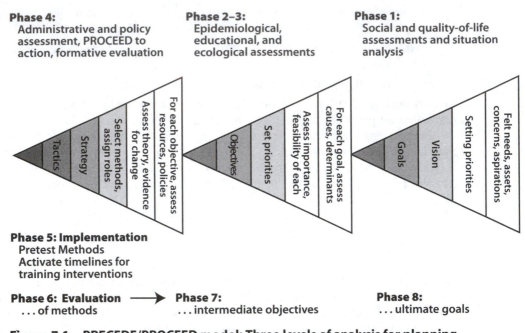

Phase 4:
Administrative and policy assessment, PROCEED to action, formative evaluation

Phase 2–3:
Epidemiological, educational, and ecological assessments

Phase 1:
Social and quality-of-life assessments and situation analysis

Phase 5: Implementation
Pretest Methods
Activate timelines for training interventions

Phase 6: Evaluation ⟶ **Phase 7:**
. . . of methods   . . . intermediate objectives

Phase 8:
. . . ultimate goals

Figure 7.1   PRECEDE/PROCEED model: Three levels of analysis for planning.

From *Health Program Planning: An Educational and Ecological Approach*, 4th ed., p. 65, by L. W. Green and M. W. Kreuter. © 2005 by McGraw-Hill. Used with permission of the McGraw-Hill Companies.

conducts assessments (see chapter 6) and/or examines findings through the lens of the vision statement. In Phase 4, Strategic Issues, the group identifies and prioritizes strategic issues that emerged from previous phases. In Phase 5, Goals/Strategies, the group creates goals and feasible strategies based on these priorities and available resources. In the final MAPP phase, Action Cycle, the group creates measurable objectives and an action plan for implementation and evaluation.

A Proposal Framework for the Planning Process

In public health and health education, planning usually includes the development of a document that contains a rationale, goals and objectives, activity descriptions, timeline, and other elements needed to develop, implement, and evaluate a program or intervention. This document may be called a program or intervention plan, an action plan, or a work plan. It may be called a proposal if you plan to submit it to decision makers from whom you are requesting resources (e.g., a grant proposal or service contract), administrative approval (e.g., a service plan for an agency), or a formal partnership agreement (e.g., with other organizations or community groups). Common components of a plan or proposal (FYI 7.1) usually reflect the basic planning elements of assessment; goals and objectives development; and intervention design, implementation, and evaluation (McKenzie et al., 2009).

If you are creating a grant proposal to submit to a specific funding agency, you will likely need to adapt your content and format to requirements described in an

FYI **7.1   General Outline for Plans and Proposals**

A proposal or program plan often contains sections similar to those listed below. You will also need a cover page/application form (for grant proposals), an executive summary (1-page overview of all components), and a table of contents. Adapt the following outline to meet specific proposal guidelines and/or your specific planning needs.

Statement of Need or Problem Statement
- Thorough discussion of problem the intervention will address
- Recommended components:
  - Review of the literature to quote national or global statistics related to the need
  - Findings from assessments conducted in local priority population
  - General living conditions, challenges, and capacities of priority population
  - Summary statement of what is needed based on information provided

Mission, Goals, and Objectives
- Program mission statement
- Program goals and measurable objectives
- Narrative if needed to explain context of proposed intervention within broader programmatic efforts

Intervention Description (Methods/Procedures)
- Overview of intervention scope and rationale
- Work plan (detailed descriptions of activity methods/procedures)
- Administrative plan (roles, responsibilities, expertise)
- Intervention timeline (Gantt chart)

Evaluation Plan (Data Collection/Analysis)
- Overview of evaluation scope and rationale
- Evaluation methods and procedures
- Evaluation timeline

Budget
- Summary table and brief narrative
- Item-line budget

Appendixes
- Reference list for all sources cited in document
- Assessment reports or summaries
- Intervention materials (marketing flyers, session/lesson plans, instruments, etc.)
- Vitas/resumes of personnel/consultants identified in administrative plan

Sources: KU Work Group, 2007c; McKenzie, Neiger, & Thackeray, 2009; Simons-Morton, Greene, & Gottlieb, 1995.

application guide. This application guide is usually called a **funding opportunity announcement** (FOA) or a request for proposals or applications. An FOA usually includes extensive requirements for format and content that should be precisely followed. Some funding agencies offer grant-writing workshops for a specific FOA and have staff members available to help guide the process.

Most funding agencies have a cover page or application form that must be submitted with the proposal. This page can be accessed through the FOA and usually requires the name and address of the responsible individual, sometimes called the **principal investigator**. It will also require the name and address of the person or organization responsible for fiscal management of the grant, the amount requested, the time period for the project, and a brief description of the agency. You will likely need to obtain signatures from designated officials in your workplace for this form, so be sure to learn about proposal-routing procedures for all organizations involved and allow time to obtain signatures prior to submission.

Some FOAs require a brief overview or **executive summary** of the entire proposal presented on one page or less. Because the executive summary is often the first (or only) part of your proposal that some decision makers read, we cannot overstate its importance. It should capture the reader's attention with a strong rationale for the need and value of the planned intervention. It should include a complete, yet concise, overview of the entire project (e.g., goals, strategies, time frame, capacities, needed resources, costs, benefits, expected outcomes), and should highlight the plan's strengths and innovative elements.

The more detailed sections of the proposal should contain information that answers the following questions.

1. What is the need in your priority population? (statement of need/rationale)
2. What is the mission of your planned intervention? (mission statement)
3. What specific changes are expected as a result of the intervention? (goals and objectives)
4. What is the general rationale and design of the intervention? (scope and sequence)
5. What specific activities will occur? (work plan methods/protocols)
6. Who will do the work? (administrative plan)
7. How will you know that you have met your goals? (evaluation plan)
8. What resources are needed to make it work? (budget)
9. How will this effort make a difference? (expected benefits and outcomes)

Some guidelines for developing a proposal are integrated into the recommended planning steps that follow.

Planning Steps

In an ideal world, all planning groups would work through a series of stress-free steps to a successful end. In the real world, that rarely happens. However, some common planning activities, when adapted and sequenced according to your specific needs, can help streamline the process, enhance productivity, and increase your chances for success. The planning steps described below and outlined in Table 7.1 can serve as a general guide. It is highly possible that your planning group will need to adapt these steps to your specific situation as part of Step 1.

Table 7.1   Planning Guide

Step 1: Establish a Shared Vision and Organize Planning Groups
1.1 Form planning and advisory groups
1.2 Develop a shared vision
1.3 Establish communication and decision-making structures
1.4 Develop work scope and action plan

Step 2: Assess Needs and Capacities
2.1 Identify existing and needed information
2.2 Collect and synthesize information
2.3 Determine priorities
2.4 Write rationale or statement of need

Step 3: Develop a Mission, Goals, and Objectives
3.1 Create a mission statement
3.2 Write goals and objectives

Step 4: Design the Intervention
4.1 Create a logic model
4.2 Select intervention strategies
4.3 Develop an intervention guide
4.4 Identify and develop needed resources
4.5 Create a budget

Sources: Green & Kreuter, 2005; KU Work Group, 2007c; McKenzie, Neiger, & Thackeray, 2009; NACCHO, 2008; Simons-Morton, Greene, & Gottlieb, 1995.

Step 1: Establish a Shared Vision and Organize Planning Groups

Partnerships and a shared vision may have already been established when planning begins. However, in some cases, those partnerships and vision may need to be more fully developed as part of the early stages of planning.

1.1 Form Planning and Advisory Groups

We recommend **participatory planning** in which "everyone who has a stake in the intervention has a voice, either in person or by representation. Staff of the organization that will run it, members of the target population, community officials, interested citizens, and people from involved agencies, schools, and other institutions all should be invited to the table" (KU Work Group, 2007b, *What is the participatory approach to planning?*, para. 1). The nature of the planning groups formed and the extent of participants' contributions will depend on interest levels, time availability, relationships between groups/organizations, and the scope of needed work.

It may be helpful to organize a **coalition**, "A group of individuals and/or organizations with a common interest who agree to work together toward a common goal" (KU Work Group, 2007b, *What is a coalition?*, para. 1). To keep your coalition vibrant and productive:

- Communicate openly and freely with everyone
- Be inclusive and participatory
- Network at every opportunity

- Set reachable goals, in order to engender success
- Hold creative meetings
- Be realistic about what you can do: don't promise more than you can accomplish, and always keep your promises
- Acknowledge and use the diversity of the group (KU Work Group, 2007b, *To sum up*, para. 5)

Continually report and celebrate progress and successes along the way so that all coalition members and the community at large are aware and appreciative of the work invested.

When no coalition exists or when your planned intervention is one of several coalition projects, you may need to form a smaller planning group of 5–12 members. This group may consist of a subset of coalition members; other stakeholders; and experts who possess needed insights and skills, will be trusted by stakeholder groups, and will work collaboratively and efficiently. McKenzie et al. (2009) recommend that you include **doers**, "people who will be willing to roll up their sleeves and do the physical work needed to see that the program is planned and implemented properly" (p. 69), and **influencers**, "those who with a single phone call or signature on a form will enlist other people to participate or will help provide the resources to facilitate the program" (p. 69). This planning group can also consult with an advisory panel of experts for technical assistance and/or a community advisory group for input about population-based needs and perspectives.

1.2 Develop a Shared Vision

A unified vision within and across groups can serve as a solid foundation for all planning activities. This vision can emerge from an examination of previously collected and/or newly implemented assessments (see Step 2) and from the collective experience and wisdom of the partnership group. Your group's **vision statement** should be futuristic and reflect a conceptualized ideal for the priority population.

> Your vision communicates what your organization believes are the ideal conditions for your community; how things would look if the issue important to you were perfectly addressed. This utopian dream is generally articulated by one or more phrases or vision statements, which are brief proclamations that convey the community's dreams for the future. In general, vision statements should be:
> - Understood and shared by members of the community
> - Broad enough to allow a diverse variety of local perspectives to be encompassed within them
> - Inspiring and uplifting to everyone involved in your effort
> - Easy to communicate—for example, they should be short enough to fit on a T-shirt
>
> Here are a few vision statements which meet the above criteria:
> - Healthy children
> - Safe streets, safe neighborhoods
> - Every house a home
> - Education for all
> - Peace on earth (KU Work Group, 2007c, *1. Vision*)

1.3 Establish Communication and Decision-Making Structures

Groups work more effectively when communication and decision-making structures are clearly understood. Group leaders, decision-making rules, and communication channels should be designated before the work begins. Decision-making procedures can include group consensus, a formal vote, or a designated executive committee that makes final decisions when consensus cannot be reached. Be consistent in how decisions are made and, whenever possible, openly communicate decision-making processes, outcomes, and rationale with all partners.

1.4 Develop Work Scope and Action Plan

Members of the planning group should agree to serve based on a clear understanding of roles and expectations. When inviting individuals to join the planning group, provide a written description of the purpose, work scope, and expected outcomes of the planning process. The established group should then refine the action plan to include planning goals and tasks, decision-making and communication channels, and other details that will guide the planning process.

Step 2: Assess Needs and Capacities

Though much of the needs and capacity assessment work may have already occurred before your planning group is formed, your group will need to examine this information in light of your planning goals. The goal of this step is to validate the need for your planned intervention.

2.1 Identify Existing and Needed Information

The MAPP and PRECEDE/PROCEED (phases 1–4) models can be used to determine the information and resources you will need to plan and implement the intervention. Your group should create a list of existing and needed information, the sources from which they have been or will be obtained, and how that information will be used in the planning process.

2.2 Collect and Synthesize Information

The assessment methods described in chapter 6 can be used to collect any additional information that may be needed. Synthesizing all information into a concise and useful format is an important part of the planning process. This synthesized information should be used to determine priorities for your planned intervention.

2.3 Determine Priorities

Your group can use a prioritization matrix (see chapter 6) to identify important and changeable factors to be addressed in the intervention. A SWOT analysis (KU Work Group, 2007e) can also be used to develop a matrix of strengths, weaknesses, opportunities, and threats (SWOT). The upper half of the matrix (see Figure 7.2 on the following page) should contain internal strengths and weaknesses of your partnership group or organization (the group that will develop and implement the intervention). These strengths and weaknesses can include a variety of elements such as existing or needed resources (e.g., equipment, supplies, and materials), levels of personnel expertise and experience, organizational structures and policies that can enable or hinder progress, or the degree to which all partners possess the needed vision and commitment.

The lower half of the matrix represents external opportunities and threats in the environment or setting in which you plan to implement the intervention. For example,

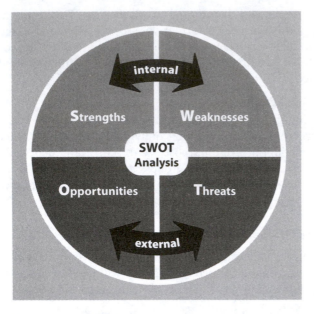

Figure 7.2   SWOT analysis matrix.
Adapted from *SWOT Analysis: Strengths, Weaknesses, Opportunities, Threats* (ch. 3, sect. 14), KU Work Group for Community Health and Development, 2007, Lawrence, KS: University of Kansas.

a recent community event that has intensified interest in issues related to your program mission could be viewed as an external opportunity for your intervention to be well received. New leadership, changes in policies or laws, or the development of new funding sources or partnering organizations can serve as external opportunities that can increase your chances for success.

It is important, however, to weigh these opportunities in light of potential threats in the environment that could hinder your progress or negatively impact your intended outcomes. In the business world, the paradigm in which the SWOT analysis concept was first developed, an external threat is often another business that competes for the same customers. In public and community health promotion, it is important to identify potentially competing programs and services and avoid unnecessary duplication. External threats can also include "competing messages" or other elements that counter or distort your health message and intended outcomes. For example, unhealthy weight-loss programs, fast food restaurants, and tobacco stores can serve as external threats to a program with a health promotion mission. Social norms that embrace risky behaviors such as unsafe sex and alcohol abuse can also be external threats. A SWOT analysis should enable your group to enhance and capitalize on internal strengths and external opportunities and address or minimize the impact of internal weaknesses and external threats.

2.4 Write Rationale or Statement of Need

A written rationale or statement of need that summarizes your findings in Steps 2.1 through 2.3 can serve as a useful communication tool for interested stakeholder groups. It can also be included in grant proposals and plans. The statement should also help your planning group develop a mission statement, goals, and objectives that match needs and capacities.

Step 3: Develop a Mission, Goals, and Objectives

Most program or intervention plans include a mission statement, goals, and objectives that frame the intervention design and planned activities. These three components should:

- Reflect prioritized needs and capacities in your priority population
- Frame the scope and specific elements of your planned intervention
- Guide the evaluation process to monitor progress and outcomes

3.1 Create a Mission Statement

A **mission statement** is a "short narrative that describes the general focus or purpose of the program" (McKenzie et al., 2009, p. 139). Where the vision statement describes a future ideal condition, the mission statement clarifies the purpose of the program or what will be done through the program to achieve that vision. Examples are listed below.

- The mission of the *BU-LiveWell Program* is to promote total well-being and health-related quality of life among Baylor University students.

- *BodyWorks* is a program designed to help parents and caregivers of adolescent girls and boys improve family eating and activity habits (Office of Women's Health, 2008, *About BodyWorks*, para. 1).

Every goal, objective, and strategy of your planned intervention should be designed to help your group achieve its stated mission.

3.2 Write Goals and Objectives

Your program goals and objectives should serve as the guide for designing, implementing, and evaluating your intervention. The first step in creating them is to clarify what your group plans to call them. In this chapter, we use the term *program mission* to refer to the overall purpose of the program. Any goal (e.g., health goal, behavioral goal) associated with your program is referred to in this chapter as a *program goal*. A **goal** is commonly a short, general statement that indicates "what will change" and the individuals or groups expected to be affected by the change. An **objective** contains detailed criteria needed to measure the degree to which you have achieved that goal (CDC, 2008j; Green & Kreuter, 2005; McKenzie et al., 2009). Because goals and objectives are so critical to effective planning, we have provided some detailed information about how to create them.

Writing goals. A goal can be written as an incomplete sentence that begins with the word "to" as in "To reduce the incidence of teen pregnancies in McLennan County" or "To increase exercise behavior among Baylor University students." Notice that these goals do not include details that would be needed to measure these intended changes. Your objectives will contain the details.

Also notice that each of our example goals focuses on only one specific change (reduced pregnancies, increased exercise behavior). There is a practical reason for this singular approach. When you begin to evaluate your program and interpret results, you will need to clearly determine and report whether you did or did not achieve each goal. If you combine two or more targeted changes in the same goal (for example, "To increase *exercise* and *healthy eating* behaviors . . ."), interpreting and reporting results can become a bit confusing, particularly if you observe an increase in one behavior but not the other. It is also easier to create measurable objectives for a goal that contains only one intended change.

There is no rule about the number of goals you will need. However, most planning groups create too few (McKenzie et al., 2009). If your planned intervention is intended to be part of a long-range community building effort, multiple goals that systematically connect the immediate results of your intervention to that broader long-term mission can be very useful. Phases 1–4 of the PRECEDE/PROCEED model are a useful framework for this systematic approach to goal development. The factor or object of interest assessed in each of those phases can be used to develop a related program goal for that factor. Figure 7.3 contains an example of possible program goals that could be developed using these four PRECEDE phases if your planning group was developing an exercise promotion program for university students. A long-range **quality of life goal** to promote wellness among students could be at least partially achieved if increased exercise activity (behavior goal) and reduced obesity (health goal) were achieved through the intervention.

To create and implement a comprehensive exercise promotion program, your planning group would likely need to create several exercise-related **health goals** (statements of intended changes in mortality, morbidity, disability, or physiological risk factors or health status indicators such as blood pressure or body fat percentage). Our sample health goal in the figure targets an intended change in the physiological risk factor of obesity as an expected outcome of our exercise intervention. But we could also have targeted changes in health problems that are commonly associated with lack of exercise and obesity such as diabetes or heart disease. We focused on obesity, a health indicator, because our program is designed for college students who may not begin to experience the chronic illnesses associated with obesity until later in life.

Quality of life and health goals are generally referred to as **outcome goals,** statements of intended changes that are often long term and far reaching. When these goals focus on long-range outcomes such as decreased mortality and morbidity rates, the emergence of observable changes can take years. To maintain morale and support for your intervention, goals that reflect more immediate successes can be an asset. In the PRECEDE/PROCEED model, **impact goals** are statements of intended change in the factors identified in Phases 2–3 of the model that impact health and quality of life. The behavioral goal (increased exercise) in our example (Figure 7.3) is a type of impact goal. Our sample **environmental goal** (create a healthy campus atmosphere) can result from an intervention that contains other goals and activities designed to impact the physical, social, and/or economic environment on campus. Figure 7.3 also contains samples of other types of impact goals designed to address the predisposing, reinforcing, and enabling factors that may influence exercise behavior and/or the campus climate. Figure 7.4 (on p. 166) contains more complete versions of our sample impact and outcome goals, along with some example objectives linked to each goal. We describe how to create measurable objectives in the following section.

Once your planning group knows *what* you want to change (stated in your impact and outcome goals), you can create goals that state *how* you will make those changes happen. These **process goals** can focus on the development, delivery, and/or quality of your planned intervention. Some process goals target the completion of specific tasks (e.g., testing educational materials, distributing a newsletter, or conducting an orientation meeting) and the delivery of health promotion sessions or services (e.g., attendance or participation). Other process goals target perceptions of program quality among program participants, staff, and other stakeholders. For goal-writing purposes, we refer to these factors that often serve as the measurement targets in process goals as

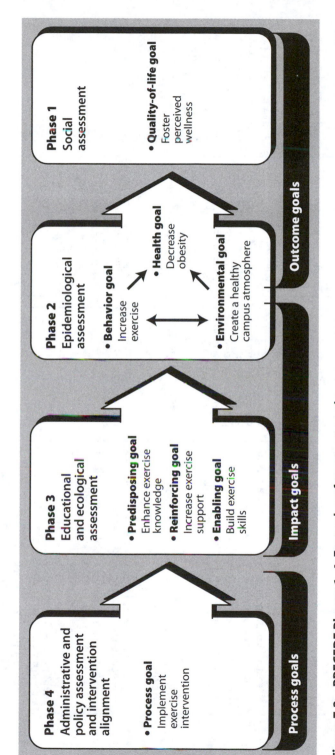

Figure 7.3   PRECEDE Phases 1–4: Examples of program goals.

Adapted from *Health Program Planning: An Educational and Ecological Approach*, 4th ed. (PRECEDE/PROCEED model), by L. W. Green and M. W. Kreuter, 2005, New York: McGraw-Hill.

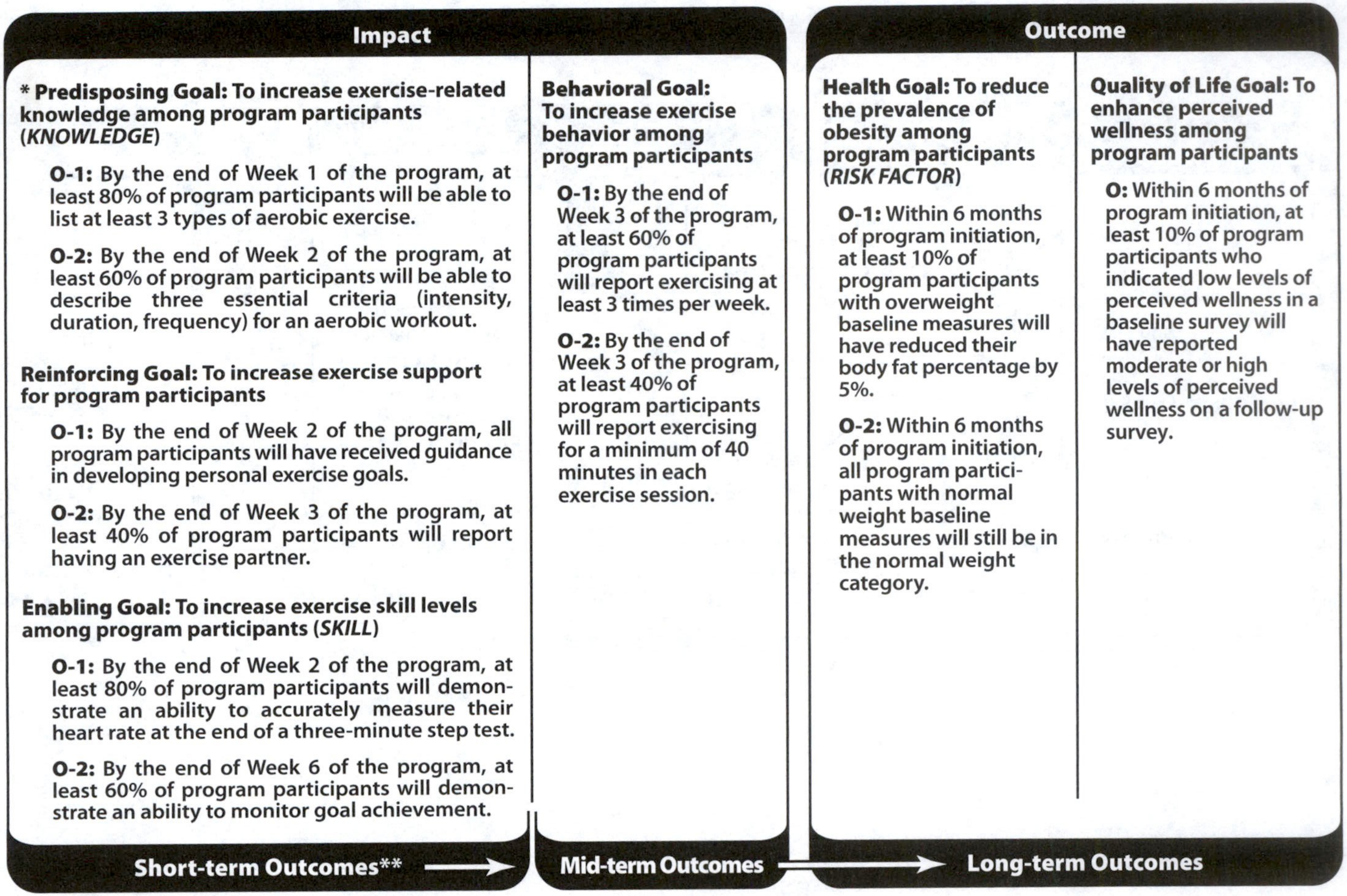

Impact

* Predisposing Goal: To increase exercise-related knowledge among program participants (KNOWLEDGE)

O-1: By the end of Week 1 of the program, at least 80% of program participants will be able to list at least 3 types of aerobic exercise.

O-2: By the end of Week 2 of the program, at least 60% of program participants will be able to describe three essential criteria (intensity, duration, frequency) for an aerobic workout.

Reinforcing Goal: To increase exercise support for program participants

O-1: By the end of Week 2 of the program, all program participants will have received guidance in developing personal exercise goals.

O-2: By the end of Week 3 of the program, at least 40% of program participants will report having an exercise partner.

Enabling Goal: To increase exercise skill levels among program participants (SKILL)

O-1: By the end of Week 2 of the program, at least 80% of program participants will demonstrate an ability to accurately measure their heart rate at the end of a three-minute step test.

O-2: By the end of Week 6 of the program, at least 60% of program participants will demonstrate an ability to monitor goal achievement.

Behavioral Goal: To increase exercise behavior among program participants

O-1: By the end of Week 3 of the program, at least 60% of program participants will report exercising at least 3 times per week.

O-2: By the end of Week 3 of the program, at least 40% of program participants will report exercising for a minimum of 40 minutes in each exercise session.

Outcome

Health Goal: To reduce the prevalence of obesity among program participants (RISK FACTOR)

O-1: Within 6 months of program initiation, at least 10% of program participants with overweight baseline measures will have reduced their body fat percentage by 5%.

O-2: Within 6 months of program initiation, all program participants with normal weight baseline measures will still be in the normal weight category.

Quality of Life Goal: To enhance perceived wellness among program participants

O: Within 6 months of program initiation, at least 10% of program participants who indicated low levels of perceived wellness in a baseline survey will have reported moderate or high levels of perceived wellness on a follow-up survey.

Short-term Outcomes** →   Mid-term Outcomes →   Long-term Outcomes

* Based on PRECEDE/PROCEED model terminology (Green & Kreuter, 2005).

** Logic model terminology (W. K. Kellogg Foundation, 2004).

Figure 7.4   Impact and outcome goals and objectives.

Sources: Green and Kreuter, 2005; W. K. Kellogg Foundation, 2004.

program delivery factors and **program quality factors.** We included examples of these two types of process goals, along with some related objectives, in Figure 7.5.

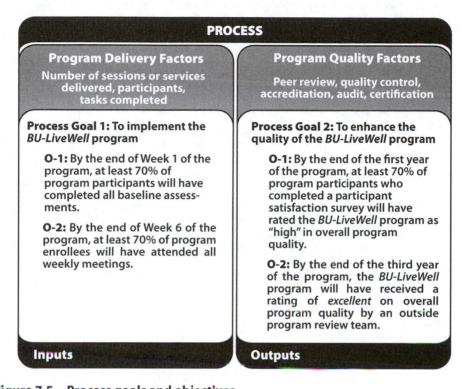

Figure 7.5   Process goals and objectives.
Source: *Logic Model Development Guide*, W. K. Kellogg Foundation, 2004.

Program objectives.   Each program goal you create should be accompanied by a set of measurable objectives similar to the examples in Figures 7.4 and 7.5. These objectives can be used to help you determine the degree to which that goal has been accomplished. For the same reason that each goal should state only one change, each objective should be designed to measure only one aspect or component of the goal. For example, if your behavioral goal is "to increase exercise behavior," you may need separate objectives to measure changes in different types of exercise behavior such as aerobic, strength-building, and flexibility activities.

Regardless of the type of objectives you write, every objective should be **SMART**: **s**pecific, **m**easurable, **a**chievable, **r**ealistic, and **t**ime bound (CDC, 2008j). In general, an objective should contain at least four elements that are described below (Green & Kreuter, 2005).

1. *Who* will change or benefit from the planned intervention?
2. *What* will change or what benefit will they receive?

3. *How much* change or how much benefit is expected?

4. *By when* will the change or benefit be evident?

Figure 7.6 illustrates needed components of a SMART objective with an example objective designed to measure changes in reported exercise behavior (what) among college students enrolled in an exercise promotion program. In the sample objective, we refer to this group as program participants (who).

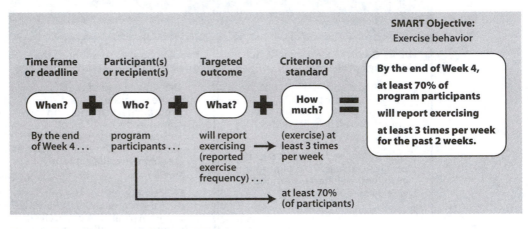

Figure 7.6   Elements of a SMART objective.
Sources: CDC, 2008j; Green and Kreuter, 2005.

Who will change? Be careful and precise in naming the "who" of your intended change or benefit. This "who" will normally be members of a specific subgroup of your priority population whose knowledge, behaviors, or health status, for example, you intend to change. However, consider the implications of naming your entire priority population as the "who" in your objective. If, for example, you name the entire target population (e.g., members of McLennan County, Baylor University students), in the objective, you just committed to measuring or having access to measures of the targeted knowledge, behavior, or health status of the entire population. In some cases, such widespread data does exist, particularly in the form of epidemiological data maintained by a government health agency, for example. But in other cases, it may be more realistic for the "who" of your objective to be defined as actual participants in your intervention so that immediate and, perhaps, long-term changes can be monitored. Either approach (a broad population group or only program participants) may be appropriate depending on your planning group's situation.

What will change? This component of the objective should state the exact factor or object of interest you plan to measure. The more specifically you describe this factor, the easier it will be to measure it. When writing a predisposing objective to measure changes in knowledge or attitudes, make sure that the verb you use to describe "what" you'll measure is observable.

For example, the two objectives listed in Figure 7.4 under the predisposing goal are knowledge objectives. These objectives are designed to measure changes in knowledge by measuring the participant's demonstrated ability to "list at least 3 types of aerobic exercise" (objective 1) and describe the essential criteria for an aerobic workout (objective 2). Note that you could observe this knowledge change by listening to the participant verbally describe the targeted knowledge or reading the participant's written description. This is what we mean by "observable" measures. Even though it may seem logical to write an objective that says participants will "understand" this information, no one can truly measure or "observe" what a person understands until that person demonstrates that understanding by describing or applying it in some way. The words listed in FYI 7.2 are but a few observable "action verbs" you can use to write objectives.

FYI 7.2   Measurable and Observable Behaviors

Cognitive (with increasing levels of cognitive ability)

Count	Express	Apply	Analyze	Assess
Define	Locate	Examine	Calculate	Judge
List	Review	Practice	Debate	Evaluate
Identify	Compute	Illustrate	Compare	Revise

Affective

Accept	Seek	Display
Observe	Complete	Discriminate

Psychomotor

Taste	Position	Copy	Create	Walk
Place	Repeat	Build	Produce	Climb

Another way to write the "what" of the objective in measurable terms is to provide more specific details about the exact type of action or behavior you will be evaluating to determine whether the objective was achieved. In our example of a SMART objective (Figure 7.6), the object of interest is "reported exercise behavior." The words "at least 3 times per week" could be viewed as further clarification of what will change in that only those participants who report exercising at least three times per week (not one or two) will be counted as having achieved this objective. This clarifying condition for inclusion could also be considered part of the "how much" component of your objective (described below).

How much will change? As already stated, the condition of having to report a frequency of at least three times per week could be considered part of the criterion or standard of achievement in your objective. Examples of other number-based measures of "how much" include percentages (e.g., 20% increase in exercise frequency), scores (e.g., minimum score of 50 points), averages or rates (average resting heart rate below 70 beats per minute). However, this standard does not necessarily have to relate to the object of interest (what) that is expected to change. In some cases, a number or percentage of the people (who) expected to change or benefit can serve as your standard for "how much" or, in this case, "how many." If it is unlikely that every participant in the intervention will achieve the stated objective, it may be more realistic for you to name a number or percentage of participants (e.g., at least 70%) as your criterion for achieving the objective.

By when will the change or benefit occur? The time frame component of your objective should serve as a benchmark or "deadline" for when your objective should be achieved. The time frame can be stated as an exact date (e.g., by February 10, 2012), a specific time period in the program or intervention (e.g., by the end of week 4), or a time frame attached to initiation or completion (e.g., within 1 year after program completion).

These stated time frames are helpful when it is time to schedule your intervention activities or plan of action on a timeline. For example, for our SMART objective example (Figure 7.6), a primary intervention activity could be group exercise three times per week. The planning group could assume that it may take a couple of weeks for all participants to adapt to this thrice weekly routine. The sample objective reflects the planning group's expectation that most participants (at least 70%) will be on track by the third week of the program. The sample objective would indicate a plan to survey all participants at the end of week 4 to determine participation levels. Activities needed to help participants meet this objective on time and a description of the actual survey event would be included in the intervention plan and timeline.

Step 4: Design the Intervention

With goals and objectives in place, your planning group is now ready to design the intervention. Decisions about the type of intervention strategies and materials used should be based on information obtained from assessments and your mission, goals, and objectives. To more readily match these elements, we recommend creating a logic model (Step 4.1) and adding relevant information resulting from Steps 4.2 and 4.3. The model can then be used to guide the development of your budget (Step 4.4) and intervention guide (Step 4.5).

4.1 Create a Logic Model

A **logic model** "is a picture of how you believe your program will work" (W.K. Kellogg Foundation, 2004, p. 1). A logic model generally illustrates the connection between your group's available resources and planned activities (your intervention) and the outcomes you expect to achieve through the intervention (reflected in your mission, goals, and objectives).

Logic models come in a variety of forms and are used for a variety of different purposes (Bartholomew, Parcel, Kok, & Gottlieb, 2006). The PRECEDE/PROCEED model, for example, is a type of logic model that can be used for assessment, planning, and evaluation of programs and interventions. Our logic model development guide in Figure 7.7 contains the generic terms often used in logic models (top row of visual), with PRECEDE/PROCEED phases and terminology inserted beneath them. In this planning step, your group could create a similar visual to brainstorm and illustrate connections between your intervention goals and planned intervention. To do so, you would replace content in the "Standards or categories" row with your actual process (Phase 6), impact (Phase 7), and outcome (Phase 8) goals. The remaining two boxes on that row (inputs and activities) would be completed through Steps 4.2 and 4.3. The resulting intervention logic model could be similar to our sample in Figure 7.8.

Logic Model Terms*	Inputs	Activities	Outputs	Short-Term Outcomes	Mid-Term Outcomes	Long-Term Outcomes	
PRECEDE/ PROCEED Phases†	Phase 4 Educational strategies, policy, regulation, organization	Phase 5 Implementation	Phase 6 Process evaluation	Phase 7 Impact Evaluation		Phase 8 Outcome Evaluation	
Objects of interest in evaluation†	Needed resources/ conditions in community to operate program**	Planned strategies/ intervention components**	Health program or intervention	Predisposing, enabling, and reinforcing factors	Protective behavior or environment	Health status	Societal benefit
Standards or categories†	• Funding • Equipment • Supplies • Personnel • Policies • Organization/ Community support	Strategy Types:‡ • Health communication • Health policy/ enforcement • Environmental change • Health-related community service • Community mobilization	Peer review, quality control, accreditation, audit, certification	Changes in knowledge, attitudes, beliefs, skills, resources, social support, policy	Changes in frequency, distribution, timing of behavior, or the quality of the environment	Changes in mortality, morbidity, disability, or risk factors	Changes in quality of life

Figure 7.7   Logic model development guide.

* Logic model terms from *Logic Model Development Guide*, W. K. Kellogg Foundation, 2004, Battle Creek, MI: Author.

** Not usually included in PRECEDE/PROCEED evaluation.

† Logic model terms from *Health Program Planning: An Educational and Ecological Approach*, 4th ed. (Figure 3-16, p. 140), by L. W. Green and M. W. Kreuter, 2005, New York: McGraw-Hill.

‡ Strategy types from *Planning, Implementing, and Evaluating Health Promotion Programs: A Primer*, 5th ed., by J. F. McKenzie, B. L. Neiger, and R. Thackeray, 2009, San Francisco: Pearson Benjamin Cummings.

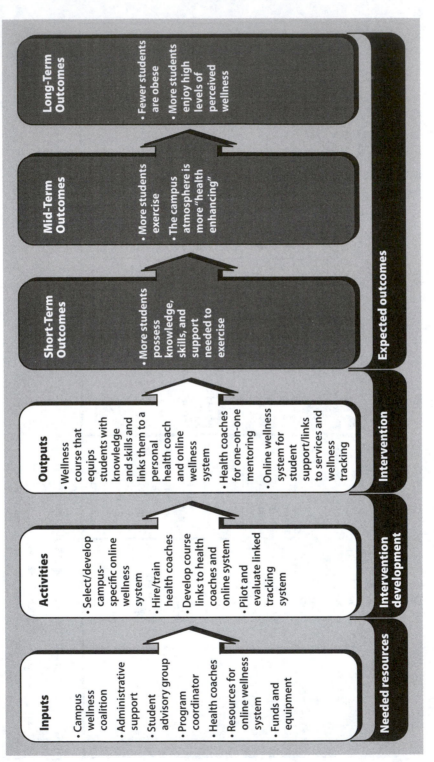

Figure 7.8   Logic model sample: Exercise promotion program.
Sources: Green and Kreuter, 2005; McKenzie et al., 2009; W. K. Kellogg Foundation, 2004.

4.2 Select Intervention Strategies

An intervention strategy is a type or category of activities designed to achieve program goals and objectives. Use your program goals and objectives and the output and outcome sections of your logic model to select the strategies needed to achieve your intended changes. These strategies can be listed as "activities" in your logic model and serve as the framework for your **intervention scope** (the breadth and depth of your intervention).

As you select intervention strategies and develop the scope, we recommend that you practice the **principle of multiplicity and comprehensiveness** (Green & Kreuter, 2005) by combining "interventions that address at least three theoretical constructs implicated in the change process: predisposing factors, enabling factors, and reinforcing factors" (p. 195) and include "educational, organizational, economic, regulatory, and other environmental change components" (p. 195). In other words, your scope of intervention strategies should be broad enough to allow you to address all of the types of program goals recommended in the PRECEDE/PROCEED model.

McKenzie et al. (2009) provide a detailed description of the six strategy types listed under "activities" in the logic model development guide (Figure 7.7). These six categories serve as a general guide for selecting strategies to be used in your intervention (see chapter 8 for more details about intervention development). Health communication strategies are often developed based on four common communication channels: intrapersonal channels (e.g., one-on-one interactions), interpersonal channels (e.g., small groups and classes), organizational and community channels (e.g., organized social and religious groups, organizations, agencies), and mass media channels (e.g., print and electronic messages and campaigns). Health education strategies promote "voluntary behavior decisions conducive to health" (Green & Kreuter, 2005, p. G-4), through structured learning experiences such as classes, workshops, and learning programs. Examples of health-related community service strategies include health screenings, treatment, and referrals provided through community-based clinics and health fairs.

Health policy/enforcement strategies include "executive orders, laws, ordinances, policies, position statements, regulations, and formal and informal rules" (McKenzie et al., 2009, p. 210). Laws or ordinances that make it illegal to drive intoxicated or smoke in public places and policies related to health service eligibility are examples. A related type of strategy, environmental change strategies, can promote or enable healthy choices and behaviors (e.g., building recreational parks, providing healthy choices in cafeterias) or protect communities from environmental hazards (e.g., environmental waste regulations, smoke-free ordinances).

Community mobilization strategies are commonly used in public and community health education to equip community members with leadership skills and resources needed to promote personal and community health (see chapter 2). Health advocacy activities aimed at health-enhancing social and political change are also examples of this type of strategy (see chapter 12).

The challenge lies in selecting or developing strategies that will work for your priority population. When considering the quality and utility of an intervention, Green and Kreuter (2005) recommend that you consider:

- **Best practices** (sometimes referred to as evidence-based practices): interventions that have been proven effective in multiple settings and populations.

- **Best experiences:** "the prior experience of other practitioners, communities, states, or national programs in addressing the same issues. Best experiences can come from prior or existing programs and from the indigenous wisdom of the local community in which the program would be implemented" (p. 206).

- **Best processes:** proven methods and strategies used to assess the population and local situation to select appropriate interventions.

Though evidence-based practices are commonly valued in clinical settings where rigorous control can produce research-based evidence, best experiences and best processes are more feasible criteria for selecting interventions in community settings (Green & Kreuter, 2005).

Green and Kreuter (2005) recommend that you "match, map, pool, and patch" (p. 125) selected strategies to integrate them into a comprehensive program that fits the needs, interests, and capacities of your priority population. In brief, this process includes matching intervention strategies to individuals or group leaders at various ecological levels (e.g., individuals at risk, organizations, communities, governments); mapping or linking proven interventions to your specific program goals (particularly, predisposing, enabling, and reinforcing); and pooling existing interventions, community-preferred interventions, and your selected/proven interventions to patch or fill gaps in current efforts.

This intervention you develop should be given a test run (see chapter 8); you can then apply the **principle of intervention specificity** to adapt the full intervention and each component to fit the unique aspects of your priority population. This adaptation process is called **tailoring** when you adapt interventions or materials for individuals and **segmentation** when you do so for specific groups within a larger population (Green & Kreuter, 2005).

4.3 Develop an Intervention Guide

We use the term **intervention guide** in this chapter to refer to a description of the general rationale and scope of the planned intervention (a general overview of strategies), a timeline for implementing all activities, and detailed descriptions of specific activities (protocols/methods, sequences, needed materials/equipment, etc.). These activities may encompass preparatory work like training personnel, developing materials, creating marketing and participant recruitment plans, orientations, and so forth, as well as activities that are actually part of your intervention strategies (e.g., awareness-building events, educational and training activities, mass media events, etc.). Though an evaluation plan is sometimes provided in a separate proposal section, the scope, methods, and instruments should be developed during this planning step and included either in the intervention guide or a separate section of your full plan or proposal.

A detailed timeline for all activities (preparation, implementation, evaluation) can be represented in one or more visuals. One of the most effective charting methods for timelines is called a Gantt chart (Figure 7.9). This type of chart helps you visualize when an activity will start, how long it will last, and which activities are overlapping.

An administrative plan with descriptions of roles and responsibilities related to tasks should be included in your intervention guide. Actual or sample materials such as marketing flyers, educational materials and lesson/session plans, and evaluation instruments should be included in an appendix of the guide or full proposal. Chapters 8 and 9 provide additional information that will help your group develop these plans and components.

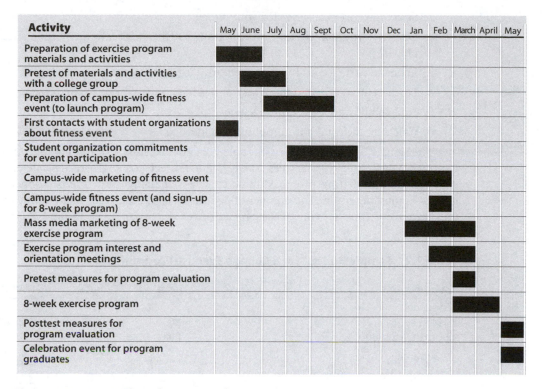

Figure 7.9 Gantt chart for an exercise program.
Although projecting an accurate timeline can be a challenge, it is a vital part of program planning. It influences all aspects of the program from start to finish.

4.4 Identify and Develop Needed Resources

With your strategies selected and intervention guide in place, your planning group can now brainstorm a list of needed and available resources for the intervention. These needed resources, often referred to as *inputs* in a logic model, can include funds, equipment, supplies, personnel, and facilities. The time needed to implement, monitor, and evaluate each strategy is also considered a resource that can help shape your descriptions of roles and responsibilities in the intervention guide (Step 4.3) and determine personnel costs for the budget. Other inputs identified in this step may include administrative support, structure, and policies as well as various types of community support and commitments needed for program development, implementation, and evaluation. A thorough approach to this step will enhance your ability to obtain all that is needed for effective implementation.

4.5 Create a Budget

Budgets are predictions of the revenues and expenses expected for the program. Budgeting is the process of developing the budget. That process includes gathering information and reviewing similar programs to identify potential program costs. According to Walter (1999), there are six basic steps in budgeting:

1. Select the cost categories for your budget.
2. Decide if you will divide your program budget into sections by time slices or phases.
3. Estimate costs for all the cost categories in your budget.
4. Document anticipated monetary or in-kind contributions to the project.
5. Add an allowance for contingencies.
6. Calculate the total amount of funding needed.

The sample budget summary in Table 7.2 contains some common budget categories: personnel, supplies, services, travel, and indirect costs. Correctly categorizing expenses and estimating projected costs can be a challenge. For the personnel category, you must determine the number of people needed, their roles and qualifications, the amount of time it will take each person to do his or her job, and the wages

Table 7.2   Sample Budget for a College Exercise Program

Budget Items	Hours	Rate	Totals
Personnel			
Health educator	960	$30	$ 28,800
Program assistant	800	20	16,000
Subtotal			$ 44,800
Personnel benefits (fringe) @20%			$ 8,960
Total personnel costs			**$53,760**
Supplies			
Printing brochure			$ 2,000
Postage (20,000 × .44)			8,800
Office supplies			300
Exercise equipment			2,400
Total supplies			**$13,500**
Services			
Telephone			$ 500
Photocopying			400
Consultants			
Data processing	25	$12	$ 300
Marketing consultant	62	75	4,650
Graphic artist	16	25	400
Total services			**$ 6,250**
Travel			
National conference ($700 air; $250 per diem)			$ 950
Total travel			**$ 950**
Total direct costs			**$74,460**
Indirect costs (20% of direct costs)			**$14,892**
Total budget estimate			**$89,352**

required for each position. Benefits are generally included if personnel will spend more than 50% of a full-time wage on the project. If a consultant is to be hired to perform a specific service and will be paid a flat fee (rather than placed on a salary with benefits), a separate consultant fee category may be needed.

The equipment category is usually reserved for durable items specifically needed for the planned intervention (e.g., blood pressure monitors, educational puppets). Some organizations separate equipment categories by cost ranges or types of equipment (e.g. computers or telephones that require ongoing service fees or technical support). Consumable supplies can include any item (e.g., paper, food items) or service (e.g., printing costs) that will be "used up" during the funding period. Some durable equipment also involves an expense for consumable supplies such as ink cartridges for computer printers or individual testing strips for glucometers (machines that measure blood glucose levels).

Depending on the budgeting practices of the organizations involved, fees charged for communication (postage, telephone services) and facility rentals may be placed in separate categories or included under consumable supplies. Travel expenses for program implementation or conference presentations are usually categorized separately and, in government-funded agencies, travel rates may be negotiated at the state level.

All of the costs previously mentioned are sometimes referred to as **direct costs** because they are specifically associated with a program and will be paid for directly with the requested grant funds. But there are also indirect costs to an institution or agency receiving funding that are not included in those direct cost categories. **Indirect costs,** also called facilities and administrative costs, include the less obvious expenses of maintaining the agency's infrastructure such as electricity and building maintenance. It is possible that the agency for which you work will have specific policies related to the addition of indirect cost coverage in a proposal budget.

If a program-planning project is large, it may be easier to break it into phases. For example, you might want to have three divisions: planning, implementing, and evaluating. Some projects for which multiple funding years are awarded require a breakdown of expenses by funding year.

Budgeting can be both fun and challenging if you approach it with a positive attitude. Because adequate funds are often essential to intervention success, we strongly encourage you to be thorough and as detailed as possible in developing a workable budget plan. Model budgets for similar projects can be a useful resource. The individuals responsible for budgets, personnel, and other fiscal management activities should be able to help you develop a budget plan.

In Conclusion

Though the steps provided in this chapter are presented in a linear sequence, in reality the planning process is rarely linear. In large-scale projects, for example, a planning group may use a linear sequence to initiate a smaller component of the intervention while continuing to collect additional assessment data to fill in information gaps. Some aspects of evaluation (discussed in chapter 9) actually occur during the planning and early implementation stages. And, no matter how hard you try to keep things organized, few interventions happen exactly the way they were planned. For these and other reasons, the key to effective planning is to use models and planning strategies as a general guide but remain flexible and fluid as the work progresses. Stay focused but do not be afraid to be creative and innovative when the situation calls for it. In the end, it is the quality of life of the people in your priority population—not the plan—that matters most.

REVIEW QUESTIONS

1. Describe the general benefits and characteristics of the planning process.
2. Explain the similarities and differences between a program and intervention.
3. Explain the purpose and characteristics of a vision, mission, goal, and objective.
4. Explain how Phases 1–4 of the PRECEDE/PROCEED model can be used in the planning process.
5. Describe the general components of the MAPP model.
6. Name the four planning steps described in this chapter. Provide examples of tasks a planning group might be doing in each step.
7. Explain the differences between and utility of process, impact, and outcome goals. Provide an example of each.
8. Describe and discuss the development of a SMART objective.
9. Describe the components of a SWOT analysis and provide a brief example for how it could be used.
10. Name and describe the general components of a proposal or program/intervention plan.
11. Provide an example of a Gantt chart that you have created.
12. List and describe the categories that are commonly used in a health program budget.

FOR YOUR APPLICATION

Writing Goals and Objectives

Practice creating goals and objectives using the PRECEDE/PROCEED model as a guide. Use a model template or create your own on a blank piece of paper by sketching the boxes of Phases 1–4 of the model (use Figure 7.3 as a guide). Choose a health problem or behavior in a specific population about which you have some knowledge (e.g., teen pregnancy, diabetes among older adults) and proceed as if you were going to develop an intervention to address that problem or behavior in that population. Refer to Step 3.2 of the recommended planning steps in this chapter to create one goal for each box in the model (e.g., quality of life goal, health goal, behavioral goal). Then use Figure 7.6 (elements of a SMART objective) as a guide to create one sample objective for each goal. Ask a friend or colleague to check your work to ensure that you have applied the steps to create feasible goals and measurable objectives.

eight

Implementation Processes

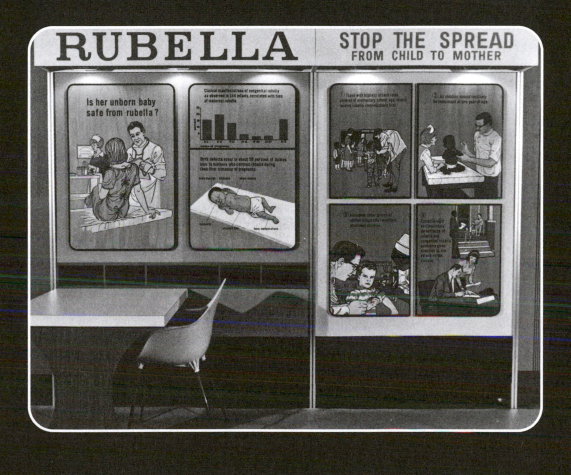

You are excited about getting started with the new program you developed for pregnant teens. You have taken all of the right steps. You conducted a needs assessment and carefully planned your program, based on the perceived and documented needs of the population or partner community. You are ready to go! But wait, there are still a few missing links. You find that you need more money than expected to conduct the program and you need to make certain that information about the program reaches the people it is meant to serve. You also have materials to develop and schedules to create. Don't let the excitement wane, because the success of the program you implement will be tied to the time you take to address these issues.

CHAPTER OBJECTIVES

1. Describe methods of social marketing.
2. List ways of assessing marketing effectiveness.
3. Discuss key considerations in the hiring and training of individuals who will deliver the health education programs.
4. Identify teaching methods that employ experiential or critical thinking activities.
5. Describe appropriate program record keeping.
6. Practice developing an action or lesson plan.
7. Analyze ways to improve health literacy.
8. Describe ways to assist individuals with barriers to use the Web.

Supplementing Funds for the Program

Program implementation (putting the program into action) requires giving attention to everything we've already discussed as well as addressing the situational issues that inevitably occur. Implementation issues range from important, difficult concerns like money to important but smaller problems like projection units that don't work correctly. Of course, money is one of the largest concerns because all programs require funding to some degree.

Adequate resources, including personnel, materials, equipment, the site, and so forth, can make or break the program. Although these issues must be addressed early in your planning, they make such an impact on program implementation that we want to discuss them a bit more in this chapter. The adequacy of program resources will depend on the available money. You learned about grant writing in the last chapter and, ideally, you will receive grants large enough to fund all of the programs you will run. If not, you may need to supplement from local funding sources.

Seeking Donations or Sponsors

If no grants are available for a particular program at a particular time, you might seek a **corporate sponsorship** or pursue donations from individuals who are likely to support your objectives and are in a position to help. With a corporate sponsorship, a business pays for a program or segment of a program. As you can probably imagine, there is no single method for seeking donations. Sometimes you write a letter; other times, you make personal contact via a face-to-face meeting or telephone call. However, there are some important things to remember, regardless of your method. For example, check with your agency about policies regarding donations. In some circumstances you won't be able to accept donations at all. In other circumstances, you will be able to receive donations but will be required to follow a well-defined set of guidelines.

If you receive approval to seek donations, make certain that other divisions in your agency aren't seeking donations from the same company or individual at the same time. It is unwise to overwhelm a corporation or individual who has been generous in the past with numerous new requests for money. If you request funds from a corporation, ask about the procedures you will be expected to follow. Most donate money frequently but have specific procedural requirements (such as submission of documents similar to a grant proposal).

Regardless of whether you will be writing letters, making phone calls, or developing a Web-based donation request, put thoughtful preparation into the project. Proofread your letters, have others read them for clarity and flow, and revise accordingly. In the case of telephone contacts, develop a script and practice before you make the call. And, of course, if you receive a donation or sponsorship, give appropriate acknowledgment. In addition to written thank-you notes, you might consider thanking donors on program handouts.

Special Event Fund-Raising

Almost any activity can be a fund-raiser. Some of the most common today include fun runs, golf tournaments, and silent auctions. Individuals pay to participate or purchase something. Fund-raisers have great potential, but they can also cause headaches if the planners are not experienced. For example, one of our local service clubs planned a chili supper fund-raiser. The planners understood promotion but did not grasp the total marketing picture. They advertised very effectively. In fact, approximately 500 people attended. However, the organizers did not assess the effectiveness of their promotion or the likelihood that so many people would attend. They cooked for only 100. Can you imagine the chaos? Although this mistake was somewhat humorous, some planning errors can be dangerous to participants. What if you planned a 6-mile run but did not offer runners water or first aid? You could easily put participants in danger. Our suggestion is that you involve an experienced special-events planner on your fund-raising committee.

Social Marketing

You may want to launch the implementation of your program with a **social marketing** campaign, which is a process of "influencing human behavior by creating, communicating, and delivering products and services to target audience members for the purpose of advancing (public health) objectives rather than for commercial profit" (Maibach, 2003 p. 41). A similar concept is **prevention marketing,** which is "CDC's adaptation of social marketing in which science-based marketing techniques and consumer-oriented health communication technologies are combined with local community involvement to plan and implement prevention programs. Essentially, prevention marketing equals social marketing plus community involvement" (CDCynergy, n.d., p.5).

Understanding Social Marketing

Social marketing uses the strategies of commercial marketing. In social marketing, decisions must be made about the product, price, place, and promotion, often called the four Ps of commercial marketing. Other Ps to consider include partnership, policy, and politics. Philip Kotler and Gerald Zaltman (1971) conceived the idea of social marketing when they realized that traditional marketing principles could apply to attitudes and behaviors that influence social issues. Prior to the development of social marketing, large social campaigns often succeeded only in increasing people's awareness of a specific health issue. On the other hand, large advertising campaigns for new products continued to effectively increase use of specific products. Today, social marketing uses the methods of commercial marketing, with differences in content and objectives.

Product

Your **product** has actually been determined before you implement your program. In social marketing, the product can range from an actual product (a physical object) to a health-related service (like your teen pregnancy program) or even an idea. Keeping this in mind, you can see that the product is actually developed during program planning. For example, some products you could market for a smoking-cessation program include a device or invention to help individuals stop smoking (like a patch), the idea that smoking is not healthful even for teens, or an actual smoking-cessation program (service).

Price

By **price** we mean more than just money. Although monetary cost is one aspect of price, other intangible things like time, effort, and risk of embarrassment must also be considered. In general, people will weigh the benefits of the product against the costs. Their use of the product will depend on a perception that benefits outweigh the costs.

Place

The means of distribution for the product defines **place**. In the traditional form of marketing, you might decide that your product would be distributed from a warehouse via trucks to retail stores. In social marketing you make decisions about the channel of communication. The channel of communication might be a newspaper, a television show or commercial, a counseling session with a physician, or face-to-face interviews.

Promotion

It is easy to confuse promotion and place in social marketing. **Promotion** deals with keeping consumers interested and motivated to use the product. It might also involve news and telephone media. But whereas place would refer to the channel or mode of communication you choose (such as a newspaper ad), the promotion aspect refers to how your message is worded to motivate or persuade the reader. The purpose differs from place; you might think of promotion as advertising and place as the medium you choose for your advertisement.

Partnership

Health-related social problems are complex. In most cases, partnership requires collaboration among health agencies. Partnerships between agencies facilitate effective decisions about price and place. However, the most important partnerships are with people from all aspects of the community.

Policy

According to Weinrich Communications (1999), "Social marketing programs can do well in motivating individual behavior change, but that is difficult to sustain unless the environment they are in supports that change for the long run. Often, **policy** (a planned course of action to guide decisions) change is needed, and media advocacy programs can be an effective complement to a social marketing program" (p. 3).

Politics

Your social marketing plan will require making decisions about the political environment. Suppose the product involved is controversial—for example, discussing birth control methods in public high schools. Unless an assessment is made of the politics surrounding the product, difficulties can snowball. Politics can destroy even the most beneficial program. There are times when it is best to wait until the political environment is more conducive to successful completion of the program.

Developing a Marketing Plan

Creating a market plan requires focusing on the people who will be using a product rather than on the product itself. Research and evaluation are the keys to an effective plan (CDCynergy, n.d.). Keeping in mind that the product has already been determined, planners must establish marketing objectives, assess the target audience, develop pricing and placing that correspond with the target population needs, and conduct promotion or advertising campaigns. Once a product has been identified during planning, we think of the acronym MAPP (Figure 8.1 on the following page) as a guide to developing a marketing plan. This process of developing a marketing plan should remind you of the PRECEDE portion of the PRECEDE/PROCEED model. As you know, assessments come first, followed by planning, implementing, and evaluating. In fact, if you have used PRECEDE, writing a marketing plan will be much easier.

Writing Marketing Objectives

Marketing objectives relate directly to the program objectives. As we stated earlier, the product is determined during program planning; therefore, those very program objectives are part of the marketing objectives. Other marketing objectives specifically address promotion. Let's look at an example of a promotion objective. "During the year 2009, center staff will improve potential participants' perception of the program by creating updated brochures with the assistance of a graphic designer."

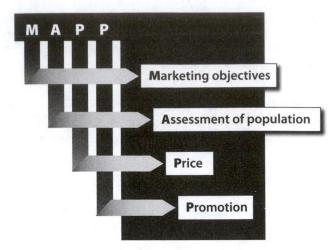

Figure 8.1   The MAPP approach to marketing.
The MAPP acronym is a simple way to remember the steps to marketing a program. Some form of marketing will be necessary for any program to be a success. Having at least a rudimentary grasp of marketing will improve your chances of success.

As you can see, the objective contains all of the components of program planning objectives. The difference is in the focus on place and promotion rather than actual programming.

Assessing the Target Audience

This aspect of the marketing plan includes knowing the demographic makeup of the audience, such as the economic status, education levels, and age structure. It also includes psychosocial information such as attitudes and beliefs. Cultural and religious beliefs and behaviors are important to understand when you are creating a social marketing plan. Fortunately, you can achieve an understanding of your target audience for marketing purposes at the same time you conduct the initial needs assessment for program planning.

Both qualitative and quantitative methods of audience assessment can be used. A combination of methods might be best. Surveys, a frequently used quantitative method, can be mailed, conducted via the telephone, or conducted in face-to-face settings. Focus groups and interviews, commonly used qualitative methods, also involve primary data collection. Can you name some secondary sources of data that might be helpful in your needs assessment and marketing research? You might have considered reviewing the professional literature or accessing previously collected morbidity and mortality data.

Determining Distribution Channels, or Place

Communications media are the most commonly used channels for distribution in social marketing. Media include television, Internet, radio, newsprint, magazines, billboards, and cinema. Other types of distribution channels are personal face-to-face communication, telephone contact, posters, direct mail, direct sales, and distribution of brochures and other written documents. The selection of the appropriate channel depends on both the target audience and the product. For example, you won't choose the business section of a local paper to provide program information that you want teens to read. Again, you must know your audience before you can determine the appropriate channel. An important theoretical basis from which to identify an appropriate channel is the theory of the diffusion of innovation.

The **theory of the diffusion of innovation** describes the ways that an innovation spreads through a population of people. An **innovation** can be anything from a product (like new athletic shoes) to an idea (like the belief that smoking kills). In marketing terms, this is considered the product. Understanding the theory can help you determine what channels to use to advertise your innovation (health program). As you can see from Figure 8.2, the theory can be depicted as a bell shaped curve. Theorists believe that consumers can be categorized into five groups by the rate at which they adopt an innovation. As you read through this information, think about where you fit along the curve. You may find that it is not easy to determine your exact speed of adoption. Each of us adopts innovations according to the type of innovation and the current environment. In other words, the speed of adoption is not necessarily a stable characteristic; however, most of us fall into patterns of adoption.

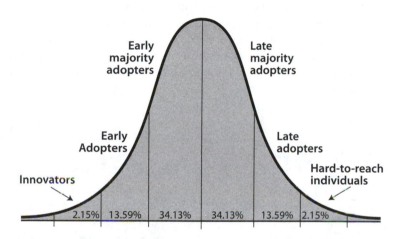

Figure 8.2   Diffusion of innovation theory.
This theory describes acceptance of change as following a bell-curve pattern. It also suggests that innovators will accept a new product or program much more quickly than individuals who are late adopters or hard to reach.

Innovators adopt change easily. In general, they are highly educated and can be reached through mass media channels. If they determine that an innovation might benefit them, they will change quickly. Suppose, for example, that we are promoting a new, effective stress-reduction strategy across the United States. For innovators, we could put an article in a national publication like *USA Today* or *Newsweek*. Innovators would be more likely than others to read the article and choose to try the new plan as a result. **Early adopters** are often public leaders and highly respected in communities. Others often follow their adoption patterns. Like innovators, they can be reached via mass media, although state or regional channels may be more effective. Again, a newspaper might be the appropriate place for dissemination of our stress-reduction plan; but, instead of an article, we might want to place an advertisement that suggests how effective the plan has been with individuals who have tried it. **Early majority adopters** accept innovations once they determine that others they respect have done so. Demonstrating the adoption patterns of innovators and early adopters is often the most effective way to reach most of the early majority adopters. For the promotion of our stress-reduction plan, we might use the same strategy that we used for early adopters, except that we would place our advertisement in a regional or local newspaper. **Late majority adopters** are somewhat skeptical of change. They will adopt an innovation most readily if they are required to do so (public law) or they believe that the change will benefit them dramatically. In order to reach late majority adopters, we might work directly with leaders in corporate worksites. Our goal would be to encourage corporations to require use of our stress-reduction plan. **Late adopters** and **hard-to-reach adopters** accept change only with difficulty. They tend to have lower levels of education and often live in poverty. One-on-one, face-to-face communication about the innovation seems to be the most effective approach with this group of individuals. For our stress-reduction plan, we might have other adopters who were initially doubtful make personal contact with late adopters.

The relative advantage, complexity, compatibility, testability, reversibility, and observability of an innovation also influence the rate of adoption (Glanz, Rimer, & Viswanath, 2008). FYI 8.1 defines some of the terms associated with the theory of the diffusion of innovation.

FYI 8.1   Diffusion of Innovation Terms

According to the theory of diffusion of innovation, there are seven characteristics of an innovation. Each will be important for you to understand when projecting how a new program or product will be accepted by the target participants.

Compatibility   When innovations are consistent with the economic, sociocultural, and philosophical value system of the adopter, adoption is more likely to take place.

Flexibility   Innovations that can be unbundled and used as separate components will be applicable in a wider variety of user settings.

Reversibility   If for any reason, the adopting individual or organization wants to revert to its previous practices, it is desirable that an innovation be capable of termination. Innovations that are not are less likely to be adopted.

Relative advantage   If an innovation appears to be beneficial when compared to current and previous methods, adoption is more likely.

Complexity   Complex innovations are more difficult to communicate and to understand and are therefore less likely to be adopted.

Cost-efficiency   For an innovation to be considered desirable, its perceived benefits, both tangible and intangible, must outweigh its perceived costs.

Risk   The degree of uncertainty introduced by an innovation helps determine its potential for adoption. Innovations that involve higher risk are less likely to be adopted.

From "Implementing Comprehensive School Health Education: Educational Innovations and Social Change," by L. J. Kolbe and D. C. Iverson, 1981, *Health Education Quarterly, 8,* 57–80. © 1981 by Sage Publications. Used with permission.

Pricing the Product

Although seemingly simple and easy to define, pricing is complex. On the one hand, price determines the accessibility of the service or product; on the other hand, price can imply credibility or quality (Alward & Camunas, 1991). People often believe that a product is not worth much unless it is associated with a high price. In order to determine the price, you must consider your objectives. FYI 8.2 discusses pricing objectives for tangible products.

Assessing Marketing Effectiveness

In chapter 9 you will read more extensively about evaluation research. We hope it is evident to you now, however, that you must always check to see if your plans are working. One of the biggest wastes of time and money comes from continuing with activities that don't work. You will learn about a number of research and evaluation methods in chapter 9; for now, we would like to suggest a few questions to ask about your marketing plan to assess its effectiveness:

- Does the product meet the needs of the population? Or, in other words, are the participants making the planned change? Do the participants perceive the program to be useful? Are people healthier as a result of the program?

FYI **8.2**   **Using Pricing Objectives for Tangible Products**

The price of your product or program will be determined by the type of outcome desired. The following provides suggestions for determining price.

Goal of Marketing	Pricing Activity	Consequence of Activity
High percentage of target population to accept health product or service	Offer product or service at a low cost	Potential perception of a product or service of low worth
Equal distribution of health product or service	Offer product or service at a flexible price structure	Individuals with high income pay more, potential perception of inequality
Expense and income are balanced	Offer product or service at a price that defrays the cost	Cost may be too high at first
Maximizing profit	Offer service or product at a price that improves the demand	Cost may be too low at first
Minimizing excessive demand of an unhealthful service or product	Offer service or product at a very high price	Negative perception of pricing

From *A Short Course in Social Marketing,* by Novartis Foundation for Sustainable Development, 1999. Retrieved September 22, 1999, from http:www.foundation.novartis.com/social_marketing.htm.

- Can the population access the product? Or, are people attending the program? Do participants perceive the price of the program to be appropriate? Do participants perceive the benefits of the program to outweigh the barriers to attending?
- Are the distribution channels effective? Or, do participants report hearing about the program through your selected channels of advertising? How did participants hear about the program?
- Do policies and politics serve as barriers or boosters to the product? Or, how do agency politics affect the program? How do local politics affect the program?

Other Aspects of Implementation

Effective implementation requires that you attend to every aspect of the program, not just money and marketing. Going with the flow, or simply letting events unfold, is not appropriate. Other aspects of program implementation that you need to address include selecting and training staff or volunteers, developing curricula and teaching methods, identifying equipment and facilities, determining program logistics, preparing materials, and program follow-up.

Selecting Staff

Randy Pennington, owner of a leadership consulting firm in Dallas, states that an effective way of viewing staff is to consider them as essential volunteers (personal communication, November 8, 1999). Adopting this attitude requires you to spend adequate time training your employees and demonstrating to them that they are valued. This approach is as necessary for retaining good employees as it is for keeping volunteers.

Staff should understand the organizational culture, have experience working with the target audience, demonstrate professionalism, and have content expertise and skills (Carnevale, Gainer, & Metzler, 1990). That said, how do you find people who fit these criteria?

Begin the process of selecting employees by asking for a portfolio and continue by interviewing those who demonstrate the knowledge and skills that you require. Many professional preparation programs encourage students to develop portfolios. As the potential employer, you can judge the potential employee's work for yourself. For example, if the individual will be asked to write pieces for a newsletter, you will want to read sample articles or other written documents that demonstrate effective written communication skills.

Begin the interview process by modeling professionalism. Be on time, prepare in advance, select appropriate attire, communicate effectively, and act with integrity. Your first meeting with the prospective employee will be your first training session. If you demonstrate a lack of preparation or ineffective communication, you are essentially giving permission for the individual to act in the same manner if hired. Remember that new employees want to do a good job and they will follow your lead.

We suggest that you ask potential employees to demonstrate their skills. If you expect your new employee to make presentations to small groups, ask applicants to do so as part of their interview. If they will be conducting program evaluations, give them an actual scenario to discuss. We also encourage you to wait for the right person rather than resorting to panic placement (selecting anyone just to get someone in the position). It may be a relief just to hire someone; but you will ultimately spend a lot more time, effort, and money if you have to start over because the individual did not match the position.

If you are seeking volunteers rather than paid employees, you should still ask for information about their educational background and skills. You want to place volunteers in an area that fits their skills and desired type of work. Unlike job applicants, volunteers are not usually turned away. But most agencies and organizations have many types of work that can be performed by volunteers, so it's wise to ensure that a volunteer's skills match the job requirements.

It addition, you need to make sure that prospective employees or volunteers do not hold beliefs that are contrary to the philosophical foundation of the agency. For example, an individual who does not approve of abortion may not support a policy that requires women to be given information about abortions. You will have the responsibility of making certain that the individuals you hire or invite to volunteer support the agency's philosophies.

Training New Employees

We asked people who had recently started new jobs to comment on their training needs. Several themes appeared in their comments. Every person noted that clear and honest descriptions of expectations were vital. Some also stated that they needed to know the extent to which they could develop their own goals. The people in our small survey indicated in various ways that they needed to understand the agency mission as well as the purpose of the specific job they would be performing. Some mentioned that explanations of their employee benefits and important agency policies were necessary. Others also valued the identification of available resources and acknowledgement of resources that were not available. Last, but not least, all of the individuals mentioned that they needed training for new skills as well as feedback on the acquisition of those skills.

Interestingly, the people we talked with regarded the training process as a reflection of the philosophical basis from which their employer worked. In other words, agencies that offered appropriate training were more likely to value their employees. And agencies that value employees provide opportunities to help them succeed rather than focus on performance problem areas. Even though our study was small, we feel that the participants targeted the major points of effective training: (a) a clear job description, (b) guidelines for developing personal professional goals, (c) guidance in following the agency mission and policies, (d) an account of available resources, (d) methods for accessing resources not readily available, (f) training for new skills, and (g) feedback meant for growth not punishment.

Facilities

The physical environment can make a major difference in people's ability to learn. Have you ever attended a lecture in a room that was very hot or very cold? How did the temperature affect your ability to listen? Room temperature, sound levels, amount of light, colors, room setup, room size, and type of furniture work synergistically to impact participants. The success of your program will be determined partially by the environment, so consider your options carefully and plan in advance.

Choosing the Site

Health programs can be conducted in many types of locations. If you do not have space available in your agency, other choices might include hotels, conference centers, universities, ships, resorts, other public buildings, and corporate settings. Your choices will depend on your budget, program objectives, size of audience, and location of potential sites. Table 8.1 provides a comparison of different types of sites.

Table 8.1   Comparison of Site Types

The type of site you select for your program will make a difference in attendance and participant satisfaction. However, the type of site also influences the cost of your program, so you will want to compare and contrast the advantages and disadvantages of different types of sites before you make a selection.

Site	Description	Advantage	Disadvantage
Hotels	Buildings that provide sleeping rooms, meeting rooms, and restaurants	Staff available to help coordinate Needs are met in one location	Possibly expensive
Convention centers	Special facilities that provide meeting rooms and resources	Able to host large groups of people Resources readily accessible	Hotels and restaurants may not be within walking distance May be expensive
Universities	Institutions with a primary purpose of educating	Rooms of various sizes available May be less costly	Distance between rooms may cause difficulties Meeting equipment may not be as readily available
Resorts	Sites designed for recreation	Provide other activities for participants	Participants may not attend meetings May be expensive

Room Size and Setup

Don't forget to plan how the tables and chairs will be placed. It may sound like busywork, but think again about your own learning experiences. Have you ever attended a small-group discussion in a classroom where you could not move the chairs? The room setup probably caused a barrier to both the discussion and the learning. Room setup should be determined only after you have decided on the method of instruction for each program. Remember the discussion of methods in chapter 7? If your program requires face-to-face interaction, you will want to make decisions about whether individual rooms are needed for each face-to-face meeting, if a table will separate you and your participants, and how many people will be able to attend. In the case of presentations to a group of individuals, there are numerous ways to set up the room. Figure 8.3 illustrates some of the most common.

The Content

In all educational environments there are two types of curriculum: planned and unplanned. According to Doll (1992), a **curriculum** is "the formal and informal content and process by which learners gain knowledge and understanding, develop skills, and alter attitudes, appreciations, and values" (p. 6). A curriculum pertains to all programs, not just those in an educational institution. As a health professional, you will

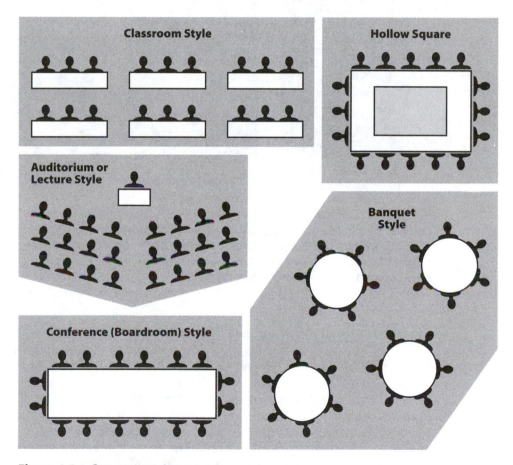

Figure 8.3   Common room setups.
Rooms can be arranged in a number of different ways. Careful consideration of the type of presentation or activity should be made before the room setup is selected. Adapted from Case Western Reserve University Room Setup Styles. Retrieved August 20, 2008, from http://studentaffairs.case.edu/thwing/facilities/setups.html

need to purposefully and thoughtfully develop your health program curriculum—this is where you build upon your planning efforts by adding substance and detail.

Developing Curricula

There are three paths you might choose for curriculum development (Figure 8.4). You might select a new idea (innovation), continue with what has been previously used in the agency, or revise the old curriculum. Make this decision early enough to allow you plenty of time to develop the content. Consider the learning tips in FYI 8.3 to help you make decisions about curriculum development.

Some like it hot—

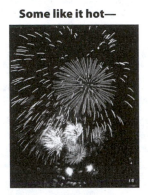

Shot through with the fireworks of innovation

Some like it cold—

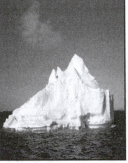

Deep-frozen in tradition and left unchanged

Some like it rebuilt, no matter how old—

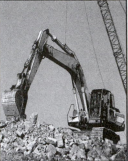

Continually inspected, revised, and changed

Figure 8.4   Curriculum development.
Curriculum development generally fits in one of three categories: hot, cold, or rebuilt. The approach chosen should be a good fit with the other elements of the program plan.
Adapted from *Curriculum Improvement: Decision Making and Process*, 9th ed., by R. C. Doll, Boston: Allyn & Bacon. © 1996 by Pearson Education. Used with permission.

Bloom's Taxonomy: The Cognitive Domain

It has long been known that providing information is not enough to promote behavior change for most people. Every education session should be based on an understanding of Bloom's taxonomy (Bloom et al., 1956), which distinguishes levels of learning. The original taxonomy contained three overlapping domains: the cognitive, psychomotor, and affective, but we are most interested in the cognitive domain. In the cognitive domain, Bloom listed six levels: knowledge, comprehension, application, analysis, synthesis, and evaluation. If you look at the words, you will note that each level requires an increasing amount of critical thinking. Anderson and Krathwohl made understanding the taxonomy easier by converting the terms into verbs:

- **Remembering:** Retrieving, recognizing, and recalling relevant knowledge from long-term memory.

- **Understanding:** Constructing meaning from oral, written, and graphic messages through interpreting, exemplifying, classifying, summarizing, inferring, comparing, and explaining.

- **Applying:** Carrying out or using a procedure through executing, or implementing.

- **Analyzing:** Breaking material into constituent parts, determining how the parts relate to one another and to an overall structure or purpose through differentiating, organizing, and attributing.

- **Evaluating:** Making judgments based on criteria and standards through checking and critiquing.

- **Creating:** Putting elements together to form a coherent or functional whole; reorganizing elements into a new pattern or structure through generating, planning, or producing. (2001, pp. 67–68)

The most effective educational programs will help participants go beyond gaining knowledge or remembering facts. The way in which information is presented to program participants will make a great difference in their level of understanding and future use of what they learn.

FYI 8.3   Learning Tips

Learning is an integral part of the process of making healthy behavior changes. Just as many aspects of a person's life affect health and wellness, many things influence learning. This list provides a few suggestions for making learning successful.

- Each person is unique.
- High stress affects learning negatively.
- Strong emotions change an individual's perceptions.
- All aspects of an individual's life influence learning (food, sleep, and exercise).
- Assistance can be given to improve information retrieval.
- Individuals learn differently; include methods for varying intelligences.
- Most individuals learn best by experiencing.
- Individuals learn from everything that happens in their environment.

Multiple Intelligences

As a student you are well aware that there are many ways to impart information. Many teachers use lectures alone, while some supplement lectures with graphics on PowerPoint slides or handouts. There is certainly nothing wrong with lecture, especially when topics are highlighted through visual aids; but lecture generally works best when used in combination with other methods. Just as there are many ways to teach, there are varied ways to learn. One theory that has been useful in many educational settings is **multiple intelligences (MI)** (Gardner, 2003). This theory suggests that many types of intelligence influence learning. Each individual will learn in different ways, depending on the dominant type of intelligence. Figure 8.5 depicts the different types of intelligences. They include being word-smart, logic-smart, picture-smart, body-smart, music-smart, people-smart, nature-smart, and self-smart (Armstrong, 1994).

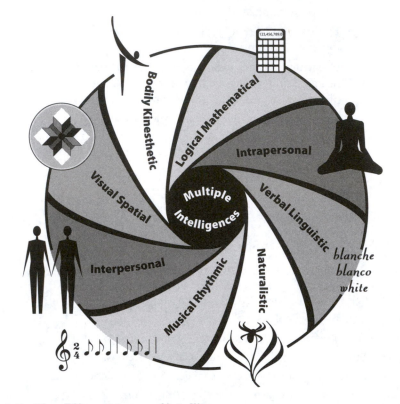

Figure 8.5   The different types of intelligence.
Each person expresses intelligence in a unique way. An individual's form of intelligence influences the way he or she will learn. It is important to use methods that make sense to individuals with varying types of intelligence.

Word-smart people learn through the use of words. They read well and understand what they read. These individuals will enjoy receiving brochures or other written material about health issues and will gather useful information from them. Logic-smart individuals use and appreciate analytical thinking in their daily lives. Understanding how health information applies to real life will help logic-smart people absorb the information you want to convey.

Picture-smart individuals have a feel for shapes, colors, and pictures. They enjoy using their hands to create visually pleasing products. Information geared to picture-smart people will incorporate visual effects. Movement is very important to those who are body-smart. They learn best if activity is part of the learning process. Music-smart individuals love sounds and learn best through auditory means. Incorporating pleasing sound as you present health information will improve the likelihood that your message will be well received.

People-smart individuals are social; they communicate and relate well with others. Providing opportunities for them to socialize while learning will enhance their learning. Self-smart individuals are strongly in tune with themselves. They understand their own feelings and express them well to others. Providing opportunities for self-smart individuals to stretch their knowledge of self while learning new information will make your program more successful. Nature-smart people relate well to their surroundings and the way their immediate environment plays a role in the larger environment (Infed Search, 2008). Nature-smart individuals will feel most successful when they participate in real-life experiences while they learn.

We encourage you to get to know your participants well enough to discover the ways in which they learn best. If this is not possible, plan programs that involve multiple intelligences. Use pleasing sounds or music as part of the program; provide activities with movement; give information in writing as well as verbally; make sure that written materials are visually pleasing and use colors, shapes, and pictures; allow opportunities for socialization within the program; and ask participants to apply the new information to real life.

Experiential Methods

Think about the environment in which you live. Would you say it is fast-paced, visual, and interactive? Most of us deal with a plethora of images, activities, and ongoing change on a daily basis. As a result, the participants in our health programs are likely to expect fast-paced programs, filled with images and activities. You will want to select methods that are creative and engaging. One of the oldest forms of teaching, providing experience, is often the most interesting and offers the greatest long-term benefit. Sometimes participants must understand a concept before they can apply it in a real-world experience. **Experiential** elements provide hands-on activities for learning concepts such as trust, teamwork, networking, and even planning.

Experiential model. The basic experiential education model presented in Figure 8.6 has five stages: (a) asking participants to set personal goals, (b) engaging participants in planned experiences, (c) facilitating the processing of the experience (helping people find personal meaning), (d) helping participants develop concepts or guidelines from the processing, and (e) guiding application of the concepts and guidelines to other situations. This model is based on three assumptions:

- Learning is most effective when the learner is personally involved in the learning experience.

- Knowledge has to be personally discovered if it is to have meaning or make a difference in behavior.

- Commitment to learning is highest when the learner sets personal learning goals and actively pursues them within a given framework.

A quick and easy experiential activity to help people understand stressors and stress reduction uses a bowl, sponge, and water. A volunteer is asked to hold a large sponge above a large bowl. A second volunteer is asked to hold a cup of water above the bowl and sponge. The other participants are told that the sponge represents the human body. They are asked to think about things in their lives that cause stress (stressors) and then to call them out. A little water is poured onto the sponge each time a stressor is called out. The instructor stops the activity when the sponge is totally waterlogged and facilitates a discussion about the activity.

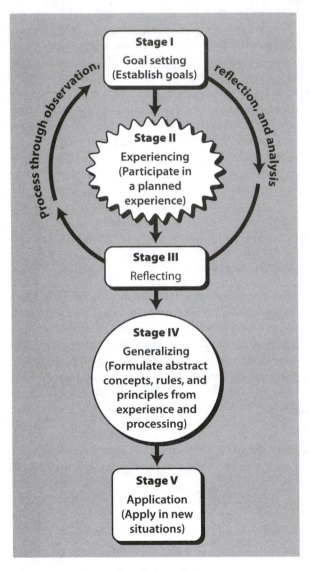

Processing the experience. As you conduct experiential activities, remember that your role is one of **facilitator**. You will help participants navigate the challenges presented to them through planned experiences and then help them integrate the learning that results into future experiences (Henry & Ward, 1999). Assisting participants as they comprehend (reflect), internalize, and transfer (generalize) the lessons learned through these experiences is called **processing.** In processing the sponge activity, the instructor would ask something like, "What happened here?" The participants would describe what they saw and probably begin relating it to real life. They might comment on how the dripping sponge represents someone who is not coping well with stress. They might also note that squeezing the sponge would represent the effective use of coping and stress reduction strategies. Rather than lecturing, the instructor *guides* the discussion so that students understand the concepts of stressors and stress reduction.

Hundreds of books contain experiential elements and activities; we hope you will check out a few. Experiential activities designed to create the same decision-making skills used in real-life experiences

Figure 8.6   Experiential model.
Experiential learning requires more than just an experience. As this model depicts, goals must be set, the experience should be planned, and participants should be allowed an opportunity to reflect, generalize, and then apply what they have learned to the "real" world.

can be very effective if the issues that arise during the activity are processed well. Participants should encounter challenges similar to those they might actually face and be given the opportunity to practice the same skills they will need to solve real-life problems. Processing the activities helps participants alter future behaviors. Failing to process the experience could negate the benefits of the activity. FYI 8.4 (on the following page) lists reflection questions and generalizing questions that a facilitator might ask to help participants maximize the processing of experiential activities.

The Action Plan

An **action plan**, called a **lesson plan** in an educational setting, is an important component of any program. Most programs have several parts; therefore, there may be more than one action plan. Programs might include a series of classes, or they might include discussion groups as well as face-to-face meetings. An action or lesson plan would be developed for each component of the program. Action plans are not lengthy; they provide just enough information to guide each part of the program. We strongly encourage you to develop them even if others in your agency don't use them. Many sample forms exist for action/lesson plans; see Figure 8.7 on p. 199 for one example.

Program Logistics

Careful attention to program logistics helps the health education program run smoothly and ensures that results are accurate. Program logistics tasks include record keeping and scheduling.

Record Keeping

Record keeping is both painful and joyful. Accurate records help you document that your program is working and that you are managing the funds adequately. This is only the case, however, if your records are consistent, accurate, and accessible. We encourage you to use a computer for your record keeping. A number of software programs provide effective tracking and organization of program data. The types of records you must keep are related to process, impact, and outcome (see chapter 7) and will relate directly to your objectives. In regard to process, you will certainly keep attendance records, but you may want to collect information about the participants' perceptions of the program, content, and learning environments. Statistical software, such as the Statistical Package for Social Sciences (www.spss.com), allows you to enter and store data easily and will produce descriptive statistics (frequencies, averages, and percentages) at a click of a button. These same programs will help you store and analyze your impact and outcome information. These are the data that will document the effectiveness of your program, so they become, in a sense, the lifeblood of the program.

Schedules

Another aspect of the program is the timing or scheduling of the activities. As always, there are a number of ways that you can illustrate and distribute your schedules. One of the most common methods involves the use of a monthly calendar as a flyer. The program activities are simply placed on the correct day of the month. Participants can then post their monthly schedules in an easily accessible location. Another method is a program-like document that lists the days and times of upcom-

FYI **8.4   Potential Processing Issues and Questions from Processing**

Allowing participants time to process their experience provides them with the opportunity to derive meaning from it. The following provide some sample questions that would maximize successful processing.

Reflection

General Opening Questions (getting the issues "out in the middle of the circle")
1. So, what just happened?
2. Tell me what you just experienced as you prepared for, moved through, this activity.
3. What were some of your thoughts and feelings during this activity?

Recognizing/Understanding/Expressing Feelings
1. Can you name a feeling you had at any point in completing the activity? Where in your body did you feel it most? Did it influence your behavior?
2. What beliefs were responsible for generating that feeling?
3. Did any of the feelings you had remind you of feelings you have experienced during stressful situations?
4. What did you do with these feelings? Were they expressed? If so, how? If not, why not?

Cooperating
1. Can you think of specific examples of when the group or specific classmates cooperated in completing the activity? Explain.
2. What does cooperation look like? Specify behaviors you saw today.
3. Were there any actions or efforts that seemed to block the group from achieving its goal? Explain.
4. What were some of the observed results of cooperating and helping others?

Appreciating Self
1. What kind of self-talk did you do during the initiative?
2. Do you sometimes put yourself down when you make a mistake? What effect might that have on your actions? On the function of the group?
3. What could you say to yourself to counteract the put-down message?

Generalizing

Transfer of Learning (essential if you want to make a difference)
1. What did you learn in this activity that you think will be helpful to you in getting through this or another class successfully?
2. Can you think of an example in school where you have faced a similar challenge as an individual? In a group situation?
3. What abilities or skills did you or your group exhibit that will help you in future courses or semesters?
4. How will you use what you learned to make school, work, and life better?

Closure Questions
1. What did you learn about yourself? What did you learn about others?
2. Was there a specific person who did something you think worthy of recognition?
3. Is there anything else you would like to say to a specific person or to the group?
4. What was the highlight of the day for you?

From "The Art and Science of Health Education," by J. Henry and S. E. Ward. Unpublished paper.

ing events. Participants receive a brochure or small booklet that provides a quick look at upcoming events. Calendars and programs can also be put on Web pages or sent in e-mails. The key is to carefully plan your schedule with regard to the characteristics of your intended participants. Keep in mind that if a schedule isn't working, it should be changed.

Activity:			
Instructor:			
Date:			
Description of participants:			
Objectives:			
Schedule	**Description of activity**	**Content to be covered**	**Resources**

Figure 8.7   Sample action plan.
As with every other aspect of program planning and implementation, individual lessons or contacts with participants should be well planned. Most professionals find it easiest to use a consistent planning tool like the action plan shown in this illustration.

Creating Materials

Every detail of a program must be planned and implemented with care. Creating materials seems straightforward—just put a few words on paper or on the Internet and present it to the participants. But to do the task well, you must take into consideration such variables as language disorders and literacy levels as well as the appearance of the materials.

Language Disorders and Literacy Levels

"The ability to read and write is strongly influenced by the ability to understand and use language. Individuals who are good listeners and speakers tend to be strong readers and writers" (American Speech-Language-Hearing Association, 1999). The term **language disorder** refers to any impairment in form, semantics, or pragmatics (American Speech-Language-Hearing, 1999). At one time or another you will have program participants with some degree of language disorder. An individual who has difficulties with form might misunderstand the information provided by word endings. Individuals who have difficulties with semantics may not understand *idiom* (a phrase or expression that cannot be understood from the ordinary meanings of the words in it); for example, describing something as the "nuts and bolts" of the program. The meaning of "nuts and bolts" in such usage is not explained by the definition of the two words as pieces of hardware. Other examples of idiom include "butterflies in the stomach," "kick the bucket," and so on. Pragmatics means using the same phrases or words for different purposes; for example, the word *cool* might indicate temperature or it might indicate a value judgment. You will need to prepare materials that are accessible to individuals with language disorders.

You will also encounter individuals with varying **literacy levels** in your programs. "How well adults can use printed and written information to function in society, to achieve their goals, and to develop their knowledge and potential is the definition of literacy" (Educational Testing Service, 2008, p. 1). Although it may not seem so, health literacy is more complex. The National Library of Medicine and National Institutes of Health define health literacy as "the degree to which individuals have the capacity to obtain, process, and understand basic health information and services needed to make appropriate health decisions" (n.d., *Quick Guide*).

If you are working with college students, you know that the **readability** level of your materials can be high; but for the general population, you will want to keep your materials between the fourth and sixth grade levels (National Library of Medicine and National Institutes of Health, 2007). Readability refers to reading ease as well as the difficulty of the material. There are many methods for determining readability, but one common procedure is the SMOG index (McLaughlin, 1969). This index assigns a grade level for written materials. Fortunately, many word-processing programs have readability indexes built into them. Unfortunately, health literacy is not so easily programmed. Keep in mind while you prepare materials that you should differentiate between medical terms that might be known to the participants and those that are unfamiliar. While difficult medical terms may raise the reading level as measured by a test like SMOG, this won't be an issue if participants are familiar with the term. For example, using the word *diabetes* might increase the reading level of a document, but if you are working among individuals with diabetes, they are less likely to have difficulty with the word (Zeng, Eunjung, & Tse, n.d). Familiarity with a word, however, does not necessarily translate into a full understanding of it. Many people will recognize the word *diabetes* but even some individuals with the disease won't truly understand it. According to the National Library of Medicine (2006), "Health information needs to be designed, written, formatted, and communicated in such a way that it is executable by the end user, including multi-media and interactive materials" (p. 9).

There are several actions you can take to develop materials that are accessible to individuals with language disorders or low literacy levels. See FYI 8.5 for a list of tips. As you can see from the list, including words with fewer syllables, writing shorter sentences, and using pictures will increase comprehension.

FYI 8.5   Tips for Developing Materials

The characteristics of the materials you select or develop will influence learning. This list will help ensure that your materials are appropriate for the audience.

- Keep the readability level between the fourth and sixth grade unless you know the specific level of your audience.
- Use pictures to supplement text. Make certain that the pictures are relevant to your audience.
- Unless the members of your audience have medical backgrounds, assume that they are not familiar with medical terms.
- Ask a member of the target population to check the language and adjust it. It should be meaningful to the people who will read it.
- Ask a second member of the target audience to read the adjusted material and describe the content. Make certain that the adjusted material still means what you intend it to.
- Provide examples that are relevant to your audience.
- Field-test your material by asking several members of the target audience to preview the materials and provide feedback.

Creating Web Pages

Web pages are excellent resources for your program. A Web page is an online informational brochure or flyer that is posted for all to see. The good news about developing Web pages is that, like other aspects of implementation, computer software makes it easy. Keep in mind that your Web pages exist to communicate information. Color, font, and format are important—but the message must be paramount. Answer the following question to get started, "What is the purpose of the Web site?" Then derive your content from the information your participants need and want.

Once your content has been selected, consider the design. The best Web pages are simple, which means they are easy to read. According to Roger Parker, the author of *Web Design and Desktop Publishing for Dummies* (1997), nine guidelines assist in Web design:

1. Design should be purposeful.
2. Design should simplify complicated information.
3. Design should provide visual contrast.
4. Design should make your program competitive.
5. Design should show how the program pieces fit together.
6. Design should help the participant know what is important.
7. Design should involve a few effective font and color changes.
8. Design should save the participant time.
9. Design should involve editing.

Individuals with special needs can have difficulty with a poorly designed Web page. FYI 8.6 provides tips for creating Web pages for individuals with special needs.

FYI 8.6   Creating Web Pages for Individuals with Special Needs

Some individuals have special needs that will require changes made to the materials they use in a program, including Web-based programs or pages. Following are some ideas for meeting the needs of individuals with barriers to Web access.

Visual Barriers
- Eliminate screen cluttering.
- Design high-contrast texts and backgrounds.
- Provide text-only options and text descriptions of pictures.

Hearing Barriers
- Explain sound clips using text.
- Provide text descriptions for all video clips that include sound.

Learning or Cognitive Barriers
- Have lots of descriptive pictures.
- Have step-by-step explanations for all instructions and commands.

Physical Barriers
- Provide compatibility with mouse substitution software such as touch screen or touch board.
- Provide compatibility for voice recognition software.

Economic Barriers
- Provide text-only options for use with slower computers.
- Provide paper alternatives.

Source: Adapted from "Web Accessibility," Alliance for Technology Access. Retrieved March 23, 2009, from http://www.atacess.org/rresources/webaccess.html

Keeping the Program Alive

One aspect of programming helps ensure its ongoing existence—ethical practices. Ethics comprises a whole host of issues, some of which we will discuss further in chapter 9. For now, think about the following characteristics of ethics: honesty, integrity, confidentiality, and communication. Honesty involves acting truthfully, integrity requires basing one's actions on a set of principles, confidentiality means ensuring that only authorized individuals have access to private information, and communication entails creating shared meaning by sending and receiving messages. When combined, these characteristics describe the basis for almost all codes of ethics. You will find the Code of Ethics for the Health Education Profession in Appendix F. Almost all professions and most agencies have codes of ethics. They have similar content, so read through Appendix F for the general feel. You will see as you read that honesty, integrity, confidentiality, and communication are reflected in every section.

In Conclusion

After completing the legwork involved in needs assessment and program planning, implementation may at first seem like the "easy" part. But it must be approached with an understanding of its importance. Ongoing funding for the program is necessary and you may need to seek supplemental funds through donations or special events. Once appropriate funding is secured, your next goal will be effective marketing. Social marketing encompasses much more than advertising. You'll revisit the needs assessment to define the market audience, address issues of place and price, and develop promotion strategies. You will also want to consider partnering with other agencies, and you'll need to review current policies and politics.

The nuts-and-bolts of the program will be fine-tuned in program implementation. Appropriate program materials and schedules should be developed with the target population in mind. Record-keeping, although not always fun, will document your ability to manage the program and produce positive impacts and outcomes. Treat program implementation seriously.

REVIEW QUESTIONS

1. List and describe the Ps in social marketing.
2. Detail the strategies you might use to select a new employee and justify your choices.
3. List tips for developing effective materials.
4. Discuss why experiential and critical thinking methods are important.
5. Describe ways to help individuals with barriers use the Web.
6. Analyze ways in which to improve health literacy.
7. Explain why ethical practice keeps a program alive.

☞ FOR YOUR APPLICATION

Select or create a format for a lesson plan. It should include space for the following categories: descriptions of the topic and target population, objectives, projected schedule, content to be covered, and needed resources. Once you have selected the format, complete the plan for one session in the program you are developing in your project. If you are not doing a project, just select a topic and target audience and develop a lesson plan for one session. Ask your instructor to review the plan and provide feedback. If you are creating a portfolio, be sure to include the updated version of your lesson plan.

Research and Evaluation

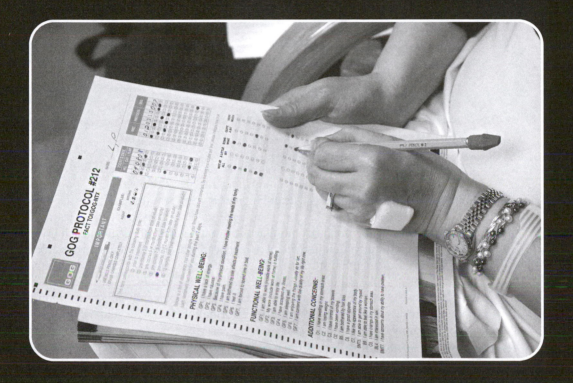

You developed a program for teen mothers in your community. You assessed their attitudes, beliefs, and perceived needs and based the program development on the assessment. Lots of teens attended the program. Everyone seemed to be having fun. Does that mean the program was effective? Can you assume that the program accomplished what it was supposed to? Did you check to see if the program had been studied in action before you used it?

CHAPTER OBJECTIVES

1. Describe the process of research.
2. Discuss developing research objectives, questions, and hypotheses.
3. Detail selected quantitative and qualitative research designs.
4. List the purposes of evaluation.
5. Create an evaluation plan.

What Is Research?

Research is a process. It provides a means for examining the reality of a circumstance, establishing patterns and relationships in aspects of a situation, or even satisfying curiosity about something. The difference between research and a casual inspection of a topic is the systematic nature of the process. Research involves a clearly defined process delineated prior to starting. There are many types of research, each involving a wide choice of study designs; all of which can be clearly defined, described, and planned in advance. Even studies that use emerging designs (such as some qualitative research designs) are planned in advance to the extent possible.

In the past, you might have been asked to write a research paper. It's important to note that research is not solely getting information from the library and writing a paper about it. A literature review—seeking information from articles written by professionals—is only one part of the research process, not the entire endeavor. The first step in the research process is to create a plan of action, sometimes called a proposal.

The Research Plan/Proposal

The research plan confirms the systematic nature of the process. In other words, the process is not one of "going with the flow" or "taking it as it comes." The plan should include carefully defined procedures that you will follow in order to conduct an effective study. It is almost like a recipe, but more prescriptive. Recipes can be adjusted to fit an individual's taste, but a research plan should be followed carefully so that others who wish to replicate the study can do so. The steps for creating a research plan and thereby fulfilling the research process involve critical analysis and include, but are not limited to, the following:

1. Determine the problem to be solved.
2. Identify information currently available about the problem (literature review).
3. Write objectives, research questions, and hypotheses.
4. Select a study design.
5. Create a timeline.
6. Establish a budget.
7. Select measurement instruments.
8. Set up implementation plans.
9. Formulate data-analysis strategies.
10. Determine a research dissemination plan.

Determining the Problem to Address

It is fairly easy to identify health-related problems throughout the world: read the newspaper, watch television, search the Internet, or simply look around. However, determining the issue to be studied in a research project requires more than just selecting a problem on which to focus. It includes analysis, prioritization, and justification. There are many considerations to resolve, not the least of which are the time and money available for the project. There is no use even contemplating a project without adequate resources. If resources are available, you can proceed to select a problem to address in a research project.

If you work for a nonprofit or voluntary health organization, research will be guided by the organizational mission. Public health agencies may be limited to programming and research that matches the national funding streams. In other words, the federal government will make monies available for selected public health issues, some of which have been determined to be national public health concerns and others that are of interest to politicians and lobbyists. In the best of all worlds, research would be determined by a partnership between community members and professionals. The problem would be analyzed and aspects of the issue would be prioritized through assessments, literature reviews, and collaborations between members of the partner community and various professionals. Justification for conducting the research would be created through the analysis and prioritization. Later in the chapter, we'll talk more about community-based participatory research, which is a process that involves the community in every phase.

Writing Objectives, Research Questions, and Hypotheses

The quality and success of a research project depends on planning. Once the research problem has been identified, the planning begins with the development of objectives, research questions, and hypotheses.

Writing Objectives

Hopefully, you have already learned the fundamentals of writing objectives and understand their importance. Basically, research objectives state what you hope to achieve with the study. There may be both general and specific objectives—that is, a broad overriding objective and several detailed objectives that when combined address the overall objective and research problem. Writing these objectives entails steps similar to those discussed in the program planning chapter. In some ways, creating research objectives is like writing a newspaper article: they should answer who, what, where, and why. For example, a broad research objective might be "To determine the effectiveness of the teen pregnancy program (we'll call our example program 'Rising Star') provided by the health education section of the local public health department." The word *effective* is not defined in this broad objective so it must be clarified in the more detailed objectives linked to it. These linked objectives might include:

1. To determine if the financial needs (what) of teen participants (who) were met through the program's social services offerings (where), for the purpose of examining the deficits (why).

2. To identify the costs incurred (what) by the public health department (who) to conduct the program (where) in order to relate the costs to the benefits of the program (why).

3. To measure the participants' (who) satisfaction (what) with the program (where) to determine if it is appropriate for them (why).

4. To compare the number of future pregnancies (what) of program participants and nonparticipant teens (who) to determine if the problem is truly being addressed (why) by the program (where).

5. To use the findings of the study (what) to improve future teen pregnancy programs (why and who) through dissemination of the results (where).

Each of these linked objectives measures a different component or aspect of the effectiveness of the program.

Writing Hypotheses and Research Questions

You may hear the phrase "research question" used in two ways. It is often used as an umbrella term for any of the questions that will be addressed in a research project, whether quantitative or qualitative. The broad questions are developed directly from the objectives that we described in the previous section. For example, one of our objectives stated, "To compare the number of future pregnancies of program participants and nonparticipant teens to determine if the problem is truly being addressed by the program." A research question based on this example objective might ask, "What are the differences in second pregnancy rates between Rising Star participants and control participants?"

The next step after writing your research question will be to develop a prediction or hypothesis regarding the question. A **hypothesis** is a prediction of the results of the study. The hypothesis will then be tested using an appropriate research design and statistical test. The hypothesis (prediction) should not be based on your hopes for the program. Instead, it should be based on your previous experience with the same program, research or program evaluation done by others using the program, or results of other programs that are similar in nature.

You may also hear the term "research question" used in qualitative research as a specific title for the questions that will be addressed in that type of study. (See the explanations of qualitative versus quantitative in the next section.) Though it is appropriate to use this term in a qualitative study, it is not appropriate to use the term "hypothesis" for this type of research. The specific title for questions in a quantitative project is "hypotheses" because a hypothesis can be tested. Hypotheses generate the use of inferential statistics (quantitative), which we discussed briefly in the epidemiology chapter. Because qualitative research questions generate words, phrases, and explanations from individuals, the results do not produce the numbers needed to test a hypothesis. So, when conducting qualitative research, you will generate research questions but not hypotheses.

Developing a Study Design

The study design will serve as a guide for data collection and analysis. Note that there is a difference between study design and data collection strategy. You must know what type of data you will be collecting in order to select your study design. The type of data needed will depend on your study objectives and research questions or hypotheses. First let's review the definitions of the broad types of data, quantitative and qualitative. Numbers are used to represent **quantitative** data. The number may be a frequency count (i.e., there are 15 men and 12 women), a score (i.e., 87 out of 100 points), the result of a mathematical computation (87%), a code to signify membership in a specified category (1 = male and 2 = female), or another numerical representation. **Qualitative** data are represented by words and phrases because the researcher wants to understand "why" something is happening. So, even though words represent the data, the meaning of the words and phrases is what is important.

Let's look at some examples of hypotheses and research questions and their relationship to types of data. Suppose your hypothesis states: "Participants in the Rising Star class will score higher on the post-program survey than control participants." This hypothesis provides three important pieces of information. First, because this is a hypothesis or a prediction that can be tested, the data will be quantitative. Second, there will be an intervention (something that will be tested, such as the program) and third, because a comparison will be made, there will be a control group. At a minimum, measurements will be taken post-intervention; preferably, pre and post. As you can see, this study design must be quantitative in nature.

However, suppose your research question asks: "What perceptions about the Rising Star program do participants hold?" It's difficult to make a prediction about this research question. If fact, it can best be answered by talking to participants and learning from their words, body language, and facial expressions. After all, think about the reason this question has been asked. You want to know what participants like or dislike and why. Knowing why people feel the way they do can help you adapt the program to their needs and interests. The data and the study design will be qualitative.

When you have determined the research questions and hypotheses, you will be able to select your study design. Your proposal or research plan should describe, in great detail, the activities that make up the design, including the data-collection strategies and the way in which study participants or study sample will be selected.

Quantitative Designs

There are more quantitative designs and their variations than we can cover in this chapter. However, we will describe a few basic designs to give you an overview. If you select an **experimental design** for your research project, you will need to identify the individuals who will be part of the study, called the study sample, with great care. In fact, you will *randomly select* the individuals who will participate and then *randomly assign* them to one of two groups, control or intervention. If you remember, random selection means giving every person in the population the same chance to be selected for the study; computer programs can be used to ensure randomness. Random assignment means that, once in the study, all participants will have equal chances to be put in the intervention or the control group. An **intervention** can be an educational program, medical treatment, marketing effort, one aspect of a program, or something else that you would like to study. One way to prove that your intervention works (or doesn't) is to use an experimental design in which two comparable groups of people receive different programs or different parts of the program (the intervention). In some cases, one group (the control group) will receive no type of programming; instead, they will complete only the pretest and posttest.

The specific behavior, knowledge level, attitude, or medical outcome that you hope will change for your participants after the intervention is the **dependent variable.** Some examples might be knowledge score, attitude rating, smoking frequency, blood pressure, and in our example, second pregnancies. The dependent variable will be measured in both groups of people (those who received the intervention and those who did not) at two times (before and after the intervention). The degree to which members of each group changed their behavior will be compared. Of course, you hope that the group who received your intervention will have the most favorable results.

If the experiment has been carefully conducted, you will be able to say that your intervention made a difference. If an intervention truly causes the effect desired, it is said to have **internal validity** (Godwin et al., 2003). In a carefully designed experiment (one that uses random selection and assignment), you can also claim **external validity**; that is, results can be generalized to other people in the population.

You will have to determine if the experimental design is appropriate and feasible for your research project. Will you be able to assemble intervention and control groups? Will you be able to make certain that the participants in each group don't talk with one another and contaminate the results? Will there be factors in the community that influence one group of participants but not the other? Experimental designs are not easy to carry out; however, the superiority of this method should encourage its use where practicable.

Some research designs that are weaker but have potential include a one-group posttest study, one-group pretest/posttest study, and post-only comparison study. Just as its name suggests, a **one-group posttest study** involves only one group and one measurement of the target behavior. All participants would be in the intervention group and would be tested after the intervention has occurred. If you select this type of research design, you look for the target behavior to be healthier after the intervention. Unfortunately, this design has some problems; can you see the flaws in it? There are many reasons, other than the intervention, for the behavior of interest to be improved after the program. The program participants might have had positive behaviors before the program even began, but you would not know because they weren't measured. Some other stimulus, like a TV show or movie, might have precipitated a change in behavior. You would never really know if your program was responsible for the positive behavior because you had no measurement of the behavior before the program started and no comparisons with individuals who did not receive the intervention.

A pretest is added in the **one-group pretest/posttest design.** With this design, you are able to measure changes in the behavior because you take measurements both before and after the intervention. But you would still not be able to say with certainty that the program itself was responsible for the change. Can you see why? Again, some other stimulus in the environment might have prompted the change. Suppose the participant read a self-help book during the same time she or he attended the program. Behavior change might be a result of the reading, not the program.

In the **post-only comparison**, you are able to measure differences in the target behavior between two groups, control and intervention, that are both tested after the intervention. Only one group has received the program, and neither has been pretested. You would find out if the post-program behaviors were healthy and how the behaviors differed between intervention and control participants. But what if the intervention group had healthier behaviors than the control group in the first place? You would not be able to determine the impact of the intervention with this study design. Figure 9.1 (on the following page) provides schematics of the quantitative study designs discussed in this chapter. Keep in mind that there are many more quantitative research designs, as well as variations of the ones we have already discussed. We encourage you to take a research design class to enhance your knowledge of this valuable and interesting topic.

Qualitative Designs

In general, qualitative research is an in-depth review and analysis of the meaning of documents, settings, relationships, and verbal communications. Like quantitative research, there are numerous qualitative designs and varied data-collection strategies that fit into those designs. We'd like to present a few broad qualitative approaches to give you an introduction to this type of research.

Ethnography. This type of research takes place in the field, not a laboratory. Detailed descriptions are made of people, places, customs, cultures, and societies with emphasis on one group of people and their culture. Nothing is studied independently; rather, the emphasis is on determining how people, places, beliefs, and behaviors fit together and influence one another (Trochim, 2006). The researcher often becomes immersed in a culture in order to study it in a technique called **participant observation.** The researcher is always an integral part of this research process because his/her analysis of the meaning of the observations ultimately tells the story of the culture.

Grounded theory. Researchers use this qualitative approach to create theory from preliminary data collection, which in turn, guides further research. This approach is an "emerging design," a phrase mentioned earlier that means data collection and analysis decisions occur while the study is progressing. Content and communication analyses are used in all phases of data collection in order to find theoretical concepts and links between them. The purpose in the end is to create a new theory that is grounded in systematic observation.

Phenomenology. Determining the lived experience of individuals regarding a specific phenomenon is the goal of this approach. Researchers conduct in-depth interviews with a number of individuals who have a shared experience; for example, very young teens who have given birth. Researchers will then look for commonalities across the interviewees in order to understand the collective lived experience with the event or phenomenon.

Case study.   A case study involves the in-depth study of one case. Many individuals, settings, documents, and communications regarding the case are reviewed and

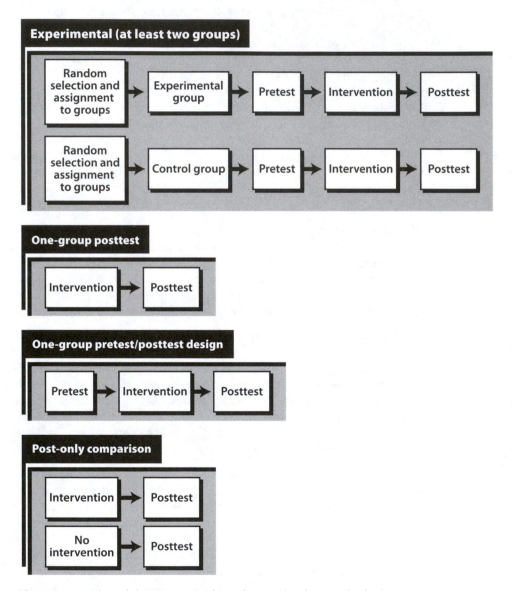

Figure 9.1   Pictorial representation of quantitative study designs.
Many types of study designs exist and often two or more types of designs will be used in one research project. This figure illustrates four types of designs.

analyzed. A variety of data-collection strategies might be used, such as interviews, content analyses, and observations.

Community Based Participatory Research

Whether you select qualitative or quantitative designs, **community based participatory research (CBPR)** provides a framework in which community members and researchers act as equal partners in the process. It begins with a health topic of interest, progresses to gathering information to increase knowledge, and ultimately applies that knowledge to improve the health of a community. The purpose of CBPR, also termed "action research," is to reach community-driven goals while collecting valuable information through research (Minkler, Blackwell, Thompson, & Tamir, 2003). The CBPR process provides an invaluable collaborative research forum, but could also play a role in improving the work of health related agencies. Nonprofit organizations and community health agencies often struggle with reaching their goals because of inadequate strategies, lack of resources, unrealistic expectations from stakeholders, and difficult timelines. CBPR may improve outcomes. Unfortunately, it's not always easy to find community members who have the requisite skills and interest in potential projects. These challenges may create a need for more time and money for the research process than might be needed for other designs. However, devoting the time and resources to this process has the potential to provide dramatic improvements in the success of programs.

According to Metzler and colleagues (2003), the activities important to developing effective community research partners include shared decision-making, defining collaboration, establishing research priorities that are meaningful to the community, and securing funding. Minkler (2004) created a framework to help develop community partners. The framework incorporates Kelly's ideas on community-based research (1986) and Jones's thoughts on understanding racism (2004). Minkler's framework helps researchers address "(a) achieving a true 'community-driven' agenda; (b) insider-outsider tensions; (c) real and perceived racism; (d) the limitations of participation; and (e) issues involving the sharing, ownership, and use of findings for action" (p. 684). We strongly encourage you to learn more about the CBPR process and to apply it when you develop a research project.

Establishing a Budget and Creating a Timeline

Each research project must have a unique budget. The steps for developing this budget are the same as those used in a program budget: selecting the categories, determining the implementation phases, estimating costs, documenting in-kind contributions, allowing for contingencies, and calculating the total funding needed. The categories for your budget will be very similar to those in the program budget. See Table 9.1 on the following page for a sample budget specific to a research project.

An exclusive timeline for the research project will be helpful as well. See Figure 9.2 (on p. 215) for a Gantt chart specific to a research project.

Table 9.1   Sample Research Budget

Budget Item	Description	Total Cost
Personnel		
Health researcher	960 hours $30/hr	$28,800
Secretary	800 hours $14/hr	11,200
Subtotal		40,000
Personnel benefits	20% of wages	8,000
Total personnel		**$48,000**
Supplies		
Printing	100,000 × .04	$ 4,000
Postage	20,000 × .44	8,800
Office supplies		500
Total supplies		**$13,300**
Services		
Telephone	$150/month	$ 1,800
Total services		**$ 1,800**
Consultants		
Data processing	25 hours $12/hr	$ 300
Graphic artist	16 hours $25/hr	400
Total consultants		**$ 700**
Contingencies		$ 500
Total contingencies		**$ 500**
Indirect costs	15% of total	$ 9,645
Total costs		**$73,945**

Selecting Measurement Instruments

Qualitative and quantitative research designs may seem to include similar data-collection strategies like surveys, interviews, or observation, but the instruments used are not the same. Quantitative instruments will collect information that is quantifiable while qualitative instruments will collect words, phrases, and observations that can be studied for meaning. Quantitative data-collection instruments include but are not limited to surveys, questionnaires, tests, medical equipment, and checklists. Qualitative data-collection instruments include but are not limited to focus groups, the Delphi method, interviews, and observations.

The instruments used in data collection must be selected, adjusted, and sometimes written. Instrument selection or development should be viewed as an integral part of the research process. If the instrument is medical equipment, for example, it must have protocols (specific procedures) for clinical measurements. The instrument might also be a paper-and-pencil questionnaire or survey.

Developing a quantitative instrument is a time-consuming and difficult process. As a result, you might tend to develop research objectives and hypotheses based on

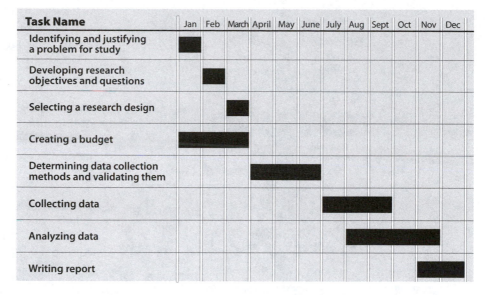

Task Name	Jan	Feb	March	April	May	June	July	Aug	Sept	Oct	Nov	Dec
Identifying and justifying a problem for study	■											
Developing research objectives and questions		■										
Selecting a research design			■									
Creating a budget	■	■	■									
Determining data collection methods and validating them				■	■							
Collecting data							■	■				
Analyzing data								■	■			
Writing report											■	■

Figure 9.2   Gantt chart for a research project.
Projecting the timeline for the whole scope of a research project will help you focus on each of the very important steps.

available instruments rather than the other way around. We agree that every attempt should be made to find an existing instrument that is appropriate, but, if it is not possible, we encourage you to use appropriate development techniques. Let's discuss instrument development as we discuss estimating validity and reliability. Figure 9.3 (on the following page) illustrates a six-step process for instrument development.

Establishing the Framework

Establishing a framework for an instrument is like building a foundation for a house. You need to decide on the best material and style for the foundation. In the case of instrument development, you might choose a theoretical base. If so, a health behavior or learning theory will guide the development process. For example, if social cognitive theory is your foundation, your intervention and the entire research project will evolve from the theory. One construct in the theory is self-efficacy. One of your intervention activities might focus on this construct. You might also choose criteria for your foundation. Perhaps study participants must achieve a standard set of behaviors (criteria). If so, the instrument would be guided by these criteria. The good news for you as a researcher is that you will keep the same framework used during intervention development. If theory guided the intervention development, then it will also guide the measurement instrument.

Developing a Skeleton

You begin by developing a first draft of your instrument. You might start by using an open-ended type of questionnaire that elicits participants' beliefs (Ajzen & Fishbein, 1977); you can talk with individuals who are expert in the measurement of your

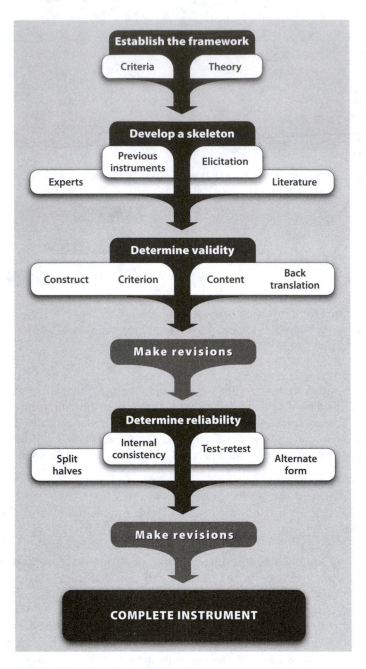

Figure 9.3   Instrument development.
Instrument development is a complex task that requires
many steps. This illustration provides a model for instrument
development.

behavior of interest; and you can review existing literature for suggested forms and formats.

Special attention must be given to both the format and wording of each item during initial drafting. The difficulty lies in creating items that accurately represent the psychosocial variables of interest (such as attitudes, perceptions, and beliefs) and are appropriate for the target populations' culture and local dialect. You will want to search the literature for scale items previously used and adapt those items, if necessary, to the proposed study. Keep in mind that you will need to get the original developer's permission to use or adjust any part of a previously existing instrument. Be sure to consider the cultural appropriateness of both the items and the instrument as a whole.

Imagine that you are asked to study a teen pregnancy program that was based on the health belief model. The purpose of one component of the program might have been to increase the likelihood that the teen mothers would select safe ways to discipline their children. You might measure their perceptions of how likely they are to choose inappropriate discipline and their perceptions of the availability of professional services. It will take a certain amount of effort on your part to select the best vocabulary for measuring components of the health belief model, specifically perceptions of susceptibility. You will have to search the literature for an existing instrument. If there is no existing instrument, you will need to find one that was used in a similar situation and adjust it. Once you have developed the skeleton format, estimating validity is the next step.

Instrument Validity

Determining instrument validity begins with attention to the brevity and clarity of the instrument. Establishing instrument brevity and clarity is particularly complicated when cultural sensitivity of the instrument is a priority. Brislin's guidelines for writing and modifying instrument items have been used widely and adapted for cross cultural instruments (Wang, Lee, & Fetzer, 2006). These guidelines suggest using short, simple sentences of less than 16 words (Brislin, 1986). This is no easy task when you should also repeat nouns instead of using pronouns, avoid metaphors and colloquialisms that could shorten the wording, and add sentences and phrases where needed to provide cultural context for key ideas. Only through collaborative community involvement in instrument development can you be sure that the instrument is sufficiently brief and effectively clear.

Once brevity and clarity have been examined, you will want to consider four major types of validity. These include criterion-related, content, construct, and back translation.

Criterion-related validity.　When the scoring of an instrument yields results similar to actual observation of the behavior of interest, the instrument is said to have **criterion-related validity.** For example, imagine that a parental discipline survey was developed as an easy way to measure the quality of a teen mother's discipline behaviors. It would have criterion-related validity if it gave the same estimate of discipline quality as did an actual observation of a teen mother disciplining her children. The observed behavior is the criterion. The process requires a statistical procedure called a *correlation* to determine if a relationship exists between a score received on the instrument and a score on the actual performance of the behavior. The resulting number is called a *validity coefficient.* The validity coefficient can range from -1 to +1. For most instruments, you should look for a moderate to high correlation (ranging between .65 and 1) before you use it.

Content validity.　If the instrument accurately reflects an area or domain of knowledge, it has **content validity**. For example, the quality-of-discipline survey would have content validity if it used the word *discipline* and other concepts appropriately. In most cases, no specific, well-defined criteria exist from which to measure content validity. Most evaluators rely on experts in the field to assess it. You would ask a panel of experts in parental discipline choices to review the instrument and suggest changes that would make the content stronger. This practice has merit as long as the people you choose truly have expertise in the content.

Construct validity.　The extent to which an instrument reflects its theoretical base is a measure of **construct validity** (Smith, 2005). Construct validation is not a matter of rapid assessment. Much research in using the instrument and follow-up analysis are required. *Factor analysis* (a statistical procedure) may provide you or your statistician with useful information about your theoretically based instrument. This statistical procedure should be used only in combination with expert knowledge of the constructs to be measured to prevent misconceptualization. Individuals with expertise in the theoretical construct being measured are normally asked to assist in establishing the construct validity of an instrument. You will want to establish a second panel of individuals (in our example, experts in the health belief model) to review your instrument and suggest changes that would help it better reflect the theory. It is important to note that professionals evaluating the construct validity of an instrument may not be familiar with the cultural norms and local dialect of the partner population. Thus, an instrument thought to be construct-valid could be virtually ineffective if a particular word distorted meaning within the targeted cultural context.

Plan to involve members of the partner culture in your instrument development. The ideal is to enlist the help of health professionals who are familiar with the construct to be measured and who understand the culture and local dialect. When this isn't possible, a combined group effort should include both construct and cultural experts.

Back translation.   An instrument designed for one cultural setting and used in a slightly different culture may cause the researcher to miss aspects of the second culture that are important to the overall picture. The resulting conclusions might then be based on concepts that are nonexistent within the targeted culture or at least partially incorrect. Thus, existing instruments should be used only after modifications are made to fit the specific culture and research situation (Brislin, 1986).

A popular method for validating a translated instrument is **back translation** (Jones, Lee, Phillips, Zhang, & Jaceldo, 2001). If you choose to have your instrument translated into another language, one bilingual individual translates from the source language to the target language. Another bilingual person then translates the resulting target-language version back to the source language. This process may be repeated several times and the first and last source-language versions compared. If the major concept survives the activity, it is regarded as *etic* (that is, readily available words and phrases exist in the two languages that facilitate concept translation). If the concept doesn't survive, it is *emic*, or expressible in only the source language.

In addition to its use when two languages are involved, the back-translation process can be used to modify an instrument to the popular jargon of a community. In this instance you would ask "bilingual" translators who understand both the local jargon and the terminology used in the original instrument to be involved in the process.

Selection of bilingual translators is a critical first step in the back-translation process. The ideal is to choose translators who are members of the partner culture and are keenly familiar with the cultural norms and local dialect of the targeted group. They must also clearly understand the original instrument language and the constructs it is intended to measure. These translators must have an ability to focus on the clear communication of concepts rather than the literal translation of words and phrases. The degree to which they understand both the original instrument and the partnered culture will affect their ability to find target-language equivalents without having to use unfamiliar terms (Jones et al., 2001).

Finding translators who meet the necessary criteria is seldom easy and the ideal is rarely achieved. Translators with differing levels and types of expertise can work as a team. Potential sources are trained professional translators identified by community gatekeepers, health professionals, or university researchers experienced in working with the population as well as members of the cultural group who are studying in a university health program. Because few bilingual individuals are trained translators, a team approach may be more effective.

The results of the back-translation process may seem inconsistent with the original instrument. The critical questions to ask in this situation are (a) whether the original instrument concepts survived the process while words and phrases changed or (b) whether the original concepts were lost in the process. Bringing the translators together with the evaluator to discuss this issue is critical. If the group concedes that the concepts remained intact, the translated instrument is now ready to be subjected to further validation procedures for readability and understandability within the partner culture. However, if the targeted concept was lost in the process, the evaluator should return to the original instrument. It may be helpful to reword the original following Brislin's guidelines and present the altered version to a new set of translators. Another alternative would be to work with the original translators to create items in the targeted language that do reflect the targeted construct. The resulting instrument can then be further validated.

The rigorous process of back translation cannot fully guarantee that resulting scales will be culturally appropriate. Further work is necessary to validate its utility within the partner culture. This work includes testing the instrument for readability and understandability with a subsample of the targeted population.

Data-Collection Strategies

Data are collected in many ways, ranging from observation to complex medical tests. If you will remember, we indicated that there is a difference between research design and data-collection strategies. When you have selected your research design, the data-collection strategy and sampling methods (methods for selecting participants) can then be determined. You will most likely be involved in collecting data through survey instruments, communication groups, or observations. As we have said, these types of strategies can be either qualitative or quantitative but the instruments themselves are designed to reflect the type of data needed. If responses from a specific strategy can be counted, the instrument is likely to be quantitative. If an open-ended response can be expected, the instrument is likely to be qualitative. We'd like to review a few common strategies in the next few paragraphs.

Focus Groups

As you know from chapter 6, a focus group consists of a small number of people who are asked to participate in a discussion. Questions are developed prior to the discussion; during the session, a trained facilitator presents the questions and keeps the discussion moving. This individual does not give opinions or participate in the discussion, other than to clarify what others have said or encourage discussion in greater depth. The participant comments are audiotaped or recorded in some fashion. A second person serves as the recorder so the facilitator can focus on the process of the discussion. Any number of focus groups can be conducted as long as different people participate in each group.

A difficult issue in a focus-group design is determining who will participate. Will you try to get everyone in the partner population to be in a focus group? If the group is too large, will you randomly select a few to participate or will you simply ask for volunteers? If you ask for volunteers, the sampling method is called *convenience sampling*. Your decisions will be based on the research objectives and design, timeline, and budget. Keep in mind that if you want a representative sample, you should include all participants or randomly select some of them.

Delphi Technique

The Delphi technique was described briefly in chapter 6. It is another group design, but participants do not meet face-to-face. It is generally used for decision making or consensus building (Raskin, 1974), which can be important evaluation processes if you are trying to determine the value of a health education program.

If you decide to use the Delphi technique, you will need to identify criteria for being included in the study. Your respondents are usually experts in the type of intervention you are delivering. They will need to commit some time to the study because they will take part in several rounds of surveys.

Round 1 is used for collecting baseline data. Participants will be asked to respond to one or more open-ended questions that reflect the research questions. When the surveys are returned, you take the responses and put them in a Likert format (items that require a rating). In round 2 participants are asked to respond to the Likert scale. When those surveys are returned, you place the items that have the highest levels of agreement in a list. During round 3 participants rank the items. You then identify the items that are most frequently ranked the highest. Your objective is to discern consensus building in the group. A fourth round may be necessary to complete the process.

Interviews

As you are probably aware by now, interviews may be formal or informal, simple or complex. A trained interviewer asks the participant at least one question and facilitates the remainder of the interview in a way that matches the data-collection protocol. If you select this strategy, you might use the same set of questions and same interview protocol for all interviewees (structured), or you might simply ask people to tell you what they think about the topic of study. If the research design is quantitative and formal, the interview questions, setting, and time will be carefully determined before data collection. Participants will be asked to stick to the questions and will be prompted in the same way. As with other data-collection strategies, you will have to make decisions about who will be interviewed. Some qualitative interview protocols use a sampling method called *snowball sampling*. In this method, a few volunteers are interviewed and they are asked to suggest others who could also be interviewed. The number of interviews thereby "snowballs." Use your research plan as your guide.

Observation

Like an interview, observations might be formal or informal, simple or complex. An observer might have specific things to look for or might note anything and everything seen. If you select this strategy, you will have to decide whether the individuals whom you are observing will be told. People who know they are being observed might change their behavior without even thinking about it. This is called **observer**

effect. You will also need to be aware of your own biases. Unless you are careful, your beliefs and attitudes will be reflected in your observation (**observer bias**).

Surveys

Surveys can be used in both quantitative and qualitative designs. The type of item or question will determine the kind of data collected. Open-ended items elicit qualitative data, while multiple-choice questions and Likert scales, for example, elicit responses that can be quantified. Surveys are very versatile; they can be used with large or small samples, and they can be conducted over the telephone, through the postal system, in a face-to-face setting, or electronically.

As with other strategies, you will have to make decisions about who will participate. One of the most difficult issues with surveys, however, is determining their appropriateness for your project. For example, surveys that collect information about behaviors, beliefs, and attitudes often use self-report responses. In other words, you are measuring the participants' perceptions, which might not match up with reality. If self-report isn't appropriate for your project, you will want to use another technique, such as an actual observation of behaviors.

Implementation

The research plan must include the implementation phase, during which the measurements (whether surveys, interviews, medical assessments, or observations) are made. The environment plays an important role in this data-collection phase. For example, if a survey is planned but there is no place to sit and write, participants may not focus well on their responses. If a medical assessment of some type is planned without a place for privacy, participants might choose not to take part. Time, place, temperature, noise level, and lighting are among the many issues that must be considered.

Coding and analysis (usually with the aid of a computer) should take place after data are collected. Coding is a way of preparing data for analysis. A simple example of coding would be assigning a 1 to the data if the participant is male and a 2 if female.

Data Analysis

Many social science researchers enjoy the data-collection process because whether the study design is qualitative or quantitative in nature, the process involves working with people. When data collection is complete, the sheer size of the results can be overwhelming even in a small study. However, data analysis provides the basis from which the researcher draws conclusions.

Quantitative Analysis

Sometimes the word *statistics* is used to mean a numerical description of an event. The frequency of accident-related deaths or incidents of violence in schools are examples of events that can be described with statistics. At other times, the word indicates mathematical procedures that are used to test hypotheses or determine reliability and validity.

These two uses of the word *statistics* actually describe two broad categories: descriptive and inferential. **Descriptive statistics** use numbers to organize data. They lend themselves to being displayed through many types of tables, charts, and graphs. Figure 9.4 presents some commonly used formats for illustrating descriptive statistics.

Pie Chart

Poliomyelitis immunization status of children age 1–4 in central cities (pop. ≥ 250,000) by financial status, United States, 1969

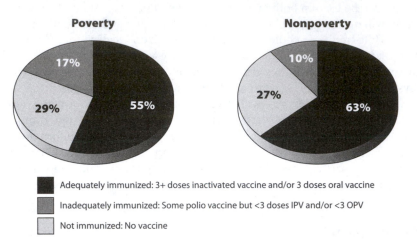

Adequately immunized: 3+ doses inactivated vaccine and/or 3 doses oral vaccine

Inadequately immunized: Some polio vaccine but <3 doses IPV and/or <3 OPV

Not immunized: No vaccine

Pictograph

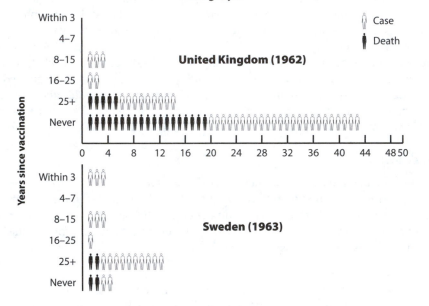

Figure 9.4   Displaying descriptive statistics.
Descriptive statistics can be illustrated for your participants or in your reports in a number of ways. The illustrations on pages 222–224 provide some examples. Careful thought should be given to the types of charts or graphs you select so that your results can be clearly understood.

Scatter Plot

**Counties reporting one or more cases
of animal rabies, United States, 1968**

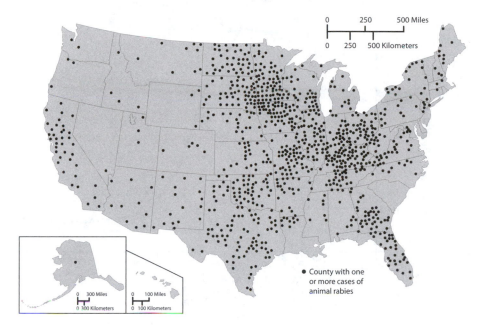

Bar Chart

**Percent of age distribution of sample population compared to
census population immunization survey, sample city, 1970**

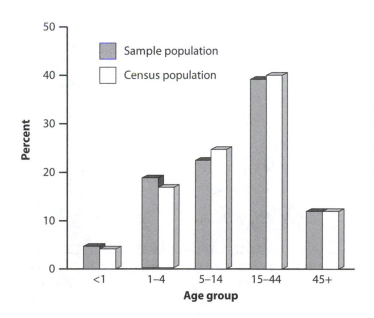

Line Graph

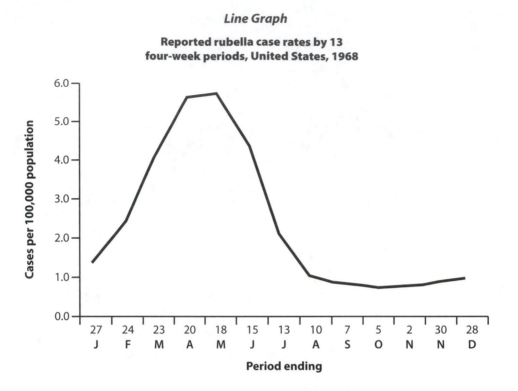

Reported rubella case rates by 13 four-week periods, United States, 1968

Block Chart

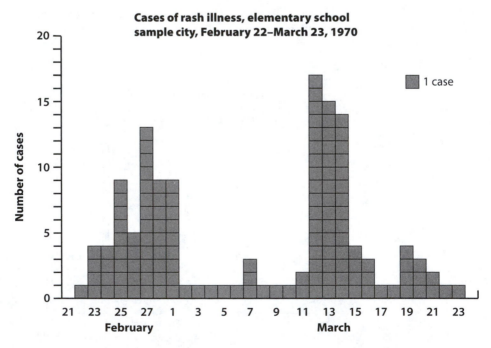

Cases of rash illness, elementary school sample city, February 22–March 23, 1970

Inferential statistics are used to make comparisons, identify relationships, and draw conclusions about data. Space prevents us from discussing these tests in sufficient detail in this chapter; but if you have not done so already, we encourage you to take a full course in basic statistics so that you are equipped to select the best ways to organize and analyze your quantitative data.

Qualitative Analysis

The type of data used in this analysis process cannot be represented well with numbers. Conversations, interviews, focus-groups discussions, open-ended survey responses, and observations are analyzed for patterns or commonalities in meaning. As mentioned earlier, numerical coding is used in quantitative data analysis but it can be used in qualitative analysis as well. The difference is that qualitative data coding could also use colors, symbols, words, or phrases.

Let us look at an example of qualitative data that might have been collected during a program for teen mothers. Suppose we asked participants to complete a survey with questions related to their satisfaction with the program. One question asks participants to describe what they liked about the program. One person wrote, "This program was fun because people I knew were in it with me." Another person wrote, "I really liked this program because I got to go with my friends." Do you see the relationship in the two responses? Both participants commented about the social aspect (friends or people I know) as a reason for liking the program. Because it looks like a pattern is emerging, "social aspects" would be given a code. You would examine all of the responses for comments related to social aspects. When you find one, the code would be placed by the statement. For example, you might use a yellow highlighter to designate comments related to social aspects or you might place a unique number beside the comments. Keep in mind that there might be many different codes so choose your coding system accordingly. If a pattern continues, you will call this a theme for the group of participants. You may even find that there are concepts or subthemes within the theme. In the end, you will report the major themes and concepts and support your findings with examples of actual statements made by the participants.

The Research Report

The reporting phase of a research project may give the appearance of being the easiest part, but it can be difficult and time consuming. Be sure to allow plenty of time. In this phase, the project must be summarized and the "results" must be articulated.

The report, which is generally prepared at the end of the project, is substantial and formal. According to the National Science Foundation (1997), the report author must consider what the readers of the report need to know, how to best organize the document, how to report conclusions that are very clear as well as those that are not as definitive, and how to protect the confidentiality of the participants in the presentation of the results.

In determining the needs of your audience, you might decide that the individuals reading the report will need sufficient detail to repeat the program in exactly the same way. If this is the case, each phase of the project must be clearly delineated and thoughtful conclusions prepared. On the other hand, perhaps the audience for the report will be the press. They may be interested primarily in a summary of results and conclusions. This type of report might be shorter but no less thought-out. Of course, when you have multiple audiences, you might be called on to do both types of report. Just be patient, collect your thoughts, and prepare the needed documents.

In general, most reports include some background information, the research objectives or questions, the data-collection strategies, a description of data analysis, a listing of the results, and a discussion of conclusions. The report should be well written and interesting to read. If you have used mixed methods (a combination of several research designs), you will want to include participant comments and observations as well as statistics. Be sure to proofread, revise, and proofread again. Small errors can detract from the importance of your message. Remember, form your conclusions carefully. If your audience is in a hurry, the conclusions will be the focus of their reading.

Evaluation: A Type of Research

Health professionals frequently assume that the health of their patients, clients, or participants automatically improves as a result of the programs designed for such purposes. However, you should be aware that some health education programs don't work, or that the hoped-for changes occur as a result of something other than the program. Evaluation must be a part of the program plan. It is also a type of research.

Definition

Green and Kreuter's 1999 definition of evaluation still remains appropriate today. They define evaluation as "the comparison of an object of interest against a standard of acceptability" (p. 220). This is more easily understood when you consider that both the *object of interest* and *standards of acceptability* are identified by your program objectives. The object of interest is the behavior and the standard of acceptability is the "how much" and "when" components of the objectives. Let's look at an example from your program for teen mothers. One of your objectives might have been, "By the end of the year-long program offered by the public health educator, participants will list at least five benefits of remaining abstinent." In the subsequent evaluation, the object of interest is "list benefits of remaining abstinent" and the standard of acceptability is "at least five."

Many individuals believe that the definitions for evaluation will change according to the purpose of conducting it. For example, if cost analysis is the major purpose of the evaluation, you might be defining evaluation in terms of **cost-effectiveness** (an assessment of the program costs and how they relate to changes in impact or outcome). On the other hand, if you want to know whether program participants are satisfied with the program, you will probably define evaluation in terms of process (the way in which the program runs).

Purposes

Some common purposes of evaluation include the following:

1. To determine if program objectives have been met.
2. To see if the appropriate participants are involved in the program.

3. To make certain that the interventions match design specifications.

4. To find out what works and what does not.

5. To determine fiscal efficiency.

6. To fulfill grant or contract requirements.

7. To provide marketing material.

8. To determine if the program will work for other people beyond program participants.

9. To contribute to scientific knowledge about health education programming.

Types of Evaluation

Regardless of the purpose, all forms of evaluation fit into two major categories: formative and summative. **Formative evaluations** occur during program development and implementation. These evaluations determine the efficacy of program development and the utility of program implementation for the purpose of program improvement (McDermott & Sarvela, 1999). **Summative evaluations** occur after program completion: immediately, after a specified waiting period, or both. As you know, most health programs use process, impact, and outcome objectives. We encourage you to review these terms if they don't seem familiar to you. The types of objectives written during program development determine the specific types of evaluation used.

Process Evaluation

In chapter 7 we defined process as "a series of actions or behaviors resulting in an end." In a health education program, processes of interest might include the adequacy of the number of people attending, the suitability of the program schedule, the acceptability of program location, and the satisfaction of program participants with the program. It's important not to confuse processes with impacts or outcomes, which are the results of the program, i.e., whether participants gained knowledge or changed behaviors. Process evaluation measures how well the program fulfills the process objectives. A sample process evaluation objective might read, "Did program participants feel that the content of the program met their personal needs?"

Can you see how important it is to write clear and measurable program objectives? Your evaluation will be directly related to those objectives.

Impact Evaluation

Impact refers to aspects of health that have changed by the end of the program. Health impacts generally occur more rapidly than health outcomes. Some examples include knowledge level (in almost any health education program), weight loss (in a weight-loss program), and number of cigarettes smoked per day (in a smoking-cessation program). Sometimes health determinants or behaviors are both impacts (short-term) and outcomes (long-term) of health programs. If you choose to conduct an impact evaluation, the short-term program effects will be measured immediately after the end of the program and analyzed.

Outcome Evaluation

A health outcome provides a broader, long-term picture of health. It might refer to determinants of health such as the social and economic environment, the physical environment, and the person's individual characteristics and behaviors (World Health Organization, 2008g) but it might also include the presence or absence of a disease. Health determinants, behaviors, and even the presence of disease can be measured. If you choose an outcome evaluation, the long-term program effects will be measured and analyzed. The major difference between impact and outcome evaluations is the length of time since the program or intervention. Impacts are short-term program results while outcomes are long-term program results.

The Evaluation Plan

The evaluation plan will have its own objectives. If you think of objectives as road maps, it is easier to understand why you might want to develop them to be specific to the type of evaluation. Your evaluation objectives will be directly related to the program objectives. Imagine that your program objective stated, "The infant safety knowledge level of Rising Star participants will increase by 25% after the four classes presented by the health educator." Can you identify the objective type? It is not a process objective; it does not describe a function or process of the program. If you said impact, you are absolutely correct. The objective describes a short-term result of the program.

The evaluation objective linked to this particular program objective might state, "Measure the percentage change in infant safety knowledge between pretest and post-test for program participants." You will have evaluation objectives that link to each of your program objectives and perhaps a few more. For example, you may want to evaluate participant perceptions of whether the program was effective because if participants didn't like it, the word will probably spread and attendance at future programs might be influenced.

The types of evaluation must be clarified (process, impact, or outcome), and the research design must be determined. From this point forward, the evaluation plan will match a research plan.

Ethics in Research

The most basic ethical consideration in research is the protection of your participants. One of the first things to do is to ask them to consent to being part of the research project. Of course, you will want them to feel free to say no. They will feel less hesitant if they understand the research process and how the information will be reported, so be sure to explain the process well. Table 9.2 summarizes risk issues that must be considered in an ethical research process.

It will be important for you to minimize risks that your participants will face. Risks include those that are physical in nature as well as psychological. For example, if you are asking questions that your participants find embarrassing, you are putting them at psychological risk. If you ask them to do something that could cause injury, this puts them at physical risk. It is up to you to protect them.

Table 9.2   Ethics and Research

Honesty	Strive for honesty in all scientific communications. Honestly report data, results, methods and procedures, and publication status. Do not fabricate, falsify, or misrepresent data. Do not deceive colleagues, granting agencies, or the public.
Objectivity	Strive to avoid bias in experimental design, data analysis, data interpretation, peer review, personnel decisions, grant writing, expert testimony, and other aspects of research where objectivity is expected or required. Avoid or minimize bias or self-deception. Disclose personal or financial interests that may affect research.
Integrity	Keep your promises and agreements; act with sincerity; strive for consistency of thought and action.
Carefulness	Avoid careless errors and negligence; carefully and critically examine your own work and the work of your peers. Keep good records of research activities, such as data collection, research design, and correspondence with agencies or journals.
Openness	Share data, results, ideas, tools, resources. Be open to criticism and new ideas.
Respect for Intellectual Property	Honor patents, copyrights, and other forms of intellectual property. Do not use unpublished data, methods, or results without permission. Give credit where credit is due. Give proper acknowledgement or credit for all contributions to research. Never plagiarize.
Confidentiality	Protect confidential communications, such as papers or grants submitted for publication, personnel records, trade or military secrets, and patient records.
Responsible Publication	Publish in order to advance research and scholarship, not to advance just your own career. Avoid wasteful and duplicative publication.
Responsible Mentoring	Help to educate, mentor, and advise students. Promote their welfare and allow them to make their own decisions.
Respect for Colleagues	Respect your colleagues and treat them fairly.
Social Responsibility	Strive to promote social good and prevent or mitigate social harms through research, public education, and advocacy.
Non-Discrimination	Avoid discrimination against colleagues or students on the basis of sex, race, ethnicity, or other factors that are not related to their scientific competence and integrity.
Competence	Maintain and improve your own professional competence and expertise through lifelong education and learning; take steps to promote competence in science as a whole.
Legality	Know and obey relevant laws and institutional and governmental policies.
Animal Care	Show proper respect and care for animals when using them in research. Do not conduct unnecessary or poorly designed animal experiments.
Human Subjects Protection	When conducting research on human subjects, minimize harms and risks and maximize benefits; respect human dignity, privacy, and autonomy; take special precautions with vulnerable populations; and strive to distribute the benefits and burdens of research fairly.

From *What is Ethics in Research & Why is It Important?* by D. B. Resnik, 2007, National Institutes of Environmental Health Sciences—National Institutes of Health. Retrieved from http://www.niehs.nih.gov/research/resources/bioethics/whatis.cfm

When you write your report, present data for a group rather than results specific to individuals. If you are presenting specific comments or observations, do not use identifying information if you can avoid doing so. If a participant can be identified, get permission first. Just remember to be honest, respect your participants, and act with integrity.

In Conclusion

Research is the cornerstone for improving health; it provides the documentation and confirmation that interventions work, that patterns created by healthy behaviors exist, for understanding why people behave the way they do, and for choosing new directions in prevention. The best health education programs are developed with evaluation research in mind. We hope you will develop an understanding of rigorousness in research, which calls for appropriate designs and data-collection strategies. When you write your research plan, pay special attention to writing objectives. They should be directly linked to the problem being addressed or, in the case of evaluation, the program objectives. As part of that plan, you will also need to create a feasible timeline and a budget. Devote as much attention to the final research report as to the rest of the research process; the report will document your work. Most importantly, let ethics be your guiding light. Every decision should be informed by both an understanding of and appreciation for ethics in research.

REVIEW QUESTIONS

1. Describe and justify the steps involved in writing a research plan.
2. Discuss the importance of the categories that might be used in a research budget.
3. Select one qualitative design and discuss its strengths and weaknesses.
4. Analyze the benefits of using an experimental design.
5. Give examples of process, impact, and outcome evaluations.

FOR YOUR APPLICATION

This activity has two parts. First, develop an evaluation plan for the program you are developing in your project. If you aren't participating in a project, select or create a simple health education program and develop an evaluation plan for it. Second, write an instrument with just a few items for your evaluation. If it is a quantitative instrument, consider how you might determine reliability and validity. Ask a few friends to take the survey and analyze the results. When your evaluation plan and instrument have been graded, revise them and put them in your portfolio if you are creating one.

PART III

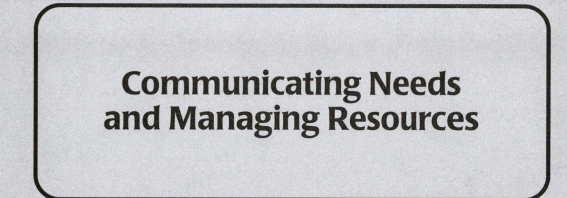

Communicating Needs and Managing Resources

Community Health Administration

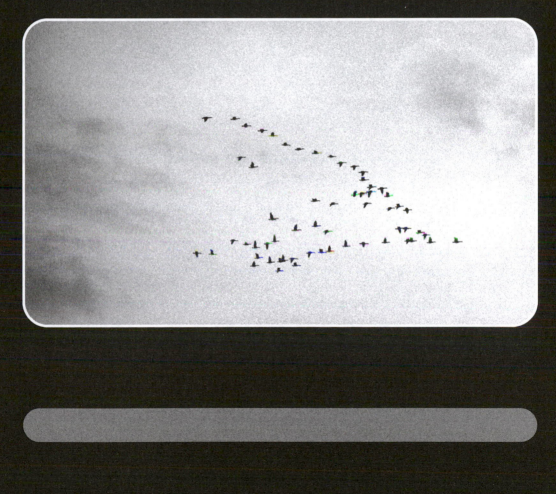

"But I thought you were going to make those phone calls!" You try to keep the exasperation out of your voice, but this is just one of many similar conversations you've had lately. It seems as though no one involved in this health program knows what anyone else is doing. What was once a good program idea, both wanted and needed by the community, is becoming an organizational nightmare. You hang up the phone and say out loud, "Where did I go wrong?" In desperation, you take out an old textbook that you never thought you'd use again. You look up the terms management, leadership, administration, and coordination.

CHAPTER OBJECTIVES

1. Detail the difference between leadership and management.
2. Identify techniques for conflict resolution.
3. Define policy and name three components.
4. Describe the difference between procedural policy and public health policy.
5. Name four federal agencies that monitor public health policy.
6. Summarize the purpose and components of the Patients' Bill of Rights.
7. Create ideas for making certain that all people have access to health care.
8. Practice writing policies.

Leadership, Management, and Administration

The magnitude of health disparities in U.S. communities, the interwoven web of causation of our most devastating diseases, and the inability of our health care system to adequately care for all of our sick underscore the importance of inspirational leadership and competent administration. John Holland of the Santa Fe Institute states that health and the health care system are "multi-layered systems largely driven by rapidly changing technology and information." He further states, "Knowing the building blocks of the organizational system and its core processes is critical. Studying the interfaces of the building blocks allows system leaders to ask questions based on the flows or patterns among the processes, identify the feedback loops, explore the interfaces, and ultimately identify an efficient system" (Holland, 2003 p. 3).

What is administration? Are leadership, administration, management, and coordination of services different terms for the same activity? Can anyone be a leader? There are a lot of questions to be answered in this chapter, and we'd like to first discuss the concept of leadership. Leaders get things started, so it's a good place for us to begin.

Leadership

Leadership research conducted in the 20th century generally focused on the leaders themselves; the traits and behaviors observed in successful leaders (Bryman,

1996). Initially, it was thought that leadership qualities were genetic. Later research seemed to indicate that leadership consisted of a set of behaviors that could be learned. Typically such behaviors focused on the transactional interaction between leaders and followers. Toward the end of the century, leadership approaches seemed to combine a number of different traits, styles, concepts, and behaviors; one of which was transformational leadership.

Transformational leadership differs from previous leadership concepts in that it focuses on the *relationship* between the leader and follower, not merely the transaction. There is an increased moral and ethical focus. Such leaders are interested in the well-being of the people being led, not just getting the job done. The transformational leader begins by determining a vision based on an understanding of the core values of the organization. Next, the leader sells the vision by developing trust with the people involved. This step may take a great deal of time, effort, and charisma. In the end, the transformational leader takes a visible role in the actual move toward the goal (Synique, 2008).

Service leadership became popular early in the 21st century. This approach utilizes a service-oriented framework in which personnel in an organization and their leaders use service activities to reach mutually determined goals. Every contact with a customer or client is seen as an opportunity to increase loyalty through providing service. Such leadership recognizes that clients are both internal and external (Gronfeldt & Strother, 2006).

In 2008, Burman and Evans published a "charter" for aviation leaders that we feel makes sense for health administrators as well. Much like health care, aviation is a field that is driven by the need for quality and excellence. According to Burman and Evans, leaders must perform the following behaviors:

• Lead by example in accordance with the company's core values.
• Build the trust and confidence of the people with whom you work.
• Continually seek improvement in methods and effectiveness.
• Keep people informed.
• Be accountable for personal actions and hold others accountable for theirs.
• Involve people, seek their views, listen actively to what they have to say and represent these views honestly.
• Be clear on what is expected, and provide feedback on progress.
• Show tolerance of people's differences and deal with their issues fairly.
• Acknowledge and recognize people for their contributions and performance.
• Weigh alternatives, consider both short- and long-term effects, and then be resolute in the decisions you make (2008, p. 10).

We believe that leadership is a fluid concept that differs by person and situation. Great leaders can be quiet and unassuming or vibrant and vocal. The two overriding traits of successful leaders are the ability to (a) envision the future and (b) motivate people into belief and action. Once a path has been selected and people are ready to move, the actual navigation is provided by managers. Managers direct people and control schedules and budgets. Leaders are not always good managers and good managers are not always leaders. Most organizations, however, need both to function effectively.

Management

Table 10.1 compares leadership and management tasks and traits. As you can see from the table, **managers** are highly involved in the day-to-day operation of an organization. They are charged with maintaining budgets, keeping schedules, maintaining optimum output, and reaching objectives. Managers are those who are responsible for the bottom line. The manager's job may be the most difficult because he or she maintains balance and flow.

Table 10.1   Leadership versus Management

Leadership	Management
Establishes vision	Controls resources
Holds a future orientation	Has a real-time orientation
Maintains a broad perspective	Focuses on details
Deals with change	Organizes activities to maintain status quo
Encourages growth	Schedules daily operations
Supports people	Directs personnel
Takes risks	Minimizes risks

Most people believe that management skills can be learned because they are task oriented. If we were to create a charter for managers, we would include the following behaviors. We hope you agree that these are skills you should have when you enter the workforce, even if you don't start as a manager.

- Manage time proficiently.
- Track activities carefully.
- Evaluate performances professionally.
- Provide clear instruction.
- Resolve disputes appropriately.
- Organize well.
- Listen actively.
- Know policies, guidelines, and rules.
- Write objectives that match organizational goals.
- Use resources efficiently.

Administration

Administration involves both leading and managing as well as coordinating support systems and activities that facilitate the effective running of an organization, institution, or program. Some of the major roles might include quality assurance, finance, human resources, facilities management, and other tasks that further the goals of the organization.

Upon graduation, most of you will work in formal organizations. These include government agencies, schools, nonprofit organizations, private practices, and health care institutions. A formal organization is one that has been established to meet a specified mission. It may consist of a small office with a few positions or numerous sites with a wide variety of departments and personnel. An organizational flow chart describes the structure of an organization, whether small or large. Figure 10.1 illustrates an organizational flow chart for a small organization.

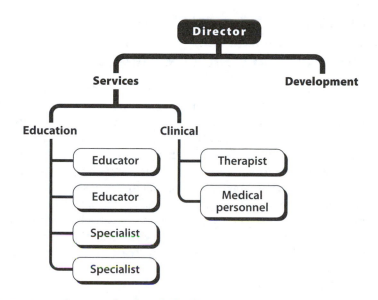

Figure 10.1   Sample organizational chart.

Viewing organizational charts and the titles of personnel can be confusing. The words *division, department, area,* and *section* may be used by different organizations to mean the same thing. On the other hand, an organization may use these terms to differentiate the size of various units or types of activities within their structure. Administrative titles are equally confusing and humorous, at times. A mid-level administrator (perhaps the administrator of a division or department) might be called *coordinator, director, manager, chair,* or even *head.* Each organization has definitions for each title. Your goal will be to understand the levels. Before you interview for a position, familiarize yourself with the organizational structure of your potential employer.

Most formal organizations exist within a bureaucratic structure in which one or more persons have been given authority to make decisions and take action. The administration of any organization may have several levels that have varying degrees of responsibility and authority. Having the authority to make decisions and take action provides power. So, power is a good thing, right? As usual, the answer is not simple. While power must be present for action to take place, power placed in the hands of an ineffective leader or manager can destroy the organization.

As you all know, there are informal organizations that exist within formal organizations. These informal groups generally represent social networks within a formal organization, and although they may not have recognized authority, they may have a great deal of power. Informal leaders may hold the key to your success as an administrator. It will be important for you to recognize and communicate with the informal leaders.

Promoting cooperation, building collaborative networks, and writing policy are important skills for administrators. We will discuss these next. Administrators also must be effective communicators. We will cover verbal and written communication in chapter 11.

Cooperation and Conflict Resolution

Promoting cooperation, enhancing collaboration, and writing policy are fundamental activities for those who administer health programming. *Cooperation* is a word most of us have heard since our early childhood, along with other phrases such as *play nicely, share, give in,* and *get along.* Most of us can probably remember a time when we were asked to cooperate, but felt that what we were really being asked was to give up some level of control and let some other person have her or his way. Because of those kinds of experiences, the idea of cooperation doesn't always excite people. Giving up control over something about which we feel strongly can be a real challenge. However, most of us can also recall a time when we received help from someone who was willing to cooperate. It's a good feeling when you experience a partnership effort that truly benefits everyone involved. It usually happens in an atmosphere of cooperation.

Promoting Cooperation

So what is cooperation? Is it really giving control to another person and following his or her lead? According to Merriam-Webster's Online (2008), **cooperation** is "to act or work with another or others: act together" or "to associate with another or others for mutual benefit." To explore the meaning of cooperation more fully, consider for a moment two important phrases in these definitions: "to act or work together/to associate" and "for mutual benefit."

If a group of people came together to build a small house, no thinking person would expect all members of the group to have the same types of house-building skills and experience. After all, an electrician who could ably wire the house would not necessarily be well-versed in plumbing. Skilled plumbers aren't always good carpenters, and carpenters may know little about applying stucco, aluminum siding, or brick to the outside walls. But each set of knowledge and skills is needed for successful house building.

These differing skills are needed at different points in the building process. One wouldn't expect the electricians to show up, for instance, until the foundation had been laid and the walls framed. If the roofers insisted on doing their job on the day the foundation was poured, we'd likely begin to worry about their competence. And though each job is important to the overall goal, each differs from the others in the length of time and amount of effort needed.

With so much diversity of effort and focus, how is the group able to achieve any common goal—much less build an entire house? In most house-building efforts, a project foreperson or contractor coordinates the project. This person usually has a blueprint of the house that illustrates how all parts are to be constructed. The contractor uses the blueprint to coordinate individual efforts, constantly checking progress in light of the master house plan. And, because the contractor is the person most aware of the contribution of each group, a full understanding and appreciation of the abilities and efforts of each is paramount to project success.

What can we learn from this illustration of cooperation in action? The concepts are very basic. First, we know that cooperation happens when everyone contributes to the project. However, oftentimes different people must do different jobs at different times, paces, and levels of effort to achieve the common goal. Misperceptions among group members about what others are contributing can lead to jealousy and resentment. A mutual understanding of group-member expectations, from the outset, is very important.

Second, we know that it helps to have a blueprint and a designated person (or group of people) responsible for coordinating the effort. This person may not necessarily complete individual tasks in the project. Nor does this person need extensive skills in all project task areas. However, the project coordinator should be someone who

- can maintain sight of the big picture and how each individual task fits
- is willing and able to maintain close contact with the project from start to finish
- has strong organization, communication, and negotiation skills
- can respectfully interact with each project contributor in a positive way

Conflict Resolution

Most of us tend to interpret the words and actions of others through the lenses of our personal values (Seelye & Seelye-James, 1996). When values and interpretations differ among individuals, misunderstandings can develop. Consider two highly qualified professionals who are collaborating on a project but have different perceptions about time and commitment. Ann tends to be task-oriented and believes that a committed professional always arrives on time. Ben highly values a cooperative approach and is less concerned about time constraints. Ann interprets Ben's late arrivals to meetings as a sign of low commitment. She decides to take a strong lead to ensure project success. Ben interprets Ann's independent decision making as controlling and aggressive. He stops attending meetings. Mistaken assumptions lead to conflict and the project flounders.

A difference in time orientation is one of the **silent value factors** that are seldom discussed but often contribute to conflict in collaborative efforts (Seelye & Seelye-James, 1996). Though such differences are often expected in cross-cultural situations, they can also influence interaction when no cultural differences are apparent. For example, using formal titles rather than first names may seem cold and distant to some people, whereas using first names can be insulting to others. Avoiding direct eye contact with a member of the other gender may seem respectful to some and devaluing to others. A lecture-based meeting presentation may appear to be the most efficient and logical approach but could cause some of your participants to suspect that you feel superior to the group and wish to control it. Understanding these potential differences is the first step to preventing **conflict**. Because time-orientation differences are a common conflict factor, we invite you to complete the checklists in FYI 10.1 as a starting point.

Resolving Differences

How can you avoid conflict that is based on value differences and misinterpretations? Communicate. Communicate clearly by using a variety of written and oral formats. Communicate often by establishing ongoing channels through which information and perceptions are exchanged. Communicate unselfishly by listening as often, or perhaps more often, than you speak. Communicate to understand. Communicate to problem-solve. Communicate to collaborate.

Communicate. But also keep in mind that, regardless of how hard you work as project coordinator to minimize the potential for conflict, it can still occur. Members

---

FYI 10.1   **Assess Your Time Orientation**

Differences in time orientation (monochronic versus polychronic) are a common conflict factor. Understanding those differences can be a first step toward conflict resolution.

How monochronic are you?

- I like to do one thing at a time.
- I concentrate on the job at hand.
- I take time commitments (deadlines, schedules) seriously.
- I am committed to the job.
- I adhere closely to plans.
- I am concerned about not disturbing others (follow rules of privacy).
- I show great respect for private property (seldom borrow or lend).
- I emphasize promptness in meetings.
- I am comfortable with short-term relationships.

How polychronic are you?

- I like to do many things at once.
- I am highly distractible and frequently interrupt what I am doing.
- I consider time commitments more of an objective to be achieved, if possible, than a quasi-legal contract.
- I am committed to people and human relationships.
- I change plans often and easily.
- I put obligations to family and friends before work concerns.
- I consider intimacy with family and friends more important than respecting their privacy.
- I borrow and lend things often and easily.
- I base the level of promptness on the particular relationship.
- I have a strong tendency to build lifetime relationships.

From *Culture Clash: Managing in a Multicultural World* (pp. 25–26), by H. N. Seelye and A. Seelye-James. © 1996. Used with permission of the McGraw-Hill Companies.

of your coalition, task force, or advisory board may agree with the overall goals of the collaborative effort, but strongly differ when it comes to decisions about how to approach a task, the time frame in which it will happen, the location of task events, or who will be involved. What do you do when the cause of the conflict isn't miscommunication but rather disagreement about the process or expected outcomes? The first step is to gain an understanding of the cause of the conflict, what motivates each person involved to disagree.

People often become involved in conflict because they are stakeholders in relation to the argument issue. A **stakeholder** is a person or organization who will likely gain or lose something as a result of the targeted health problem and the efforts made to reduce it. In decision-making situations, most stakeholders are motivated at least in part by what they and the people they represent stand to gain or lose through the decision. That isn't necessarily a bad thing. A diverse representation of community stakeholders can serve as a healthy set of checks and balances in the decision-making process. The protected welfare of various community groups often depends on advocates who look out for their interests. It is likely, however, that some members of such a diverse decision-making group will disagree from time to time. When that happens, your goal as project coordinator will be to facilitate appropriate discussions and negotiations so that the project progresses and, to the extent possible, all groups benefit.

How strong are your negotiation skills? Have you ever attempted to resolve differences between people you care about? If so, you may have concluded that at least one person seemed more interested in personal well-being than the good of all involved. Getting someone like that person to cooperate can be an intellectually and emotionally draining task and you may be tempted to use some choice adjectives such as *stubborn, selfish,* and *impossible* in the process.

If you've had a similar experience, you can probably relate to the dilemma some project coordinators face. The ideal is to resolve the conflict in a way that allows all parties involved to reach a mutually satisfying solution. FYI 10.2 contains tips for conflict resolution (Espinoza, personal communication, August 2008). One step refers to a technique known as **active listening**, or **reflective listening**. In this technique,

FYI 10.2   Tips for Dispute Resolution

DO	DON'T
• Know that conflict is normal and healthy.	• Think that everyone responds to conflict in the same way.
• Realize that differences may not be as great as perceived.	• Respond purely on emotion.
• Try on the other hat—listen.	• Suppose that you know everything.
• Be creative in considering resolutions.	• Deem that your truth is the only truth.
• Watch for potential conflict and understand it before it escalates.	• Believe that conflict resolution is simple.

each person involved in the discussion is required to orally paraphrase or repeat back what was just said by the other person. The purpose of this exercise is for each person to focus on the thoughts and feelings of others rather than on his or her own personal reactions or interpretations. The person whose statements have been paraphrased is then given the opportunity to correct mistaken interpretations and elaborate for deeper understanding.

In our example, Ann and Ben could use active listening to discuss their frustrations and seek conflict resolution. For instance, Ann might say, "Ben, I don't think you are really committed to this project and it frustrates me." Ben's reflective response could be, "You don't think I care about the project? What makes you think that?" Ann might then launch into a description of how Ben is always late for meetings and doesn't seem to care about deadlines. At this point, Ben could respond in at least two different ways. He could abandon the active listening technique, become defensive, and react. On the other had, he could take a deep breath and attempt to focus on Ann's reasoning and feelings rather than his own. In doing so, his response could be more reflective. "Ann, until now, I didn't realize that my 'late arrivals' irritated you. It isn't because I don't care. It's just that traffic holds me up. Besides, I've been thinking that you don't really want my input on this."

It would then be Ann's turn to paraphrase rather than react. A reflective response would be, "Why do you think I don't want your input?" This would allow Ben to explain how hurt he felt when Ann moved ahead on decisions without him, and two mature professionals would have the opportunity to view the situation through the eyes of the other.

Their new appreciation for each other's perspective could then be applied in the next resolution step, finding mutual ground for agreement. In our example, both individuals agree on the importance of the project, which implies that they share mutual goals. A return to common goals reminds individuals that they are partners rather than adversaries. Competition can then give way to flexible collaboration.

Because Ben and Ann share a common goal, they can collaborate in order to reach it. They might, for example, alter meeting schedules and locations to reduce Ben's traffic barriers. Ben could commit to leaving his home earlier and Ann could agree to be more flexible and work on other projects should Ben be late. The two could agree to identify and work toward important deadlines, but adopt a more flexible approach to less time-dependent tasks.

The individual strengths of each person could also be applied more effectively to different aspects of the project. Ben's strengths might be in interacting with other people who are important to project success, while Ann might prefer to take on greater responsibility for needed organizational aspects. The two could learn to trust each other more in these responsibilities, respect and appreciate the asset inherent in their differences, and communicate more freely to prevent future misunderstandings. The approach would not guarantee consistently smooth interaction, but effective collaboration could hardly occur without it. The same concepts of individual collaboration and conflict resolution can be applied to group and community settings. Although the processes become more complex in broader interactive settings, some of the same principles apply.

Community Development

Think back for a moment to other chapters in which we've discussed the definitions and roles of communities in health education. By now you have had the opportunity to explore concepts of how individuals within a community form bonds driven by values, interests, needs, and capacities. We hope you appreciate how important it is to partner with the community from the earliest stages of the needs assessment and to maintain community connections throughout program planning, implementation, and evaluation. If so, you may have reached the same conclusion that many in our profession hold: A community that has the power to create its own solutions is the most likely to have success in improving the quality of life of its members.

If community building and empowerment are so important, can they be fostered? The health professionals involved must hold the philosophy that community connectedness serves as a foundation. The strategies selected must be geared toward building community, not just isolating a problem or two in the community as targets for health programs. And, significantly, the community must possess the capacity to become involved in the process. One of your first goals may be to help the community become aware of its existing competencies so that it can capitalize on strengths and rectify gaps. Community-based participatory research or action research, discussed in chapter 9, may be an effective method for identifying community strengths. Other practical community building and organization suggestions are listed in FYI 10.3 on the following page.

But, wait a minute! Didn't we tell you in an earlier chapter that the health problems you are hired to address will likely be dictated by agency missions and available grant money? How can you reconcile the need to target pre-designated goals with what we've said here about beginning with community concerns? It is possible that the agency decision makers who set those targets are quite aware of the need for community ownership and, before you were hired, set the wheels in motion for effective community partnerships. You should be able to learn a lot by talking to your superiors and coworkers, along with community members, to understand how decisions were made.

If you find that the community was not involved in the decision-making process, the concepts and methods of community organization and building should still be applied. You can begin talking about the targeted health problem with various community groups and gatekeepers, along with representatives of other agencies and community health organizations. Ask for their perceptions about the extent of the problem and potential community-based solutions. If awareness of the problem is lacking, awareness-building messages can be disseminated through the media, town hall meetings, pamphlets, health fairs, presentations to organizations, and focus groups. The time and effort you invest to gain community support will be well worth it in the long run. Without it, your programs may be viewed in the community as just another come-and-go event that is best ignored.

Coalitions

Once community support is in place, there are other steps you can take to further develop community organization and foster community building. The asset-mapping and capacity-building efforts should help identify community agencies and organiza-

FYI 10.3   **Community Building and Organization Suggestions**

Following these community building and organization suggestions can help a community identify its own health problems and potential solutions.

Support community issues	Start where the community is, and let community members make the decisions. Be a catalyst or facilitator of those decisions, not a decision maker.
Foster issue awareness	Talk with various groups of community members to raise awareness levels. Offer ideas for how community members might convert concerns into action.
Expedite information collection	Provide information about where to access resources. If needed, be willing to research information and pass it on to community members.
Develop community competence	Identify natural leaders and helpers within the community. Help them identify and tap into their own networks of support. Encourage and support collective problem solving and resource development. Emphasize capacity building and assets mapping.
Advocate for the community	In staff meetings or other settings in which community members are not present, speak on their behalf in a supportive, respectful manner.
Mediate when negotiation is needed	When needed, help resolve differences between community stakeholders by emphasizing the mutual benefits of cooperation and negotiating mutually acceptable compromise to reach common goals.

Derived from *Community Health Education: Settings, Tools, and Skills for the 21st Century,* by D. J. Breckon, J. R. Harvey, and R. B. Lancaster, 1998, Gaithersburg, MD: Aspen; and "Improving Health Through Community Organization and Community Building," by M. Winkler and N. Wallerstein, 1997, in K. Glanz, F. M. Lewis, and B. K. Rimer, *Health Behavior and Health Education: Theory, Research, and Practice* (pp. 241–269), San Francisco: Jossey-Bass.

tions other than the one in which you work that could contribute to and benefit from collaborating on community health projects. Shared ideas and resources can streamline costs, reduce duplication, and improve the quality of resulting programs (Payne, 1999). For these reasons, we encourage you to consider forming a coalition.

A health **coalition** is a "group of individuals and/or organizations with a common interest who agree to work together toward a common goal" (KU Work Group, 2007b). Coalitions are often formally structured with written goals and designated responsibilities (Parker et al., 1998). They can be useful throughout all aspects of a community health effort, offering guidelines and resources for everything from needs assessment to program evaluation (KU Work Group, 2007b). It is important, however, that specific coalition tasks remain consistent with designated goals.

One way of using a coalition in an effective manner is to ask its members to brainstorm a list of immediate and long-range objectives and tasks that, if accomplished, can help the coalition meet its goals. For example, consider a fictitious coalition whose primary goal is to reduce the incidence of HIV infection among adolescents in the community. There are several different tasks or projects a coalition could initiate to help accomplish this goal. Among them could be a needs assessment to identify HIV/AIDS-related attitudes, knowledge, and risk behaviors among local adolescents; an HIV/AIDS awareness campaign through local newspapers and radio and television stations; a telephone AIDS hotline to which adolescents could call to ask questions; and an HIV testing and referral program that adolescents could readily access. Each of these activities would match the coalition goal of reducing the incidence of HIV infection. Each could be carried out over time and, in some cases, simultaneously if varying clusters of coalition members served as leaders and members of subgroup task forces.

A coalition of this breadth would require careful coordination and consistent communication among coalition members. Each task force would need clearly communicated directives, specific objectives, and designated deadlines by which a particular task objective should be met. Consistent periodic coalition meetings, with task-force reports requested at each meeting, provide the accountability check needed to encourage progress. The person asked to coordinate this effort could be you.

Keep in mind that coalitions aren't always a good choice. Coalitions can help you accomplish more than you could within the capacity of your single agency and community contacts. However, coordinating a coalition usurps a large amount of time, energy, and resources. And barriers to progress can arise within coalitions if individual members push personal agendas or continue to react negatively to earlier problems with other coalition members. So, before you form one, carefully consider its usefulness and cost in light of your community's intended objectives. Invest the time needed to learn all you can about potential coalition members and how they are viewed by the community before inviting them to the table.

Partnerships

In some instances, a coalition may be deemed less desirable than a simpler partnership established between your agency and a single community group or organization. The political lines and historical perspectives are often less complicated in these types of partnerships. Thus, progress on designated tasks can, in some ways, advance more quickly. However, the simpler partnership approach can also reduce the scope of what you are able to accomplish because you will have fewer resources and contacts.

A partnership with a community organization is a good place to start when the goal can be adequately accomplished through the partnership capacities. You and your partner organization can establish clearly stated objectives and initiate important tasks. Then, as the work progresses and the need for broader involvement arises, other groups can be invited to join in your well-established efforts. The guidelines in Figure 10.2 can help you establish a strong partnership from the beginning.

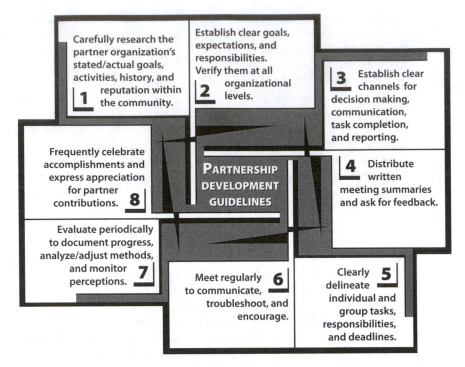

Figure 10.2   Guidelines for establishing effective partnerships.
These guidelines can facilitate mutually beneficial outcomes.

The Role of Policy in Administration and Coordination

When was the last time you heard someone mention the word *policy* in a conversation? You might have been in a department store attempting to return some merchandise. Or you could have been in your supervisor's office asking why changes couldn't be made. If you've ever been told you couldn't do something because it would violate a policy, you may be tempted to think the purpose of any policy is to make life difficult. Yet, despite occasional frustrations, most of us recognize that, when needed, a carefully developed and applied policy has its merits.

Policy Defined

Westerinen (2003) defines **policy** as "a definite goal, course, or method of action to guide and determine present and future directions" (p. 3). This definition is relatively easy to use because it touches on two important characteristics of a policy: goals and guidance. Policies provide the guidance or direction for reaching goals.

Procedural Policy

An organization's **procedural policy** is the set of rules and regulations by which an institution or organization operates. Procedural policy serves as a guideline for *how* things are accomplished. For example, suppose you worked in a hospital patient education program and had a great idea for a health education program you'd like to develop for the hospital's employees. How would you go about gaining permission to develop it? And, if permission were granted, would there be rules about using hospital time versus your own time to work on it? Where would you go to gain access to supplies and other resources? Who would need to see memos about its development and who would sign off on important papers and contracts? The answers to such questions would depend on organizational regulations, the procedural policies that guide such things as how decisions are made, resources are requisitioned, tasks are accomplished, and reports are disseminated.

Procedural policies often focus only on how tasks are to be accomplished. They don't always explain *why* the task should be initiated in the first place. Examining the reason for the task or health program takes us back to Westerinen's policy definition, which included goals as part of a policy's driving force. Adding an objective component to the definition creates a more complete perspective on policies and policy development. Objectives that are clearly stated in an organization's written policies help justify the health services and promotion programs provided by that organization. They help organizational decision makers stay on track as they make choices about how they will use precious resources to improve health and quality of life in their communities.

Public Health Policy

Developing policy to help decision makers stay on track also works at the national level. Many national initiatives to enhance the well-being of U.S. citizens begin as national policies. National policies do not have to be health-specific to have an impact on our nation's health. Policies that affect housing, education, and crime control, for example, influence the health and well-being of U.S. citizens.

Federal Policy Makers

Specific components of the federal government direct and monitor health-specific policy development. As we have stated in previous chapters, the Department of Health and Human Services holds primary responsibility for national health services and initiatives in the United States. The department's programs are administered by eleven operating divisions, including eight agencies in the U.S. Public Health Service and three human services agencies. National health policies are largely generated and maintained within this organization through its agencies. One of those, the Health Resources and Services Administration (HRSA), directs health policy initiatives and service programs to underserved and special-needs populations, through six bureaus and twelve offices. "HRSA is the nation's access agency—improving health and saving lives by making sure the right services are available in the right places at the right time" (HRSA, n.d.).

The Centers for Disease Control and Prevention promote health policy as it relates to prevention initiatives for specific health issues, such as chronic disease prevention, environmental health, and injury prevention. CDC works directly with health departments and other partners to research public health concerns that could impact health policy issues. They respond to federal policy makers with the following services: "rapid and reliable response to congressional requests for information; congressional briefings on broad public health issues and specific CDC programs; technical assistance on public health policy and legislative initiatives; CDC materials, services, and tours of facilities, including new state-of-the-art labs; discussions with scientific experts on programs of interest; participation by agency leadership and scientific experts in local public health-related events; and e-mail updates on key CDC topics" (CDC, 2006b).

The Agency for Healthcare Research and Quality (AHRQ) supports research and subsequent policy development that improves the quality of health care, reduces health care costs, and broadens health service access. It also provides evidence-based information on health care outcomes and quality of care. AHRQ's User Liaison Program helps state and local health policy makers by providing research results through various formats such as workshops, electronic courses, and teleconferences. FYI 10.4 summarizes an online education program for new legislators offered by AHRQ.

The United States Food and Drug Administration (FDA) works to keep foods, drugs, medical instruments, and other products safe. The Center for Food Safety and Applied Nutrition (CFSAN), part of the FDA, oversees a research program that provides information for regulatory decisions and the development of policies (FDA, n.d.). Information about other agencies can be found in Appendix E.

FYI **10.4**   **Educational Program Offered by the Agency for Healthcare Research and Quality (AHRQ)**

Introduction to State Health Policy: A Seminar for New State Legislators

This nonpartisan seminar was designed to provide an overview of major health policy issues facing state legislators who are new to health policy issues.

Presentations

Session 1: Roles of State Legislatures and State Government in Determining Health Policy

Session 2: State Roles in Regulating Health Care Markets: Balancing Cost, Access, and Quality

Session 3: Quality and Cost: Achieving Value in Today's Health Care System

Session 4: Understanding the Importance of Public Health

Session 5: Providing Access to Care, Part I: The Uninsured and the Health Care Safety Net

Session 6: Hot Issues in Health Care: Focus on Medicaid and SCHIP

Session 7: Health Care Workforce Issues

Session 8: The Crisis in Medical Malpractice Insurance

Session 9: Prescription Drugs

Session 10: Cost, Quality, and Access: Providing Long-term Care Services to an Increasingly Elderly and Chronically Ill Population

From Agency for Healthcare Research and Quality, n.d., "Introduction to State Health Policy: A Seminar for New State Legislators," held March 31–April 3, 2005. Retrieved August 8, 2008, from http://www.ahrq.gov/news/ulpix.htm

Policies and the Legislature

Public policies are often put into effect as a law, ordinance, or resolution (Breckon, 1997). Ideas for legislated health policy initiatives can originate from a variety of sources, including members of Congress, the executive branch, committees, government health agencies, voluntary health agencies, special interest groups, and many other sources.

Once introduced as a bill, a health-related policy initiative will be submitted to a legislative committee that will likely conduct hearings on the proposed bill and, subsequently, rewrite, amend, approve, or reject the bill. A bill that has been approved by a committee is then placed before the Senate or House of Representatives for consideration. A number of health agencies and organizations are actively involved in efforts to influence health policy legislation. In chapter 12 we will explore this advocacy process in more detail.

Patients' Bill of Rights

A health policy concern that received national attention was the concept of protecting patients' rights in relation to health care (Reardon, 1999). In 1998, President Clinton directed the Department of Health and Human Services and other federal agencies to comply with the Consumer or Patients' Bill of Rights (USDHHS, 1998). As can be noted in FYI 10.5 (on the following page), these rights focus on accessibility to quality health care. Late in the 20th century there appeared to be a growing sentiment that current managed health care initiatives were not working and that drastic measures were needed to return the power of health care decision making to the doctor and patient rather than health maintenance organizations (HMOs) (Online News-Hour, 1999; Reardon, 1999). Congress passed a law in 1999 to allow patients to sue their HMOs if they were refused needed health care. In the wake of that legislation, some HMOs voluntarily relinquished the health care decision-making power back to physicians (Online NewsHour, 1999).

The Uninsured

A current concern for policy makers lies with the number of employers who are dropping or decreasing health insurance benefits. According to the Kaiser Family Foundation (2004), "Almost 45 million Americans were uninsured in 2003, growing by 1.4 million from the previous year and a total over 5 million since 2000. The proportion of Americans with employer-sponsored insurance continued to decline for the fourth consecutive year in 2003, driving both the share and number who are uninsured upward." Unfortunately, uninsured individuals are the most likely to be in poor health (Kaiser Family Foundation, 2004). Lack of insurance promotes delays in seeking medical attention, a lower likelihood of filling prescriptions or taking medications as frequently as prescribed, and fewer expenditures on preventive strategies. Health professionals and political leaders alike need to create policies that will impact health insurance issues in ways that will produce tangible health benefits.

The Process of Policy Development

National public health policies serve as guidelines for establishing health program priorities in the United States. For instance, a law that provides health insurance for

FYI 10.5   Patients' Bill of Rights

The Patients' Bill of Rights focuses on accessibility to quality health care among health care consumers.

1. Consumers have the right to receive accurate, easily understood information and some require assistance in making informed health care decisions about their health plans, professionals, and facilities.

2. Consumers have the right to a choice of health care providers that is sufficient to ensure access to appropriate high-quality health care.

3. Consumers have the right to access emergency health services when and where the need arises.

4. Consumers have the right and responsibility to fully participate in all decisions related to their health care.

5. Consumers have the right to considerate, respectful care from all members of the health care system at all times and under all circumstances.

6. Consumers must not be discriminated against in the delivery of health care services consistent with the benefits covered in their policy or as required by law based on race, ethnicity, national origin, religion, sex, age, mental or physical disability, sexual orientation, genetic information, or source of payment.

7. Consumers who are eligible for coverage . . . must not be discriminated against in marketing and enrollment practices based on race, ethnicity, national origin, religion, sex, age, mental or physical disability, sexual orientation, genetic information, or source of payment.

8. Consumers have the right to communicate with health care providers in confidence and to have the confidentiality of their individually identifiable health care information protected.

9. Consumers have the right to a fair and efficient process for resolving differences with their health plans, health care providers, and the institutions that serve them, including a rigorous system of internal review and an independent system of external review.

From *Report to the Vice President of the United States: Status of Implementation of the Consumer Bill of Rights and Responsibilities in the Department of Health and Human Services*, U.S. Dept. of Health and Human Services, 1998 (Nov. 2). Retrieved November 15, 1999, from http://aspe.os.dhhs./gov/health/vpreport.htm

uninsured American children (State Children's Health Insurance Program administered by the Centers for Medicare and Medicaid Services), is a direct outcome of public health policies. But why do those specific policies exist and how were they developed?

Decision Making

The *Healthy People* 2000, 2010, and 2020 goals, described in chapter 1, are products of national health policies. But why did the policy developers target the specific health problems described in those documents? Health policies have historically been driven by economic, social, and political concerns (Ibrahim, 1985). Epidemiological statistics such as mortality and morbidity rates are often categorized by demographic characteristics (such as age, gender, ethnicity, and socioeconomic status) to identify groups at risk. The impact of existing health services and programs on the health status of these groups is also considered. And, in some instances, a politically influential figure can be instrumental in swaying policy decisions (Ibrahim, 1985). These three components (existing needs, current program impact, and available support) are important considerations in any effort to develop health policies.

Most new policies are developed because someone perceived a need for change. Perhaps you have recently benefited from a new university policy that expanded library operation hours. Why would university officials put such a policy in effect when they know it will cost more money? It is because they have considered your needs. But how did they know you needed those changes? We hope they didn't guess. The appropriate approach would have been to survey a representative sample of students to find out about library access needs and interests, consult with library administrators to assess their perceptions of need and feasibility, and test the newly designed service to observe the degree to which the change would make a difference. These actions would be taken before the proposed policy was officially enacted to ensure a *cost-effective* approach.

In the same manner, health policy development should be based on sound needs-assessment efforts and careful interpretation of the results. A scientific investigation into existing health status and needs in a population is the first critical component of policy development. Perceived needs among population members and the professionals who deliver health programs should be identified in this step.

Second, the availability of resources and the feasibility of being able to maintain the proposed policies must also be considered. The overwhelming list of needs within some communities can confuse policy developers. The goal is to develop policies that reflect a balanced perspective, one that considers actual and perceived needs in light of service feasibility.

This balanced perspective can then help you move to the third component of policy development, that of soliciting support from those who have the resources and political influence to assist with policy adoption. We will discuss this issue more fully in chapter 12 when we address advocacy concepts. For now, it is sufficient to know that political power is a critical component of policy development and adoption.

Writing Policy

Green and Kreuter (1999) state that a well-written policy has three components: "(a) the clear statement of a problem (or potential problems) that needs attention, (b) a goal to mitigate or prevent that problem, and (c) a set of strategic actions to accomplish that goal" (p. 386). With those three requirements in mind, where would you begin in the process of policy development? Assume, for a moment, that you work for a large manufacturing company where many of the employees smoke cigarettes. The company decision makers have already identified the problem, which is that employees are smoking on the job. You've been asked to write a policy that addresses the problem.

Your statement of the problem could be written in a number of ways, as long as it identifies the problem of smoking employees. The second part of the policy, a goal to mitigate or reduce the problem, would likely include a statement about reducing the frequency of smoking on the job or creating a smoke-free environment. The third part, the set of strategic actions needed to accomplish that goal, would likely be difficult to put into effect, especially if you realized that any policy you created could upset some of the employees.

The nature of the policy you would develop and strategies used to implement it would greatly depend on your philosophy and goal. If your ultimate goal is to have no smokers on the payroll, your strategic approach could embrace quick, drastic action, such as posting no-smoking signs throughout the building and automatically firing any employee caught violating the rule. If, on the other hand, you desire to keep smokers in your employ but still maintain a smoke-free environment, you might take a more gradual approach that provides advance notice to employees, designated smoking areas, and smoking cessation classes for employees who smoke. Your goal would dictate your policy and how you applied it.

In Conclusion

Whether or not your title is that of manager, we encourage you to continually build skills in the areas of time management, project tracking, dispute resolution, organizing, listening, interpreting policy, and allocating resources. These are skills that will help you succeed in any job. When it comes time for you to assume a leadership role, we hope you will lead by example, build trust, tolerate differences, communicate effectively, recognize accomplishments, assure quality, and make resolute decisions.

The concept of synergism illustrates how we view the connection between leadership, cooperation, and policy development; that is, the combined partnership efforts of collaborating parties produces a greater result than the sum of efforts independently exerted by each party. Effective coordination of health programs and services is dependent on a collaborative effort toward policy development and goal attainment. Your efforts toward these goals may not always produce the desired effect and, even when they do, the results sometimes emerge very slowly. However, even in small, gradual increments, collaboration can be effective.

REVIEW QUESTIONS

1. Write an essay that compares and contrasts leadership and management and explains why they are both important.
2. Describe the process of cooperation and how to promote it.
3. Identify techniques for conflict resolution.
4. List ways in which coalitions and partnerships can be developed.
5. Define policy and name its three components.
6. Describe the difference between procedural and public health policy.
7. Name four federal agencies that monitor public health policy.
8. Summarize the purpose and components of the Patients' Bill of Rights.
9. Write a procedural or public health policy for your community.

☞ FOR YOUR APPLICATION

Creating a Community Coalition

Select a local age- or ethnicity-specific community and a health problem it faces. Use your project community if applicable. Create a proposal for a coalition whose primary goal would be to address the health problem in the community you selected. Your proposal should include:

- A coalition mission statement and goals. Each goal should represent a specific project or task needed to accomplish the stated mission.
- A list of potential strategies needed to accomplish each goal.
- A list of national and/or state organizations or agencies that could provide support.
- A list of local organizations, agencies, institutions, and other community groups that could provide support.
- A timeline for the coalition to follow in completing designated tasks.

When your coalition assignment has been graded and revised, place it in your portfolio if you are preparing a portfolio.

Communicating
Health Information

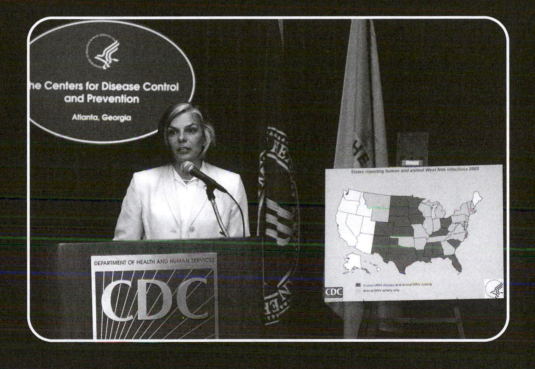

The teenager shifts her baby to the other hip and opens the pamphlet you just handed to her. "Oh, how she needs this information," you think to yourself. But will the pamphlet convince her to get her baby immunized? Did the explanation you gave make sense to her? She's so young and has much to learn about parenting. There are other needs in her life that impact the decisions she makes about the health of her child. The few minutes you have to convince her to come back next week are fading, and it appears that it is the information you can share verbally that will truly make an impact. You feel that every word counts. So, what do you say and how do you say it effectively?

CHAPTER OBJECTIVES

1. Specify the skills necessary for effective communication.
2. Practice effective communication skills.
3. Name and describe each component of the health communication model.
4. Name and give an example of each of the six stages of health communication.
5. Explain the difference between persuasive communication and coercion.
6. Discuss the role media advocacy plays in health education.
7. Explore reasons why health literacy is so important.
8. Critique examples of health education print materials.
9. Practice using the SMOG technique to determine the reading level of text-based health education materials.
10. Develop a plan for health communication.
11. Describe effective writing tips.
12. Identify effective speaking techniques.

Effective Communication

"This is your brain. This is your brain on drugs." You might be old enough to remember this common slogan from the 1987 national antinarcotics campaign by Partnership for a Drug-Free America (PDFA). The campaign used television and print ads to communicate an antidrug message to millions of young people. The PDFA's first 15-second television PSA (public service announcement) showed a woman who held up an egg and said, "This is your brain," before picking up a frying pan and adding, "This is drugs." She then cracks open the egg, fries the contents, and says, "This is your brain on drugs." Finally she looks up at the camera and asks, "Any questions?" A shorter version of this, simply showing a close-up of an egg dropping into a frying pan and the sound of it sizzling in the pan, was used a few years later. The phrase "this is your brain . . ." worked its way into popular culture and was aired on MTV, parodied on popular sitcoms of the times like *Married with Children*, and mimicked on shows like *Saturday Night Live* and cartoons like *The Far Side*. The "Fried Egg" TV message was so popular it was printed and spoofed on T-shirts, record labels, posters, and bumper stickers (PDFA, 2006). Although some teens felt "turned off" by the scare tactic approach (Alexander, 2000), the message had staying power in the media and it evolved into a more sophisticated PSA in 1998, showing how drugs could destroy individuals both emotionally and physically (see FYI 11.1).

FYI **11.1** **The PDFA's Behind-the-Scenes Look at the Creation of the Campaign Advertisement for "The Egg" PSA**

The Partnership's "Fried Egg" spot, *"This is your brain. This is your brain on drugs. Any questions?"* has been updated by Margeotes/Fertitta Partners, Inc., for PDFA. While the original spot (created in 1987) was aimed at general drug use, the strategy behind the new version is to deglamorize the use of heroin. Graham Turner, creative director at Margeotes/Fertitta Partners, Inc., calls the endeavor, "a good idea made great—all for free."

In "Frying Pan," a young woman holding a cast-iron pan says, 'This is your brain." She places an egg on a kitchen counter saying, "This is heroin." Lifting the pan over her head, she continues, "This is what happens to your brain after snorting heroin." After she smashes the egg with the frying pan, she proceeds to destroy dishes, glasses and everything else in her way as she screams, "This is what your family goes through, and your friends, and your money, and your job and your self-respect and your future." Tossing the frying pan back onto the stove she looks directly into the camera and, of course, asks, "Any questions?"

Though the spot was originally written with a male actor in mind, the director, Eden Tyler, decided it would be more powerful with an actress. Rachel Leigh Cook, Tyler says, "wanted to get on board because it was such a great cause." The spot was shot in Los Feliz, CA, in one day. "We went through a lot of glassware and clocks, we trashed the house and had a lot of fun," said Tyler. "It was an honor to revitalize the original concept."

From the Spring 1998 newsletter of the National Youth Anti-Drug Media Campaign. Accessed April 12, 2008, from http://www.mediacampaign.org/newsletter/spring98/update-04.html. © Partnership for a Drug-Free America.

Partnership for a Drug Free America won several honors for its creative "Fried Egg" campaign (Alexander, 2000). With a short, straightforward message, its creators were able to heighten awareness of the physical and psychological impact of drugs on the brain and the human spirit. This example demonstrates the power of communication and how clear, concise, and relevant health messages can "mobilize communities and individuals to adopt healthy behaviors, direct policy makers' attention to important health issues, and frame those issues for public debate and resolution" (Harvard School of Public Health, n.d., para. 1).

As we've mentioned in previous chapters, effective communication plays a vital role in the diffusion of a health behavior or innovation. Moreover, it is pivotal in collaboration and conflict-resolution efforts. We've also discussed the usefulness of careful and culturally sensitive communication in a variety of health education efforts (see FYI 11.2). However, we have not yet addressed the issue of what communication *is* and how you can use it to be an effective health educator.

FYI **11.2   Health Communication: Related Topics in This Text**

Chapter	Health Communication Topic
2, 4	Communication styles (of traditional cultures)
6	Community participation and capacity building
8	Social marketing, health literacy, multiple intelligences, and theory of the diffusion of innovation
9	Research reports
10	Collaboration and conflict resolution
11	Communication models, communication strategies and principles, cultural communication, and health literacy
12	Advocating for health
13	Obtaining accurate information from resources

Communication Defined

Communication is the process of transmitting ideas and information (KU Work Group, 2007f). Communication is a vital component of community health, especially as it relates to health education. It permeates every area of responsibility and can become your most valuable tool as you interact with community members to conduct needs assessments and plan, implement, and evaluate programs. It is particularly important in the process of community capacity building, which we described in chapters 2 and 6, because you may need it to help community members raise community awareness about an existing health problem, influence public opinion about the need to address the problem, and mobilize support from institutional, political, and community leaders and stakeholders (Harvard School of Public Health, n.d., para. 1).

Accurate Communication

"I communicated to him that I was going to finish the job. He just didn't listen!" You can probably imagine the tone of frustration that accompanied this statement. Few things are more irritating than to believe you have successfully communicated with another person, only to later discover that the person didn't understand at all. Do you think whomever our speaker is referring to simply didn't listen? It's possible. Picture two people, Vanessa and Tyson, who are busily putting away groceries. Vanessa talks as she works. Tyson interjects a few "um-hums" here and there as he places cans on a shelf. What Vanessa doesn't realize is that, for some reason, Tyson isn't hearing what she thinks he hears. Days later, Vanessa discovers through a friend that Tyson did not believe she had told him about her plans and reacted negatively when she carried them out. Miscommunication led to misunderstanding, and problems resulted.

There could be a number of reasons for this miscommunication, including the actions, thoughts, and cultural norms of both people involved. True communication depends on both the giver and the receiver of a message. The absence of clear communication can quickly lead you astray when you are attempting to serve as a resource person or program coordinator (Seelye & Seelye-James, 1996). Miscommunication can foster frustration and resentment and destroy important working relationships. It can result in wasted time and resources when you have to backtrack and reconstruct project components. It can also affect your credibility in the community and reduce community members' motivation to become involved.

Accurate, effective communication is also important within the context of the basic philosophies of community health that we discussed in earlier chapters. If the primary goal of community health was to force people to do what we believe is best for them, the communication process would be simple. We would merely need to clearly state what we expect from people and graphically describe the consequences for those who do not comply. We would not need an entire chapter focused on communication because most people are already familiar with how direct orders are communicated.

We do need this chapter, however, because community health is not primarily about enforcing directives. It is, instead, about helping people to help themselves. From this perspective, the focus isn't on you, the health professional, and your expectations. *The decision-making power lies in the hands of the people you serve.* Their beliefs, expectations, values, desires, and concerns will ultimately dictate their health-related behavior. Your role is to facilitate healthy decisions by providing information, resource access, and guidance as needed. And, in some instances, you may also discover a need to persuade, motivate, and encourage healthy choices.

That's why community health professionals rely on effective communication. Designing something intended to communicate—like the immunization pamphlet given to the young mother in our opening scenario—can be a challenge. How do you persuade a young woman whose life views are different from yours that the temporary discomfort of an injection is a good thing if it protects her baby from disease? You already know the answer. It begins with effective communication. Effective communication depends not only on the people involved but also on the nature and quality of the message itself and the channel through which the message is delivered. The process is a bit more complex than it first appears. To understand it more clearly, we introduce you to a useful model.

Health Communication Model

Jerrold Greenberg (2003) is a well-known health educator who has contributed much to what is known in the field about the process of health communication. His **health communication model** illustrates how communication works (Figure 11.1). On the surface, the communication process seems simple. The *sender* (Vanessa in our illustration) attempts to convey a *message* (that she plans to do something) through a communication *medium,* or channel of message delivery (orally, as she puts away groceries), to the *receiver* (Tyson). That sounds straightforward enough, doesn't it? How-

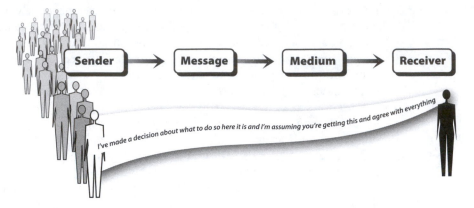

Figure 11.1 Health communication model.
This model shows a linear flow of health communication that reminds us to consider factors that influence each component and shape the degree to which clear, effective communication occurs. Adapted from *Health Education: Learner-Centered Instructional Strategies*, 5th ed., by J. S. Greenberg, 2003, New York: McGraw-Hill.

ever, if the process is so simple, why does miscommunication occur? Let's explore the possibilities as they relate to each of the four model components.

Sender

Have you ever been totally certain that you said something in a particular way only to discover later that what you said and what you thought you said were two different things? Perhaps you made a statement in conversation and immediately realized that your wording conveyed something other than what you intended. Such situations can be embarrassing, but they are a useful example of how the sender plays an important role in the communication process.

How the sender processes information, decides upon the message to be conveyed, and formulates the message to be expressed are critical to message development. Possible contributing factors to the miscommunication in our illustration may have included inconsistencies between what Vanessa intended to say or believed she said and what she actually stated. A clearly communicated message begins with careful decision making and message construction on the part of the sender.

Before we move on to the second component of the model, let's discuss who the sender is in most health situations. Greenberg (2003) points out that most community health educators think of themselves as the message senders. After all, we are the ones hired to communicate health education messages. But isn't the sender also considered the originator of the message? The sender in our illustration certainly originated her message about her plans. But are community health professionals truly the originators of health education messages about, for example, the effect of exercise and diet on one's health? Or are we simply the messenger, the deliverer, the medium through which the message is sent? Greenberg (2003) maintains that society is the true health education message sender and that we, as health professionals, are the message conduit. Understanding that difference serves as a reminder that we must carefully consider the accuracy and quality of the message we are sending before we send it.

Message

In our example involving the two grocery-bearing friends, we know little about the message itself. We know only that it was about some decision Vanessa had made about something she planned to do. Whether that decision was a good idea and how it would affect others seems irrelevant to our discussion about how it was miscommunicated. However, as a health professional, the nature of the messages you will be asked to convey is a critical issue. It's important to consider message accuracy and message appropriateness.

Many confusing health-related messages are transmitted to our society through the news media, infomercials, books, magazines, and the Internet. Many of them are products of sensationalized half-truths, money-making schemes, or misguided individuals who mean well but mistakenly believe and spread inaccurate health information. As a health professional, you are responsible for the accuracy of the health messages you deliver. That is why it is important for you to understand research methodology and the difference between evidence-based fact and opinion. In chapter 13, we will discuss the importance of knowing where to go for accurate information as a resource person. For each message you send, you will need to first consider who originated that message and on what research evidence it was based.

Message appropriateness is another important aspect to be considered. For example, the message that regular exercise can positively contribute to one's health may be accurate. But the term "regular exercise" can mean different things to different people. What is considered an appropriate exercise type, frequency, and intensity for one person might place another at risk of injury. We need only compare the exercise needs of an Olympic athlete to those of a sedentary 80-year-old adult to understand the importance of adapted messages. Another example relates to pregnancy prevention. It would be necessary to understand the cultural values and religious beliefs of your audience before you demonstrate how to unroll a condom on an anatomical model of a penis or before even using the word "condom." In fact, the word "contraception" could be offensive to some groups who do not endorse contraceptive use. The phrase "family planning" may be a more appropriate choice. Both examples underscore how health messages should be presented in a way that is appropriately tailored to match the needs, cultural values, and abilities of the message receivers.

As we stated in chapter 8 when we discussed social marketing and the diffusion of innovation theory, presenting the message in a way that appropriately appeals to individual values, culture, and readiness for change increases the chance that the message will be accepted. Some individuals in our society suffer from what is referred to as **iatrogenic health education disease** (IHED) (Greenberg, 2003). Though IHED isn't truly a diagnosable disease, the phrase is used to describe a state of mind in which a person feels overwhelmed by the onslaught of health-risk messages. As a result, the person believes that trying to live a healthy lifestyle is futile and gives up on trying to maintain healthy behaviors (Greenberg, 2003). If you have ever heard someone say, "We all have to die of *something!*" or "Oh, *everything* causes cancer!" you may have been listening to a person suffering from IHED. To guard against this, your messages should be appropriately tailored to the receiver's sense of what is reasonable and worthwhile.

Medium

As we stated earlier, Greenberg (2003) would likely contend that you, the health professional, are the message medium, the channel through which the health message is delivered. From a different perspective, pamphlets, Web pages, oral presentations, newspaper articles, and PSAs could also be considered examples of message mediums. Whether you consider yourself or these message delivery channels as the medium, it is important that you pay close attention to how health messages are delivered.

You may have noted in our miscommunication illustration that both parties were busily putting away groceries as the message was delivered. Can you imagine Vanessa bending down to put something on a bottom shelf just as she began her message about her plans? While her back was turned Tyson could have momentarily stepped into a closet pantry and never even heard her statement. Or, through the noise and shuffle of activity, he may have heard only part of what she said. In either event, one could conclude that the chosen message channel left a lot to be desired.

This is why the selected message medium or channel is so important. Your message can be accurate and appropriately adapted to your intended audience. It may be worded in a way that effectively appeals to audience needs, values, and levels of readiness for acceptance. Yet, with all those important components in place, the communication process still may break down due to a faulty message medium. That medium must be a consistently reliable channel to the audience, one that can be depended upon to deliver the message to the right place at the right time.

Receiver

Finally, we arrive at the place where blame was placed in the beginning. Vanessa's comment that "He just didn't listen!" placed all the blame at Tyson's feet. We've already considered the possibility that it wasn't Tyson's fault—that the problem could lie with the sender, message, or medium. But let's reconsider. After all, Tyson was providing some indication that he was listening with each "um-hum" he offered. It is possible that Vanessa clearly stated her plans in an audible format, and Tyson was there all along to receive every word, but didn't. He may not have been really listening at all. Or he may have been listening but didn't really place importance on what she said and, thus, quickly forgot it. Or he may have listened carefully but, because he and Vanessa process information differently, may have placed an entirely different interpretation on what she said.

The receiver obviously plays a vital role in the message communication process. In health education settings, the receiver could be the person whose health needs you are attempting to assess and address with health programs. It could also be the community gatekeeper or stakeholder whose support you need for your assessment and programming efforts. The receiver could be someone whose resources you hope to attain for use in your efforts through grants, donations, or volunteered services. In each of these situations, knowing your communication goal is important.

The Communication Effect

Before developing a specific message and choosing an audience-appropriate medium or message channel, the message sender should carefully consider the desired communication effect, or outcome. For instance, is the purpose of a message to simply provide information, or is it intended to persuade the message receiver to adopt a particular health attitude or behavior? The difference between these two goals could drastically alter your communication approach.

There was a time when public health educators believed that we needed only to impart health-related knowledge to bring about positive changes in health behavior. If we simply told people, for example, that smoking causes cancer and regular exercise can help prevent heart disease, then people would automatically stop smoking and start exercising—or so it was believed. Thus, we needed only to bridge knowledge gaps with informative health messages, and all people everywhere would live healthier lives. Right? Wrong!

You may recall our discussions in previous chapters about the multitude of factors that influence health attitudes and behaviors. You may also remember that knowledge about health is only one factor, which, in the face of all those other influences (such as values, habits, peer pressure), carries very little weight on its own in health-related decisions. That is why developing effective health communication messages is such a challenge. In addition to providing needed health information in a format that is easily understood, the messages you send must also appeal to the message receiver's value system. They must motivate your receivers to overcome any perceived barriers that might prevent them from adopting healthy attitudes and behaviors.

Persuasive Communication

If health communication focused only on developing clearly stated health information, health educators might not be needed. After all, many professional disciplines train their members to clearly present information. However, there is a real art to knowing how to assess and adapt health-related messages to the needs and values of a variety of audiences and to package those messages in ways that can persuade receivers to change attitudes and behaviors.

This art is known as **persuasive communication**. A return to our discussion in chapter 8 about the theory of diffusion of innovation could be helpful in understanding this art within the context of mass communication. We encourage you to develop persuasive communication skills and seek opportunities to practice applying them through a variety of media (see "For Your Application" at the end of this chapter). Never forget, however, that persuasive communication is not the same thing as **coercion**, which means manipulating or even forcing people to do what you want. The decision to adopt or reject a health-related attitude or behavior is not yours. Your job is to provide needed information, training, and resources for positive health behavior change and to attempt to respectfully persuade and encourage the adoption of attitudes and behaviors that are clearly in the best interests of your audience. However, the decision belongs to the message receiver, not you. Adopt a respectful approach in your health communication efforts and you will likely avoid crossing the line between the professionally appropriate tone of persuasive communication and inappropriate coercion.

Regardless of whether your message is intended to inform or persuade, the receiver is the pivotal component in the communication process. The receiver is the component over which you have the least amount of control. For that reason, it is critical that you learn all you can about the receiver's thought processes, needs, values, and preferred communication channels.

Learning Styles and Information Processing

People think in different ways, and that's why communication can sometimes be a challenge. The ideas formulated by the message sender do not always match the thought processes of the receiver. What may seem to you to be a perfectly clear pamphlet about the need for immunizations may not make any sense at all to another person. Or perhaps your pamphlet helps clarify the issue for one mother, but she would achieve full understanding more readily by listening to oral testimony from another teenage mother who provides the same information but in story form.

Differences in learning and information-processing (cognitive) styles have been researched for years (Anderson & Adams, 1992; Bean, 1996; Gardner 1993), and much of this information is reflected in the multiple intelligences model we described in chapter 8. Here we wish to add only that understanding the differences in individual information processing represented in the model will greatly enhance your communication efforts.

Some controversy exists in the literature about whether learning and communication-style differences can be detected across cultures. Numerous studies have been cited as growing evidence that distinct *cultural* differences exist in relation to these styles (Anderson & Adams, 1992; Cushner, 1994). Others argue that such studies do not provide conclusive evidence (Kitano, 1997). As with other cultural differences, these distinctions appear to emerge among groups of individuals who closely adhere to their cultural roots. In fact, some scholars suggest that culture shapes not only *what* one thinks, but also *how* one thinks and learns (Cushner, 1994). We call this to your

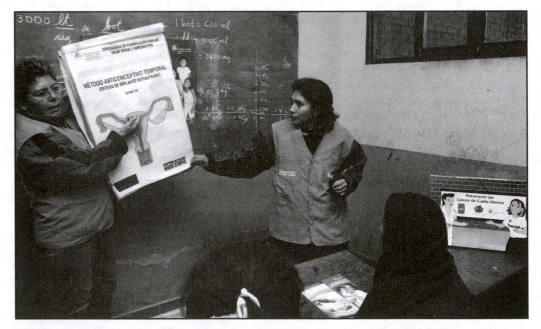

Effective health communication should be clear, accurate, persuasive, and culturally appropriate.
(© Richard Lord/The Image Works.)

attention to make two points. First, as the cultural diversity of our society expands, so will the need to offer your communication message in multiple formats and channels. Second, we caution you to carefully consider both sides of the cultural distinction argument so that you don't make the mistake of either ignoring culture-specific differences or of stereotyping those who share certain cultural characteristics. Whenever time and resources allow, a balanced, multiple-strategy approach is a good idea. In order to work effectively as a community health professional, you will need to not only communicate effectively, but be able to deliver your message cross-culturally. This takes time and effort on your part to learn a different perspective as well as practice skills that can help you deliver your message to a variety of audiences. You may wish to further your knowledge of effective cross-cultural communication by enrolling in a course at your local university or participating in online training through a local agency in your community. FYI 11.3 contains a comparison of cultural values, while strategies for effective cross-cultural communication are included in FYI 11.4 (on pp. 266–267). We encourage you to practice these strategies as well as seek out additional opportunities to strive for cultural competency in your everyday life.

FYI **11.3**   **Comparing Cultural Values**

Values Typical of Some Cultures	Anglo-American Values
Fate	Personal control over the environment
Tradition	Change
Human interaction dominates	Time dominates
Hierarchy/Rank/Status	Human equity
Group welfare	Individualism
Birthright inheritance	Self-help
Cooperation	Competition
Past orientation	Future orientation
"Being" orientation	Action/Goal/Work orientation
Formality	Informality
Indirectness/Ritual/Privacy	Directness/Flexibility/Openness
Spiritualism/Detachment	Materialism

Adapted from *Community Health Education and Promotion: A Guide to Program Design and Evaluation*, by N. Di Lima and C. Schust, 1997, Gaithersburg, MD: Aspen Publishers.

Communication Strategies and Principles

Now that you have a firm understanding of the communication process and your role and purposes in health communication, we can begin to explore methods that have been proven to enhance the likelihood of successful communication. We first

FYI 11.4   Enhancing Cross-Cultural Communication

Messages are conveyed both verbally and nonverbally. A tilt of the head or a certain inflection can give a message a whole new meaning. You should be aware of variations in nonverbal and verbal communication to avoid misunderstandings or unintentional insults when working with individuals and families.

Nonverbal Communication	Interpretations
Silence	You may find silence is awkward, intimidating, or a waste of time. However, many cultures value silence and view it as a normal part of a conversation. Conversely, some cultures find it socially appropriate to talk over another person or begin talking before the other person has finished. Being aware of the other person's natural pauses and interruptions will enhance the communication process and help foster respect.
Distance	The appropriate physical distance between people in a social setting varies from culture to culture. Provide people with options for space preference, such as saying, "Please have a seat wherever you feel comfortable."
Eye Contact	The amount of eye contact that is comfortable also varies from culture to culture. Do not be offended if some individuals do not hold your gaze; this could actually be a cultural sign of respect, not disinterest.
Emotional Expression	Expression of emotion may also be influenced by culture. Some cultures value stoicism, while other cultures are more accepting of displays of emotion. Varying beliefs about the origins and treatment of pain may also influence emotional expression from culture to culture.
Body Language	Gestures, motions, and positioning of the body can be interpreted differently depending on the culture. A hand signal commonly used as a funny expression in one culture can be an offensive insult in others. Conservative use of body language is prudent when you are uncertain of cultural norms relating to body language.
Oral Communication	
Greetings and Formality	In some cultures, it may be okay to greet your new female client with "Hey, Mary," while in others, a "Señora Hernandez" would be most appropriate. Do not assume that a first-name basis is appropriate for all client relationships. It could be inferred as disrespect, and you will lose credibility with your client. Avoid terms of endearment such as "dear" or "honey," and do not refer to adults as "boy" or "girl." If you're unsure how to address your client, simply ask what they would prefer.

Rapport	It's important to establish some form of trust with your client, even if you've just met. You can use small talk to demonstrate that you're open and friendly, and then transition into more pointed, open-ended questions such as, "How are you?" and "How may I help you?" If the client is not very responsive, you can always offer some suggestions and options. Be sensitive to personal boundaries; some questions could be viewed as invasive. Be sure not to interpret a client's non-response or silence as disrespect. Patience will go a long way toward building relationships in a short amount of time.
Subject Matter	Do not ever assume that because you are a health professional that people will be willing to discuss their health behaviors with you. Certain subject matter may simply not be culturally appropriate to discuss. For example, asking about family, sexual orientation, spouses, or religious beliefs may be taboo depending on one's culture and gender. Consider phrasing questions so they are less pointed; or, you can simply reassure clients that they "do not have to answer if they do not feel comfortable."
Translating	Language is a common barrier for health professionals trying to work with diverse populations. Working with a translator will help you deliver the health message in the most direct way. The translator could be a bilingual colleague, or it could be your client's family member. However, children are not always the most appropriate translators because the subject matter or ideas may be beyond their understanding or maturity. While working with the translator, avoid slang terms, lengthy sentences, or complex ideas. Instruct interpreters to use the client's own words instead of paraphrasing and ask for further clarification if a word or phrase is unclear. Allow sufficient time for the client to hear and formulate answers to questions.

Adapted from *Community Health Education and Promotion: A Guide to Program Design and Evaluation*, by N. Di Lima and C. Schust, 1997, Gaithersburg, MD: Aspen Publishers.

present some general strategies for the development and implementation of health communication. We follow that with some broad communication principles and strategies that can be adapted to most media. In subsequent sections, we also provide basic guidelines for selected media.

Stages of Health Communication

The circle in Figure 11.2 illustrates six stages of health communication (NIH, 2002) that can help you develop effective messages. Note that the first three stages, shaded in gray, are steps you should take before the communication is implemented.

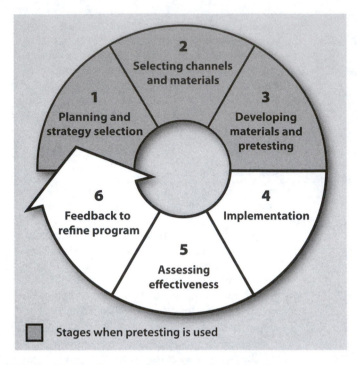

Figure 11.2 Stages of health communication.
Adapted from *Making Health Communication Programs Work: A Planner's Guide*, National Institutes of Health, U.S. Dept. of Health and Human Services, 2002. Retrieved August 28, 2008, from http://www.cancer.gov/pinkbook

After reading the earlier chapters in this book, you should be able to anticipate that a thorough needs assessment and detailed plan are recommended before any health education effort begins. This includes efforts toward effective health communication.

Let's suppose for a moment that you work in the community education division of a nonprofit refugee assistance program for Sudanese immigrants in your city. You've been asked to enhance awareness in the local refugee community about the need for annual well-woman checkups and the availability of free cervical screenings at the grant-funded refugee clinic nearby. You begin with stage 1, planning and strategy selection, which entails a preliminary needs assessment. As with any needs assessment, you first study existing data and then collect new data to fill in any information gaps. The goal is to identify specific beliefs and norms within the Sudanese refugee community that may serve as either barriers to or promoters of the likelihood that Sudanese women will obtain screenings and routine follow-ups. (Return to chapter 6 for a reminder of needs-assessment components and strategies.) Stage 1 would end with clearly defined communication goals and objectives that are designed to address influencing factors.

You would then be ready to move on to stage 2, to select communication channels and materials that best match your selected audience's needs and preferred information sources (such as specific radio stations, local eating establishments, newspapers, and organizational newsletters). We encourage you to solicit as much input as possible from community members; in doing so, expect to receive a variety of suggestions about channels and formats. Individuals who share similarities or group titles do not necessarily access the same communication channels. Find out about communication channels that have been used in the past to reach members of the community, and analyze existing communication materials to determine strengths and weaknesses of past and current efforts.

Communication channels for refugees can be very complex due to within-group diversity and the fact that acculturation may impact individuals in different ways. For example, Sudanese women who have lived in the U.S. for more than five years may still live in the same area of town, but may think very differently than those who have just arrived. The definition of the "Sudanese refugee community" follows the same distinctions and limitations we discussed in earlier chapters when attempting to identify other recognized community groups. You may, for instance, be able to access some Sudanese refugee women through other organizations whose specific purpose is to provide service to and support for the community. However some Sudanese refugee women, especially those that have lived in the U.S. longer, may not choose to access information through these organizations any longer. They may have developed a sense of distrust or no longer feel they need assistance. They may, however, receive your message about the need for annual checkups via their friends who do participate in those organizations. Or you may more readily reach these women through churches, grocery stores, the local health department, or through respected community leaders.

It is a good idea to draft and test (stage 3) several different message channels (such as brochures, videos, or public service announcements on radio). Ask community gatekeepers and health experts with knowledge about local Sudanese culture to critique each and provide suggestions. Then do a **pilot test** of the revised message formats and channels and obtain feedback from representatives of the intended audience. Ask those representatives to give you their honest impressions of the message and its format, the degree to which the message could be understood, recalled, and accepted as important and culturally appropriate. Make revisions based on their feedback.

In our example, let us assume that the outcome of the first three stages was the development of a flyer in the Zaghawa language and Arabic to distribute in the Sudanese refugee community. The flyer encourages women to seek well-woman checkups offered at the nearby free clinic and attempts to overcome barriers that often prevent these women from obtaining the checkups. Your flyer also contains the contact information of the free clinic as well as the names and phone numbers of contact individuals there. You also train volunteers from the community to present this information at local organizational meetings and worship centers that specifically serve the Sudanese refugee community. In addition, you decide to develop a public service announcement for the small radio station that is run by, and serves, Sudanese refugees. In the message, a woman identifies herself as a Sudanese woman who arrived in the U.S. two years ago. She describes how the free well-woman exam her sister received detected an early form of cervical cancer and saved her sister's life. She describes the care and respect her sister was given at the clinic and from the local refugee agency that helped her find the financial means to cover her treatment. The woman encourages women to join her as she, too, will seek the screening. The last few seconds of the PSA provide a heartfelt appeal to the listener to break through the barriers and schedule a checkup. Listeners are then given the clinic's phone number, which is also provided on the flyer.

You now have implemented three different communication channels (stage 4). The radio PSA serves as one. The volunteer presenters who distribute the pamphlet serve as a second channel. And, if the presenters' audiences respond to the appeal, the flyer alone may serve as a third channel as it finds its way into the hands of other Sudanese refugee women who never hear the presentation. How will you know whether any of the three channels is working and whether you should continue to invest time and money into some, none, or all three? That's where stages 5 and 6 come in. You won't know unless you track the messages.

You can choose from several tracking strategies. You could ask the volunteer presenters to keep records of the frequency, location, and date of each presentation; the number of people who attend them; and the number of pamphlets distributed at the end of each meeting. You could also record the number of times the PSA was aired with dates and time of day noted. But those counts would only tell you how often you presented the message. They would tell you nothing about whether you achieved the intended communication outcome and if so, which channel was responsible. That is, did the communication increase the frequency of annual well-woman checkups among targeted members of the Sudanese refugee community?

Measuring the communication effect would require a different kind of tracking, one that would allow you to survey those who received the message to learn how they perceived the message and whether it motivated them to complete an annual checkup. After your campaign begins, you could also survey those who visited the clinic to determine whether any were motivated to make an appointment by one of the communication channels and, if so, which one. A review of chapter 9 will help you generate other evaluation possibilities. For our purposes here, note that evaluation and revision are important components of health communication.

General Communication Principles

The National Cancer Institute (1999), part of NIH, provided an overview of how the public commonly perceives health messages (FYI 11.5). Understanding these perceptions can help you shape your health messages so that they are more likely to be accepted. First, the NCI points out that few people understand the concept of *health risk*. That is why the public is more likely to react strongly to such low-risk possibilities as homicides and accidental deaths that are often sensationalized by the news media, yet may ignore information about chronic diseases (such as heart disease, stroke, diabetes) that represent a greater health risk (are a more likely possibility) for most Americans.

To counter this imbalance, it might seem logical to focus our communication efforts on risk-awareness messages. However, messages that frighten the audience can backfire by producing feelings of helplessness and denial. When someone says, "Everything causes cancer," it underscores the dangers of using fear tactics in your communications. A well-balanced message can include an explanation of related health risks, but should not target fear as the intended outcome.

In the same sense that few people understand health risk, the general public has little confidence in or understanding of scientific research (NIH, 1999). People tend to embrace easy solutions and absolute answers and expect to find them in scientific research results; they have little patience with discussions about the need to replicate studies over time to test for consistency. Few understand how variability in study participant numbers and characteristics, methods used, and research settings can bias results. Even fewer know the difference between an association that only proves two factors coexist and a well-designed cause-and-effect study. For this reason, oversimplified news media coverage of a man who drank throughout his life and lived to be 100

FYI **11.5   Public Perceptions about Health Messages and Suggested Communication Strategies**

These suggested communication strategies (right column) are based on what is known about common public perceptions (left column) and how they affect people's acceptance of health messages.

Common Public Perceptions	Suggested Communication Strategies
• Few people understand the concept of health risk.	• People personalize new information.
• Fear tactics sometimes backfire.	• Focus on positive outcomes of positive behaviors. (Avoid fear tactics.)
• The public may not believe or understand science.	• Minimize use of scientific jargon.
• People respond to easy solutions and absolute answers.	• Keep messages simple.
• People tend to live for today, not tomorrow.	• Accentuate immediate health and nonhealth benefits.
• Health may not be a priority.	• Personalize messages.
• Individuals do not feel personally susceptible.	• Suggest "do-able" first-step solutions.
• The public holds contradictory beliefs.	

From "How the Public Perceives Health Messages," in *Health Communication Processes That Work*, National Cancer Institute, 1999. Retrieved April 11, 2008, from http://rex.nci.nih.gov/NCI_Pub_Interface/HCPW/HOME.HTM.

years old, for instance, can quickly become accepted as conclusive evidence that alcohol intake increases longevity.

The irony in this is that few people dwell on the future; long-range health risks and related information are seldom a priority (NIH, 1999). These tendencies apply especially to the younger members of our society and to those at lower socioeconomic levels. But no matter who your audience is, your health messages should emphasize immediate health and nonhealth benefits to adopting healthy lifestyles. An example would be to explain how regular exercise results in immediate stress reduction and weight management benefits, to show that people who exercise report more positive perceptions about life and are more productive. These short-range, nonhealth benefits may create a greater message appeal and have greater impact than would a discussion about how exercise can reduce risk of long-range heart disease.

Our perceptions about personal susceptibility to a particular health problem are usually lower than our actual risk rates (NIH, 1999). Yet individuals can also hold contradictory beliefs about how people, in the abstract, are susceptible to a multitude of health dangers. To return to an earlier example, picture a smoker who doesn't believe he or she is at personal risk of developing lung cancer but insists that all things cause cancer. The smoker may believe that we will all eventually die of cancer anyway and that quitting smoking will do little to change that. To counter low levels of perceived susceptibility and contradictory beliefs, design your messages in a way that personalizes the issue and provides clear, simple suggestions that won't overwhelm your message receiver.

Mediums for Communicating Health Information

There are various mediums used to communicate health messages. Public service announcements (PSAs) and brochures were mentioned earlier. Radio ads, press releases, news features, flyers, billboards, and interviews are other ways to deliver your message (see FYIs 11.6 and 11.7). An exhaustive discussion of all of these mediums would fill an entire book. Therefore, let us recommend a very helpful Web site sponsored by the University of Kansas called the Community Toolbox (**http://ctb.ku.edu/en/**). This Web site is a "living document" developed by a number of professional community groups, organizations, and foundations whose members are interested in promoting community health and community development (KU Work Group, 2007). From it, you can

FYI **11.6   Tips for Creating Appealing Posters and Flyers**

Posters and flyers are common channels for health communication. They rely on words and images to get their main point across. When creating your poster or flyer, consider the following:

- Simplicity is key—try not to have too many different elements vying for the reader or the viewer's attention.
- Large, colorful images will grab your reader's attention. Lots of contrast helps, too.
- A novel image is another good way to catch your audience's eye.
- Make sure that your images are culturally appropriate and do not lead to stereotyping.
- Your poster should be easy to read from a distance.
- Colors can have different effects: greens, blues, and purples tend to be soothing while red, orange, and yellow tend to excite and attract attention.

Mistakes to Avoid

- Visual clutter—too much of "a good thing" is not necessarily good. Keep it simple.
- Unclear and misunderstood wording can confuse (or even anger) the reader.
- Typos or spelling errors—can discredit the source and look unprofessional.
- Poor quality photo or artwork is bad for your organization's public image.

Adapted from KU Work Group for Community Health and Development, 2007, Chap. 6, Sect. 11: *Creating Posters and Flyers*. Lawrence: University of Kansas. Retrieved April 11, 2008, from http://ctb.ku.edu/tools//sub_section_main_1069.htm. Copyright © 2007 by the University of Kansas for all materials provided via the World Wide Web in the ctb.ku.edu domain.

FYI **11.7   Arranging and Developing News Stories**

There are many good reasons for publicizing your organization or event on television or in the newspaper. Benefits may include gaining increased publicity, heightening community awareness and support, and attracting not only attention but possible funding.

Consider the following when arranging for a news story:

- Timing: schedule your news story to appear around the time of your event and take advantage of national dates and awareness campaigns (e.g. National Health Education Week).

- Contact a local health or feature reporter. Keep in good contact with this individual as he or she may serve as a continual contact for future events.

- Take a human angle. People love human interest stories.

- Prepare a press release (FYI 11.8).

- Include pictures in your news story.

- Provide contact information for your organization.

Adapted from KU Work Group for Community Health and Development, 2007, Chap. 6, Sect. 4: *Arranging News and Feature Stories*. Lawrence: University of Kansas. Retrieved April 11, 2008, from http://ctb.ku.edu/tools//sub_section_main_1062.htm. Copyright © 2007 by the University of Kansas for all materials provided via the World Wide Web in the ctb.ku.edu domain.

download skill-building information on more than 150 community health topics. Among those topics are a variety of practical "how to" articles that relate to the development and use of professional presentations, fact sheets, pamphlets, PSAs, and grant proposals. The Web site provides a much broader array of resources than what we have mentioned here. We invite you to visit this site for more detailed information about how to effectively apply health communication theory, principles, and skills when selecting and using such mediums. Tips for writing an effective press release are covered in FYI 11.8 on the following page, with an example in FYI 11.9 (p. 275).

Writing for Success

An important first step in good writing is knowing *why* you are writing and for *whom* the message is intended. Then create an outline or cognitive map of your intended message so that you have a clear vision of the major points you wish to communicate. A number of different types of writing styles and formats could be appropriate, depending on your writing purpose and audience. These can range in complexity and length from single-statement public service announcements to brief informational brochures and flyers to full articles intended for a general audience or a professional community. Across these formats, however, there are some general rules of thumb you can follow for effective writing (FYI 11.10 on p. 276).

In many cases, the most powerful, thought-provoking statements are those that are clear and concise. Marketers have known for years that people tend to respond to short slogans they can easily remember. We need only to watch an evening of television and pay attention to the myriad of commercial jingles to find examples of that concept. Good writers follow the same guideline by deleting unnecessary words or phrases and simplifying sentence structure. Imagine if the concise slogan from the "Fried Egg" antidrug campaign, *"This is your brain. This is your brain on drugs"* was transformed into something like, *"This is what drugs can do to you physically and emotion-*

FYI 11.8   Writing a Press Release

Headline Is in Title Case Meaning You Capitalize Every Word Except for Prepositions and Articles of Three Letters or Less and Short; Ideally It Is Not More Than 170 Characters and Does Not Take a Period

The summary paragraph is a synopsis of the press release in regular sentence form. It doesn't merely repeat the headline or opening paragraph. It just tells the story in a different way. The summary paragraph is mandatory at FPRC.

City, State (FPRC) Month 1, 2005—The first paragraph, known as the "lead," contains the most important information. You need to grab your reader's attention here. And you can't assume that they have read the headline or summary paragraph; the lead should stand on its own.

A press release, like a news story, keeps sentences and paragraphs short, about three or four lines per paragraph. The first couple of paragraphs should cover the who, what, when, where, why, and how questions. A press release is usually no more than 250 words.

The rest of the news release expounds on the information provided in the lead paragraph. It includes quotes from key staff, customers, or subject matter experts. It contains more details about the news you have to tell, which can be about something unique or controversial or about a prominent person, place, or thing.

"You should include a quote for that human touch," said Gary Sims, CEO of the Free Press Release Center. "And you should use the last paragraph to restate and summarize the key points."

This is the example press release template for use at the Free Press Release Center. The last paragraph can also include details on product availability, trademark acknowledgment, etc.

About ABC Company:

Include a short corporate backgrounder about the company or the person who is newsworthy before you list the contact person's name and phone number. Do not include an e-mail address in the body of the release. Your e-mail address goes only in the "Contact Email" box when you submit your press release. To stop spam, your address will not appear on the site, but rather people will be able to contact you via a special contact link displayed with your press release.

Contact:
David Brown, Director of Public Relations
ABC Inc.
555-555-5555
http://www.YourWebAddress.com

From Free Press Release Center. (n.d.). *Sample Press Release*. Retrieved on April 11, 2008, from http://www.free-press-release-center.info/sample-press-release.html

ally as well as to your family." Do you see how the addition of just a few words changes the overall effect of this message?

Three additional tips for concise writing are to avoid excessive use of prepositional phrases, delete unnecessary words, and use verbs in an active voice. Consider the statement, "The attitudes of the community are so powerfully strong that the program offered by our agency will need to focus on them." The phrases "the attitudes of the community" and "the program offered by our agency" could be shortened to "community attitudes" and "agency program." The words "so powerfully" in the

---

FYI **11.9   Sample Press Release**

A Broken Engagement Could Bring Relief for Orphans in Sierra Leone

Spanaway, WA (PRWeb) November 16, 2006—International charity, All As One, is hopeful that the upcoming Warner Bros. film, *Blood Diamond*, will raise awareness about the decade-long war in Sierra Leone and the children who are still suffering its effects. One supporter of the cause will be auctioning his diamond ring from a broken engagement and donating the proceeds to All As One, in an effort to shine a light on the continuing issue of "conflict" diamonds, while benefiting the children of Sierra Leone in the process.

The civil war in Sierra Leone, funded by corruption and the "blood" diamond trade, was devastating to the people and economy of the country. Though the conflict ended in 2002, it is the children who are still suffering the most. Operating by donations from individuals across the world, All As One's Children's Center in Freetown provides shelter, food, clothes, education, and medical care for orphaned and destitute children, who would otherwise be living on the streets.

Deanna Wallace, a resident of Washington and founder of All As One, is a mother of twelve—ten of whom came to her through adoption, both internationally and domestically. She says, "In Sierra Leone's past, orphans were raised by their extended families. But the war has ravaged the country, destroyed villages, and left Sierra Leone's citizens in poverty. The government simply does not have the resources to begin implementing child welfare programs or orphanages." Complicated adoption procedures and restrictions, many imposed by the U.S. government, make the need for organizations like All As One even greater. "For many of these children, this is the first, and possibly the only, home they will have" Wallace says. "But they are thriving at the Children's Center—here, they have a chance to learn, play, and just be kids."

The eBay auction will run from December 5–15, to coincide with the December release of the film. Wallace hopes the film and the auction will bring needed attention and support to a country much of the world has forgotten.

For additional information about All As One or the upcoming auction, contact:

Jen Brauer, Public Relations/Media Contact, US
jen@allasone.org
511-923-3632
or visit http://www.allasone.org

Photos are available upon request.

From All As One (allasone.org). Used with permission.

FYI 11.10   Rules for Good Writing

Practicing these rules will enhance the efficacy of your health education messages.

To prepare for writing:

- Identify why you are writing.
- Identify your audience.
- Create a message outline or cognitive map.

To write concisely:

- Use active voice.
- Delete unnecessary words.
- Avoid strings of prepositional phrases.

To adapt materials to the intended audience:

- Use SMOG or your word-processing program to determine reading levels.
- Use back translation to determine cultural appropriateness.

To correct mistakes and evaluate finished products:

- Edit more than once.
- Have a "fresh" pair of eyes review the final draft.
- Pilot test materials.

phrase "so powerfully strong" could be deleted without losing meaning. Sentences should always be in the *active voice;* make the organization or person who will do the action (the agency) the subject of the sentence and use a verb in the active voice. Thus, a shorter statement could be "The agency program should focus on the strong community attitudes." The "For Your Application" at the end of the chapter contains an editing exercise that will allow you to practice this simplification process.

The **SMOG formula** presented in Figure 11.3 can be used to adapt your written materials to specific audience reading levels. More specific guidelines for its application can be accessed through the Community Toolbox Web page. Your word processing program probably has a feature that can help you assess readability. The back translation process described in chapter 9 can help you adapt your message to a culturally appropriate format. Because you will likely have spent a great deal of time working with the material at this point, you will need to submit the final draft to people who can read it with a fresh eye and suggest further changes. Don't skip this step! A final edit by other health experts and community leaders, followed by a pilot test among community members, can save you the cost and embarrassment of distributing materials that contain misspelled words, incomplete sentences, or confusing text. The Community Toolbox Web site also contains specific guidelines for materials development and pretesting.

The SMOG readability formula is commonly used to determine the reading level of written materials. To calculate the SMOG reading grade level, begin with the entire written work that is being assessed and follow these four steps:

1

Pick 30 sentences,* 10 each from near the beginning, in the middle, and near the end of the text.

2

From the sample of 30 sentences, circle all of the words containing three or more syllables (polysyllabic words), including repetitions of the same words, and total the number of words circled.

3

Estimate the square root of the total number of polysyllabic words counted. This is done by finding the nearest perfect square and taking its square root.

4

Finally, add a constant of 3 to the square root. This number gives the SMOG grade, or the reading grade level that a person must have reached if he or she is to fully understand the text being assessed.

SMOG Conversion Table**

Total Polysyllabic Word Counts	Approximate Grade Level
0–2	4
3–6	5
7–12	6
11–20	7
21–30	8
31–42	9
43–56	10
57–72	11
73–90	12
91–110	13
111–112	14
113–157	15
157–192	16
193–210	17
211–240	18

* Visit the NIH Web site for details about pamphlets and fact sheets. http://rex.nci.nih.gov

** Developed by Harold C. McGraw, Office of Educational Research, Baltimore County Schools, Towson, MD.

From *Making Health Communication Programs Work: A Planner's Guide,* National Institutes of Health, U.S. Dept. of Health and Human Services, 2002, NIH Pub. 92-1493.

Figure 11.3   The SMOG readability formula.

Informational Pieces for Lay Newsletters

We encourage you to consider regular newsletter mailings to keep community members apprised of agency or program activities and related national and local news. A number of word-processing programs contain newsletter templates that are simple to use. Access to the Internet for late-breaking health news and graphics makes newsletter production a straightforward task. Before you develop your own, study newsletter content and layouts from a variety of sources and apply the tips for good writing provided in FYI 11.10. Advice from a graphic artist or journalist can improve the quality of your product.

Brochures and Pamphlets

An effective brochure or pamphlet should have a single theme. You cannot cover all aspects of a particular health topic in one brochure. As stated earlier, use an outline and keep the message simple. For example, if the purpose of your brochure or pamphlet is to convince a teenage mother to obtain immunizations for her baby, limit your message to reasons why she should get them and where she can get them. Don't get bogged down in related but unnecessary details about, for example, the human immune system or symptoms of childhood diseases. Apply the rules of thumb listed in FYI 11.10 and use bulleted lists where appropriate. Enlist the help of an experienced graphic artist or photographer for advice about layout, graphics/visuals, typefaces, and paper. We live in a fast-paced, visually stimulated society, so visual appeal is extremely important.

In preparing your work, talk to people from the intended audience to understand some of their perceptions and attitudes about the topic. This will help you better understand your intended audience and help you focus on presenting what is most relevant. When you're finished designing your materials, pretest them with members of your intended audience to make sure that the wording, images, and content are appropriate. **Pretesting** allows you to gain initial feedback from your audience before the final version is created. This preview allows your intended audience to offer you suggestions for refining your work so that it creates the impact you had hoped.

Public Service Announcements

Public service announcements are short video or audio messages provided to radio and television stations. Generally, PSAs are sent as ready-to-air audio or videotapes, although radio stations (especially community or public stations, such as campus radio, PBS, and National Public Radio) sometimes prefer a script that their announcers can read live on the air. PSAs are usually 30 seconds or less and can be as simple as a person talking into the TV camera, urging someone to not drink and drive, or they can be elaborate productions that are scripted with actors, music, and story lines.

Broadcast media—radio and television—are required by the Federal Communications Commission (FCC) to serve "in the public interest." Most stations use PSAs as one way to meet this requirement. While they aren't required to donate a fixed percentage of air time per day to PSAs, stations do have to state in their licensing and renewal applications how much air time they plan to devote to PSAs. Most stations donate about a third of their commercial spots to noncommercial causes; in other words, if a station has 18 minutes of commercials in a given hour, six minutes of that will probably be devoted to PSAs (KU Work Group, 2007f).

PSAs require a bit of work on your part, and they tend to be ineffective at influencing policy. Consider using them when you have a specific action you want the viewer or listener to take, or when they can be coordinated with other activities designed to influence people's behavior. FYI 11.11 provides some suggestions for creating an effective PSA.

FYI **11.11**   **Creating a Public Service Announcement**

Here are some key points to remember when writing a PSA:

- Keep the language simple and vivid since you will often have 30 seconds or less to get your message across.
- Use "hooks," words or phrases that grab attention, to attract and sustain your audience.
- The PSA should request a specific action, such as calling a number to get more information.
- Choose points to focus on—don't overload the viewer or listener with too many different messages.
- Brainstorm: Get together with your colleagues and toss around ideas about ways to illustrate your points. You may want to look at other PSAs for ideas.
- Check your facts. It's very important your PSA is accurate.

For 10 second spots, keep word length to 20–25; for 15 seconds, 30–35, and for 30 seconds, 60–75 words.

Adapted from KU Work Group for Community Health and Development, 2007, Chap. 7, Sect. 8: *Preparing Public Service Announcements*. Lawrence: University of Kansas. Retrieved April 11, 2008, from http://ctb.ku.edu/tools//sub_section_main_1065.htm. Copyright © 2007 by the University of Kansas for all materials provided via the World Wide Web in the ctb.ku.edu domain.

Letters and Memos

Frequent letters and memos sent through the postal service or e-mail can be an effective tool for keeping a variety of team members apprised of your progress and plans. As with other written materials, brevity is important. Try to limit letters to one page and memos to one or two paragraphs. When appropriate, use a business-style heading that lists "Date," "To," "From," and "Re" so that readers can quickly identify the purpose and content of the letter or memo.

Professional Articles

Most professional journal articles follow a thesis-based structure, meaning that they begin by introducing the reader to a specific question, problem, or issue. The introduction explains why the question or issue is significant by reviewing and citing professional literature on the subject. If the paper is a *scientific article,* meaning that it describes and reports the results of an experiment or applied program, a description of the methods or program implemented should follow the introduction section. Next comes the description of the results or outcomes, a discussion of the strengths and weaknesses of the study or program, and the author's interpretations and conclusions (Garrard, 1999). The article must also include a bibliographical format that allows you to cite each source used. Each journal has its own author guidelines, usually printed in every issue, that describe how to format a manuscript you plan to submit. Pay careful attention to these guidelines and study several past volumes of your target journal to note commonly published topics and writing styles.

Manuscripts submitted for publication in professional journals are usually subjected to a rigorous review process before they are placed in print. The journal editor who receives your manuscript will first read it to determine whether your manuscript topic matches journal goals and readership interest. If the editor believes so, he or she will then send out copies of your manuscript to journal reviewers who have knowledge about your manuscript topic. Each reviewer will submit a recommendation about whether the manuscript should be rejected, accepted for publication as written, or accepted if certain revisions are made. In the case of the last recommendation, the reviewer will also provide directions for suggested manuscript changes. The editor will then synthesize responses from all reviewers and make a decision about rejection or acceptance of your manuscript for publication in the journal. If "accepted with revisions," you may ask the editor to clarify suggestions before submitting a revised manuscript. It sometimes takes as long as a year or two for a manuscript to progress from your seed of an idea through manuscript development and submission to a printed journal article. Writing for publication takes lots of practice, patience, and persistence. We recommend that you begin by looking for opportunities to be a co-author with professors who have publication experience.

Speaking for Success

Think back to the last time you heard a good speaker deliver a message. What made you think the speaker was so effective? It probably had something to do with your degree of interest in the speech topic. However, an interesting topic isn't the only characteristic of a good speech. A skilled speaker can make almost any topic sound interesting. But public-speaking skills do not come naturally to most people; if you've ever attended a banquet or wedding reception you can attest to this. Rather, accomplished speakers have honed their skills over time. FYI 11.12 lists some qualities of a good speaker, many of which you can develop with practice. What other qualities are missing from this list?

Telephone Voice

The tone of voice you use in a telephone survey or business conversation can make a difference in how well your words are accepted. In most cases, using a slightly lower and deeper tone than you usually use in common conversation can convey warmth and confidence. Practice speaking in a calm, carefully concise manner and enunciate your words distinctly. Adopt a cheerful telephone demeanor, even when talking to a difficult person, and you will be surprised with the results.

Presenting for Lay Audiences

Three key elements to a successful community presentation are the right background conditions, the right preparation, and the right delivery (KU Work Group,

FYI **11.12**   **Qualities of an Effective Speaker**

The qualities of an effective speaker go beyond good preparation and include skills related to verbal and nonverbal communication.

An effective speaker:

- begins the speech with an attention-catching statement or story.
- tells the audience what to expect in the speech.
- limits the speech to 3 or 4 main points.
- includes the whole audience through frequent eye contact.
- uses stories and illustrations where appropriate.
- uses pleasant and appropriately animated facial expressions.
- uses an outline to enhance flow.
- never reads notes to the audience.
- projects the voice to the back of the room.
- uses differing voice inflections and appropriate nonverbal body language.
- speaks slowly, clearly, and concisely.
- uses visuals to illustrate major points.
- involves the audience as much as possible.
- summarizes the speech by reiterating its major points.
- limits the speech to the designated time frame.

2007f). You can gain understanding and some control over the background conditions by studying your prospective audience. Ask questions about their demographics (for example, age, socioeconomic status, ethnicity), knowledge about and attitudes toward the presentation topic, and their expectations of you and your presentation. Consider recruiting key stakeholders and community gatekeepers to attend the presentation to help them recognize the need for community action. Whenever possible, study the presentation setting ahead of time to check room size, temperature, acoustics, seating arrangements, and audiovisual equipment. Find out in advance who will be present to help you with last-minute adjustments if needed.

Good preparation begins with a clear presentation objective. Let's return to our earlier example in which you were asked to address the need for well-woman check-ups among members of the Sudanese immigrant community. Suppose that you are preparing to make one of the community presentations we described, and let's work through some basic preparation steps (FYI 11.13 on the following page).

Your written objective might state that you wish to convince members of the audience to get an annual well-woman checkup and encourage others in the community to do the same. Your main presentation points should contain information designed to persuade your audience (that is, reach your presentation objective). For example, your points could include a brief description of the risks involved in bypassing annual

FYI **11.13   Preparing for a Presentation**

Following these simple presentation preparation steps can strengthen message delivery and acceptance:

- Write a clear, brief presentation objective.
- Develop a presentation outline.
- Select supporting materials.
- Create visual aids.
- Practice.

Adapted from KU Work Group for Community Health and Development, 2007, Chap. 4, Sect. 5: *Making Community Presentations*. Lawrence: University of Kansas. Retrieved April 11, 2008, from http://ctb.ku.edu/en/tablecontents/section_1029.htm. Copyright © 2007 by the University of Kansas for all materials provided via the World Wide Web in the ctb.ku.edu domain.

well-woman checkups, an acknowledgment of past barriers to checkups for members of the Sudanese immigrant community, a summary of how some women's health clinics have begun to address the problem and are accessible, a list of the benefits of participating, and directions for calling to set up an appointment. You could then create bulleted lists under each of your main points that would contain key subpoints. From there, you could expand your outline into a full presentation.

We recommend that you use a software program for slide presentations (such as Microsoft PowerPoint) to develop your outline. Most programs will allow you to add detailed notes beneath each slide created, and you can then convert the results to a variety of visual formats, including computerized slides projected onto a screen with a data projector, 35mm slides for a more traditional slide projector, overhead transparencies, or even paper printouts for poster displays. FYI 11.14 contains valuable design tips for any visual format used (and you can use multiple formats in the same presentation).

Don't forget to practice your presentation and delivery! What looks good on paper doesn't always sound good in an oral format, and the length of time needed for the presentation will likely be important. Begin with an opening sentence that will grab your audience's attention. At the end, summarize the main points you just delivered and appeal to your audience's values and concerns as they relate to your presentation topic. Memorize the key points of the presentation so you can concentrate on a professional delivery, but plan to use your presentation notes to help you stay focused.

As you practice your presentation, visualize speaking to your audience or stand in front of a mirror. Concentrate on projecting your voice to the back of the room, but in a relaxed, expressive tone that exudes appropriate levels of enthusiasm and confidence. Work on including all members of the audience through frequent eye contact and avoid turning your back to the audience when referring to visual aids. Instead, stand to the side of the visual and face the audience as you describe the visual.

FYI **11.14   Tips for Creating Effective Visual Aids**

These tips for creating effective visual aids improve the appearance and acceptance of the health message:

- Limit each visual to one main idea.
- Use no more than 6–8 lines of text per graphic or slide.
- Use bulleted lists and key phrases rather than sentences.
- Use plain language; avoid jargon.
- Double-space between text lines.
- Use large, bold, crisp fonts.
- Check for visibility from the back of the room.
- Only show information you plan to discuss.
- Plan to quote and clarify each graphic or slide.
- Turn off the projector lights when you have no slides to project.
- Cover the next graphic or slide until you are ready to address it.
- Use chart formats effectively:
  + Horizontal bars: to compare categories
  + Vertical bars: to show change over time
  + Line graphs: to show trends across time periods
  + Pie charts: to show amounts as a percentage of the total

Adapted from KU Work Group for Community Health and Development, 2007, Chap. 4, Sect. 5: *Making Community Presentations*. Lawrence: University of Kansas. Retrieved April 11, 2008, from http://ctb.ku.edu/en/tablecontents/section_1029.htm. Copyright © 2007 by the University of Kansas for all materials provided via the World Wide Web in the ctb.ku.edu domain.

Presenting for Professional Audiences

Much of what we recommend for community presentations also holds true when presenting to professional audiences. However, whereas professional and technical terminology is considered jargon and should be avoided in community presentations, it is more likely to be understood and expected among professional audiences. We suggest that you use professional terminology among your professional peers to enhance your credibility as well as audience understanding. This does not mean your language will be obscure or your meaning hard to discern. Your primary goal should still be communication. Professional audiences are also more likely to expect and appreciate your knowledge of the professional literature and how your work relates to other studies and theories. We encourage you to develop a strong research and theory-based understanding of your work so that you can convey to your professional peers how your work contributes to universal understandings. When presenting at professional conferences, it often helps to provide a handout to your audience that contains an abstract of your presentation and a list of references or recommended readings. Expect some audience members to want to contact you later to learn more about your work and explore future collaborative efforts. Maintaining contact with your professional peers through conferences and seminars can be your professional lifeline. We highly encourage you to participate in professional meetings and present your work so that others may learn from and add to your understanding.

Health Literacy

As we mentioned in chapter 8, one of the most pressing community health issues today is health literacy (see pp. 200–201). Factors relating to poor health literacy in the U.S. include the consistent finding that the literacy demands of most printed health materials exceed the reading abilities of the average American adult (Weiner et al., 2004). With up to 25% of the American population having difficulty with everyday reading tasks such as reviewing medication instructions, interpreting food labels, or filling out health forms at a doctor's office or clinic (Weiner et al., 2004), there has never been a greater need for you to learn more about how to develop health communication materials that are easily understood by those who have less than a sixth-grade reading ability. This starts with knowing and understanding your intended audience and assessing factors that impact decision making among this group (see chapter 6). In order to create health communication materials like the ones described in this chapter for those with lower literacy skills, you may need to attend a workshop, a professional conference, or visit some Web sites such as the Center for Health Communication at the Harvard School of Public Health (www.hsph.harvard.edu/chc) to get a better understanding of what works when designing for this special population.

As explained in FYI 11.15, using more pictures and less text, eliminating jargon or slang terms, and curtailing the use of polysyllabic words (3 syllables or more) in your text will help (Weiner et al., 2004). However, learning to effectively communicate information that often is complicated takes practice. We urge you to explore ways to improve your health communication skills as you further your professional development.

In Conclusion

Communicating effectively is at the crux of community health. Whether you are communicating with people face-to-face in personal conversations or group presentations, through written media, or via public service announcements, the basic concepts remain the same. State your message clearly and concisely. Remember that simple statements and messages are often powerful motivators. Use visuals and illustrations whenever appropriate, and communicate your message in a variety of formats as frequently as possible. Communicate to inform. Communicate to empower. Communicate to progress. We encourage you to begin developing these skills immediately and practice them as often as possible. "For Your Application" provides a suggestion that will help you incorporate several communication formats into one experience and document them in your professional portfolio.

FYI **11.15   Designing Health Materials for Those with
Lower Literacy Skills**

1. **Culture is key.** Know your audience. Pay special attention to their preferences, values, language, and dialect. Talk to individuals from your audience, and talk to a variety of people. Ask for feedback from your audience before you publish or distribute your materials. Revise if necessary.

2. **Present the information in a simple manner.** When preparing the written content:
   - Write as if you are speaking to the reader.
   - Present only the most important information.
   - Use headings and subheadings to signal to the reader about upcoming information. Break up large amounts of information into easy-to-read sections.
   - Use short sentences and short paragraphs. Sentences should be no more than 25 words, and paragraphs should be no more than 60 words.
   - With audiences for whom English is a second language, it is preferable to write in their native language. If that is not possible, consider using materials written for lower literacy levels in their second language.
   - Set quotes or phrases off to the side of the main body of text. Use buzzwords to draw the reader in or to notify them of information.
   - Leave an adequate amount of white space along the margins and throughout the publication. This is especially important for low-literacy audiences. Avoid overcrowding each page with words.

3. **Use photos and graphics.** Many times, a picture really *is* worth 1000 words! A well-designed graphic can clarify the message being presented or even replace large blocks of text.
   - Avoid stereotyping by carefully selecting images. Again, culture and audience preference play an important role in deciding what is an acceptable image or graphic to include.
   - Seek specific feedback regarding potential images you intend to include in your publication.
   - Show various types of families in your publications. Include pictures of two-parent families, single-parent families, multi-racial families, and families that depict grandparents raising grandchildren, among others.
   - Show images that reflect a variety of different types of residences.
   - Show people in a variety of occupations, including those that are nontraditional. An example might include a male nurse, a female engineer, or a person with a disability in a job most often held by people without visible disabilities.

4. **Keep the reading level below a 6th grade level.**
   - Avoid using polysyllabic words (more than 3 syllables).
   - Do not use slang or jargon.
   - Use SMOG or another readability formula to check the complexity.

Sources: "Tips for Designing Publications for Underrepresented Audiences," by P. D. Ingram, M. H. Dorsey, and S. Smith, 2004, *Journal of Extension,* Vol. 42 (4). Retrieved August 31, 2008, from http://www.joe.org/joe/2004august/tt2.shtml; *Making Health Communication Programs Work: A Planner's Guide,* National Institutes of Health, U.S. Dept. of Health and Human Services, 2002. Retrieved August 28, 2008, from http://www.cancer.gov/pinkbook

REVIEW QUESTIONS

1. Describe some skills that are necessary for effective communication.
2. Name and describe each component of the health communication model.
3. Explain what is meant by iatrogenic health education disease.
4. Differentiate between persuasive communication and coercion.
5. Name and give an example of each of the six stages of health communication.
6. Provide at least four strategies for improving cross-cultural communication.
7. List at least five effective writing tips.
8. Explain how each of the following communication mediums could be used to help deliver a health message to your intended audience: press release, PSA, news story, and brochure.
9. Name at least six characteristics of a good speaker.
10. List at least four tips for developing health communication for those with lower literacy skills.
11. Analyze why health literacy is a pressing community health issue.

FOR YOUR APPLICATION

Learning to Write Concisely

Convert each of the following sentences into a more concise statement by rewriting to avoid excessive prepositional phrases, delete unnecessary words, and use active voice. Ask a friend to do the same and compare your results.

1. The incredibly high incidence of hypertension among males of African American descent has been reduced by education programs.
2. The common opinion that AIDS is something that happens only to members of the gay community is held by students who attend the local high school.
3. Educational programs that prevent needless accidental injuries have been designed by a large number of the employees of the agency.
4. Preventive health services that are available and affordable were already mandated by the members of the community.

Gaining Communication Experience

Volunteer to deliver a health education presentation to a local community group. Thoroughly research the professional literature and use Internet resources listed in Appendix A of this text to obtain the information you need and ideas about how to communicate it. Create a slide presentation, poster, and/or informational pamphlet or flyer to be distributed to your audience at the end of the presentation. Ask the audience and, if possible, an experienced presenter to evaluate your presentation and materials.

Observing Health Communication Delivery

Attend at least two health-related events or presentations in your community and take notes on the delivery of each presentation. Design an evaluation form based on the content of this chapter and additional resources you find, evaluate each presentation and presenter, and reflect on the presentations' strengths and weaknesses. How could the delivery of the information be improved? (Note: Instead of attending a presentation, you could choose to evaluate print material such as a brochure or Internet sources, such as a Web site).

Developing Print Materials for Low Literacy Populations

Obtain an existing health-related brochure from a local clinic, grocery store, health department, or nonprofit agency. Assess the reading level of the brochure using the SMOG formula or your word-processing language tool, and revise this brochure to appeal to a group with lower literacy skills. Justify your changes based on what you've read in this chapter as well as other credible sources.

Advocating for Community Health Needs

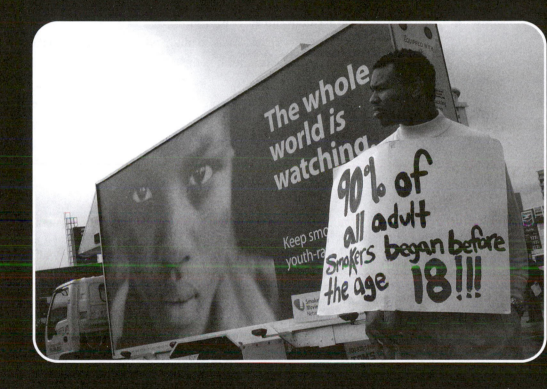

In an effort to collect data for a community needs assessment you are preparing for a local non-profit, you come across some unsettling information on the county's Web site. Over 33% of children in your county are overweight or obese! As a health professional, parent, and resident of the county, you feel the need to advocate for change, but you don't know where to start. How do you convince other parents, policy makers, educators, and other health professionals to support your cause? With little experience in policy making or politics, how do you advocate for legislative action and garner community support? How do you get people to care about the health needs in your community?

CHAPTER OBJECTIVES

1. Define advocacy.
2. Identify methods of advocating for health issues.
3. Discuss the importance of health advocacy.
4. List tips for writing advocacy letters, using media, and visiting policy makers.
5. Identify organizations that advocate for health.
6. Outline advocacy survival skills.
7. Practice developing advocacy materials specific to a particular health issue.

What Is Advocacy?

Have you ever encountered a situation where you thought "That's just not right! There ought to be a law!"? That's how advocacy begins. **Advocacy** is defined as "the pursuit of influencing public-policy and resource-allocation decisions that directly impact people's lives within political, economic, social systems and institutions" (Cohen, de la Vega, and Watson, 2001, p. 7). Advocacy extends beyond the bounds of this definition, however. Advocacy is actively working to change the social, political, legal, economical, and medical environments; it is working to make a change in society. It is actively participating in the democratic process and expressing your rights as a citizen of the United States. It is also standing up for individuals who cannot speak for themselves. When used effectively, advocacy can have a tremendous impact on public health. FYI 12.1 provides a more thorough description of advocacy and what it commonly entails.

Skills for Successful Advocacy

Leaders in the field of community health increasingly recognize that the discipline's mission is to address not just individual health but also the social, political, and economic structures that serve as barriers to community health and well-being. Health edu-

FYI 12.1 **Examples of Advocacy**

- Advocacy is *active* promotion of a cause or principle.
- Advocacy involves *actions* that lead to a selected goal.
- Advocacy is one of many possible strategies, or ways to approach a problem.
- Advocacy can be used as part of a community initiative, nested in with other components.
- Advocacy is *not* direct service.
- Advocacy does not necessarily involve confrontation or conflict.
- Some examples may help clarify just what advocacy is:
  + You join a group that helps build houses for the poor—that's wonderful, but it's not advocacy (it's a service).
  + You organize and agitate to get a proportion of apartments in a new development designated as low to moderate income housing—that's advocacy.
  + You spend your Saturday handing out information for the American Lung Association—that's not advocacy (it's a service).
  + You hear that the local recycling center is going to be closed down and you band together with many others to get the city to preserve this site, or find you a new one. Some of you even think about blocking the bulldozers, if necessary. That's advocacy.

Adapted from KU Work Group for Community Health and Development, 2007, chap. 5, sect. 4: *Systems Advocacy and Community Organizing*. Lawrence: University of Kansas. Retrieved from http://ctb.ku.edu

cators and community health professionals serve as leaders in addressing conditions that diminish health. However, many community health workers go through professional preparation programs that do not provide any information or training in advocacy (Ward & Koontz, 1999). There are several key components to effective advocacy that health educators must be aware of in order to achieve the intended goal. These include:

- "rightness" of the cause
- power of the advocates (i.e., more of them is much better than less)
- thoroughness with which the advocates researched the issues, the opposition, and the climate of opinion about the issue in the community
- skill in using the advocacy tools available (including the media)
- selection of effective strategies and tactics (KU Work Group, 2007d)

The process of advocacy is many things to many people. It might be lobbying on Capitol Hill in Washington, D.C., with the purpose of educating and influencing policy makers; encouraging insurance companies to cover prevention services; or standing up at a school board meeting to campaign for a comprehensive health education curriculum. Advocacy can be local or national, can be directed toward policy makers of all kinds, and can be used to change many environments. See FYI 12.2 for some terms you may come across while participating in or researching advocacy.

FYI 12.2   **Advocacy Terms**

Following are some of the common terms used in the advocacy process.

Advocacy	Actively working to change the social, political, legal, economical, and medical environments; making a change in society.
Lobbying	To conduct activities aimed at influencing public officials and especially members of a legislative body on legislation.
Appropriations	Money that has been set aside by formal action for a specific purpose.
Entitlements	A government program providing benefits to members of a specified group or the funds supporting or distributed by such a program.
Discretion	The power of free decision or latitude of choice within certain legal bounds.
Constituent	One who authorizes another to act as agent.

Source: Definitions for *lobbying, appropriations, entitlements, discretion,* and *constituents* are from *Merriam-Webster's Collegiate Dictionary,* 11th ed. 2003, Springfield, MA: Merriam-Webster. Cited in "Putting Advocacy into Action" by S. E. Ward and N. Koontz, 1999. *Eta Sigma Gamma Monograph,* 17(2), 36–40.

Basic Tools of Advocacy

Among the basic tools of advocacy are knowledge, coalitions and partnerships, lobbying, grassroots activities, media, personal communication or legislative advocacy, and technology.

Knowledge

Information, of course, is the basis of knowledge. We have talked about information gathering in several chapters. We have discussed assessing individual and community needs through various methods, and we have discussed libraries, local health departments, voluntary health organizations, the Internet, and many other sources of information. In the case of advocacy, information and knowledge provide you with the power to affect others. We are not suggesting that to be an advocate you have to be an expert. But you do need sufficient knowledge about an issue to be able to provide adequate decision-making information for those to whom you are advocating.

Coalitions and Partnerships

As mentioned in chapter 10, coalitions involve coordinating individuals or organizations into a team that can work toward a common goal. Good examples include the child protection teams that many cities have formed. Such teams consist of individuals from all of the agencies in the city that are in a position to help abused children. In chapter 10 we included some strategies for building coalitions; FYI 12.3 provides a short summary of key steps.

FYI 12.3   **Building a Coalition**

Coalitions are groups of individuals (generally representing agencies that can provide resources) working toward a common goal. Building a coalition should be done with thoughtful planning. Below is a list of helpful steps for building a successful coalition, excerpted from the APHA's *Legislative Advocacy Handbook*.

1. Define your objectives and needs.

2. Secure resources.

3. Identify potential members.

4. Get the ball rolling by inviting individuals and representatives of the chosen organizations to join the coalition.

5. Convene the coalition's first meeting to develop an action plan.

6. Establish an identity for the coalition.

7. Follow up with coalition members and potential members.

8. Develop coalition materials.

9. Keep the ball moving. Be sure to maintain momentum and interest by keeping participants posted on progress or action in the issue area.

10. Keep the lines of communication open.

Excerpted from *APHA Legislative Advocacy Handbook: A Guide for Effective Public Health Advocacy*, p. 41, Washington, DC: Author. © American Public Health Association. Used with permission.

Lobbying

Lobbying is a form of advocacy. The difference between the two is sometimes subtle yet important. Lobbying refers specifically to *paid* advocacy efforts that attempt to influence legislation. On the other hand, when nonprofit organizations advocate on their own behalf, they seek to affect some aspect of society, whether they appeal to individuals about their behavior, employers about their rules, or the government about its laws (Connecticut Association of Nonprofits Advocacy, 2003). This distinction is helpful to keep in mind because it means that laws limiting the lobbying done by nonprofit organizations do not govern other advocacy activities. Advocacy can be focused but is generally broader, covering more issues. You need to be aware that if you are employed by a state or federal agency, you cannot represent that organization through lobbying. You may advocate for health issues as an individual, but you cannot serve as a paid lobbyist. The American School Health Association and other professional organizations hire lobbyists to talk with policy makers about health issues.

Grassroots Activities

These are activities for which the impetus comes from the people rather than city officials or even local health educators. You can help individuals or groups within your community mobilize to effect change in health-related policies. The Vision Project in Denton, Texas, is an outstanding example of grassroots activity. A few individuals wanted to improve and strengthen the city. They knew they could not do it by themselves, and they knew that city officials could not accomplish what they had in mind. They realized they needed input and help from a wide variety of people. They wanted to hear what others thought would make the city of Denton better. The organizers held focus groups where anyone could participate and offer suggestions. Hundreds of people participated, and dozens of ideas were shared, many of which were health related. Eventually, planning and action teams took the ideas, developed objectives, and carried them forward. As a result, the city of Denton is now home to the Denton Family Resource Center, which helps families access health education and services (http://www.dfrc.org).

Media

Daniel Schorr, a commentator for National Public Radio, once stated, "If you don't exist in the media, for all practical purposes, you don't exist" (Bernhardt, 2006). One of the most powerful ways to advocate for health is by using media and "The Media." The potential for media to promote awareness of health issues is evident every day as you turn on the TV, listen to the radio, open up a magazine, or surf the Internet. As Smith and Wakefield (2005) note, media

> shape attitudes and beliefs, act as agents of public education, and play an important role in determining the policy agenda. They serve as a forum for the elucidation of concepts such that they are subject to public consideration and comment, influencing which issues people think about and how people think about the issues. (p. 472)

Media advocacy is "the strategic use of any form of media to help advance an organization's objectives or goals" (U.S. Administration on Aging, 2008, para. 1). Community health organizations and health professionals now recognize the importance of media advocacy in promoting their health issues, missions, and/or agendas. On a daily basis, an average American is bombarded with more than 3,000 commercial messages, most of them counter to healthy living (Kilbourne, 2003). In order to compete with this barrage as a health professional, you will need to know how to effectively package and deliver your message so that it has the biggest impact. Examples of media advocacy include:

- A *press release* highlighting a "no cell phone zone" call to action, sponsored by a local parent organization that seeks to ban the use of cell phones in school zones.
- A *letter to the editor* of a newspaper from the director of a women's health organization highlighting a popular misconception or factual errors cited in the previous newspaper report on the HPV vaccine. The letter provides a link to the organization's Web site, which lists facts, supporting sources, and contact information.
- A *blog* sponsored by the American College Health Association about the need to legislate "smoke-free" campuses across the United States.
- A *radio interview* with a representative from a local breast health organization about the need to change medical coverage of mammography for those under 40 who have a family history of breast cancer.

- A *public service announcement* (PSA) sponsored by Mothers Against Drunk Driving that urges people to vote against lowering the federal legal drinking age.

- A *Web site* like the Health Education Advocate that educates the public on the need for health care reform in the United States (www.healtheducationadvocate.org).

- A *social networking group site*, such as TWU Pioneers for the Cure, that encourages Facebook users interested in breast health to join the group and share the message of breast health with others.

Each format can be used effectively in health advocacy. See FYIs 12.4 and 12.5 for specific suggestions relating to each type of media.

FYI **12.4   Traditional Media Formats for Advocacy**

There are many different ways you can use the media in advocacy. You can hold news conferences, write letters to the editor, give interviews or arrange editorial board meetings. The method you choose should be the best one to promote your issue.

Media Format	Tips
News Release	Standard format includes: • Organization's name • Contact information • Release date • Headline • Body Your release should follow the inverted pyramid style: • The first paragraph, the lead, should be the most powerful • Keep your sentences and paragraphs short and use plain language • Use quotes if possible • Finish your release with a "tag" • End
Letter to the Editor	Follow these general tips: • Be brief and concise • Refer to other stories • Include contact information
Op-ed	Before you submit your Op-ed, you will want to: • Obtain guidelines • Talk to the editor • Localize it—adopt a local angle, even on national issues
Editorial board meeting	Here are some tips on arranging a meeting: • Call the editorial page editor • Prepare for the meeting • Present your issue • Follow up

(continued)

Media Format	Tips
Interview	Here are some tips on arranging and preparing for an interview: • Arrange an appearance • Familiarize yourself with the program • Prepare for the interview Keep the following in mind to help the interview go smoothly: • Speak in a natural, audible tone • Avoid jargon and acronyms • State your message • Be concise • Tape yourself When being interviewed for television, remember the following: • Appropriate clothing • Look at the interviewer • Sit straight • You're always "on"
Media Event	The two most common are the press briefing and news conference: • Location—You will want to find a well-known location that is convenient for journalists to get to. • Timing—Plan around competing events, holidays, or other activities that may impede journalists from attending your event. • Contacting the media—Send a media advisory several days to a week in advance if you have the luxury of time. If not, e-mail and fax the advisory. • Materials—You will want to have material at your press event to give out to the media. • Prepare—Set up the room for the number of people you invited. • Resource people—Have extra people from your staff available to assist at the event. • Presenting—Make your formal statement as brief as possible—15 or 20 minutes. • Interviews—Allow time at the conclusion of the event to take personal interviews, arrange photos, or answer more detailed questions. • Follow up—After the event, than reporters for attending. • Feedback—Respond in writing to any news stories your event or media outreach garners.

FYI **12.5** **Electronic Media Formats for Advocacy**

Media Format	Tips
Web sites	• Be findable—make sure your URL makes sense and is memorable.
	• Be navigable—good organization is key; good labeling is also important. Keep it simple, consistent, and user friendly.
	• Be relevant and readable—make sure content is helpful and timely. Put a date on materials and keep information current. Provide resources and links to other sites. Keep word choice and readability at about a sixth-grade reading level.
Blogs	• Blogging is an inexpensive way to reach a large number of people, so understand the population you want to reach.
	• Allow people to comment and "have a voice."
	• Advertise events and organizations that are relevant to your topic.
	• Monitor your blogs frequently and respond to queries.
	• Keep it current.
	• Block "hate" messages.

Legislative Advocacy

Legislative advocacy is actually a form of personal communication with legislators (local, state, or federal). You can communicate with your legislators by writing letters, calling, visiting, or e-mailing. In general, you want to know about the person with whom you will be communicating—his or her philosophies and voting records on health issues. After all, if your legislator is a smoker and is heavily supported financially by tobacco companies, you probably won't gain much by discussing tobacco control with him or her. It is important to establish a positive working relationship with your legislator by contacting the office before you visit and providing some preliminary information. You will probably talk with a staff member during this preliminary call and perhaps even during the visit. Don't be put off by this. Staff members will take your information to the legislator, especially if you provide accurate information succinctly and in a straightforward fashion.

The timing of your visit or letter determines the potential impact. A letter or visit that provides information after a vote has been made is meaningless, even if the information would have changed the vote. On the other hand, a letter or visit immediately before an impending vote might play an important role in changing the vote. In order to time your communication well, you need to learn about the legislative process and keep abreast of the issues that are being addressed. The Internet can help you stay up-to-date.

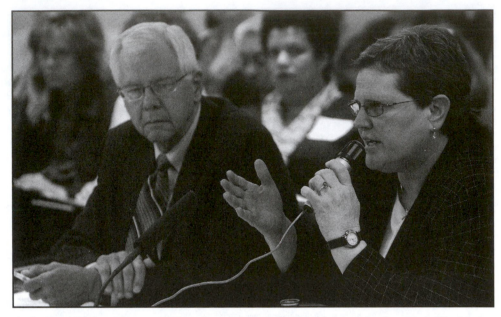

Actively working to change public policy with regard to health issues is a key goal of legislative advocacy. (AP Photo/The Albuquerque Journal, Adolphe Pierre-Louis)

Writing Your Legislator

Letters can be effective means of influencing legislation. Your letters can be sent via postal mail, fax, or e-mail. The same guidelines apply to each format. See FYI 12.6 for tips for writing your policy maker.

Calling or Visiting Your Legislator

Making a personal phone call or visiting your legislator's office can have a powerful impact on policy decisions. Legislators want to know how their constituents feel about the issues being addressed. Your visit will be more impressive if a large group of you contact a number of legislators about the same issue. FYIs 12.7 (p. 300) and 12.8 (p. 301) present tips for calling or making a personal visit to your policy maker.

Survival Skills for Advocacy

The work involved in advocacy is not for the faint of heart! It takes ongoing commitment and energy to drive forward policy and social action. Add to your skills arsenal by adopting some of the "advocacy survival skills" from the Community Toolbox (KU Work Group, 2007d) outlined below.

Accentuate the Positive!

Keep your eyes open for positive events that happen in conjunction with or as the result of your community initiative.

- When you notice something positive happening, even if it's something small, recognize it publicly. Call a local media representative or construct a press release.

- Thank others for their efforts. Pay them public compliments. This will help motivate people to contribute in the future, knowing that you appreciate their involvement!

- Being conscientious about thanking people will help set you apart from other groups that only complain.

FYI 12.6   Tips for Writing to Policy Makers

Your policy maker will pay attention when he or she receives a number of letters about the same issue. Some member of your coalition may be hesitant to write a letter to a policy maker and will need your encouragement. The following tips from the American Public Health Association's *Legislative Advocacy Handbook* will provide some assistance. Keep them in mind as your correspond with your policy makers.

- **Accuracy and attention to detail.** Be sure to use the proper form of address and correct spelling of the policy maker's name.
- Whenever possible and appropriate, use your **organization's letterhead**.
- Remember to identify yourself as a **constituent**.
- **Identify yourself as a public health professional in the text of your letter.** Whenever possible, give your official title and any professional degrees, following your signature.
- **Short letters are best**—try to keep them to one page. Be sure not to use jargon or confusing technical terms.
- **Concentrate on a single issue.** Letters should cover only one topic or bill and be timed to arrive while the issue is still alive.
- **Praise, praise, praise.** If your legislator pleases you by supporting a public health issue, write and tell him/her so. In addition, there are important points to remember regarding the substance of your letter.
- **State your purpose for writing at the outset.**
- **Correctly identify the legislation.** If you are writing about a specific bill, remember to describe it by its official title and number, as well as by its popular name.
- **Tell your legislator how the issue would affect you and the rest of his/her constituents.** Your own personal experience and district-specific information are the best supporting evidence. In addition, data and research supporting your position are important.
- **Be sure that your facts and assertions are accurate.** Often legislators use constituent mail to make points during speeches or debates and to convince fellow legislators of their position.
- **As your policy maker for his/her position on the issue.** Indicate that you look forward to hearing from him/her on the issue.

Excerpted from *APHA Legislative Advocacy Handbook: A Guide for Effective Public Health Advocacy*, p. 28, Washington, DC: Author. © American Public Health Association. Used with permission.

FYI **12.7   Tips for Calling Policy Makers**

Legislative offices in home districts, state capitols, and Washington, DC, can provide you with services and information. Call your legislator's office to learn the status of legislation, to convey your opinions, or to find out the legislator's opinion on an issue.

A phone call to your legislator can be very effective in influencing the outcome of a piece of legislation. You can call the offices of any of your policy makers—congressional representative, state senator, governor, or the president—and ask to have a message delivered to him or her. Some policy makers have hotlines that allow constituents to voice their opinions on legislation. Legislators regularly ask their staff to report on the opinions of constituents calling the office, and some offices keep track of the numbers of constituents weighing in on either side of a particular issue.

Making the Connection:

- Call the U.S. Capitol Switchboard (202) 224-3121 and ask for the office of Senator/Representative _____. Or,

- Call the White House comment line at (202) 456-1111 and leave your comments.

- "Hello, I would like to leave a message for Senator/Representative/President _____."

- Start your call by saying, "My name is _____, and I am from _____." End your call by saying, "Thank you." (Some offices may ask for your full name and mailing address so they can follow up with you on the issue).

- "Please let the senator/representative/president know that I support/oppose (bill number and title)." For your information, you may want to ask what the legislator's opinion is on this issue.

- You can then offer your position by stating, "I would like to urge him/her to vote for/against this provision because: (give one or two reasons)."

- If you would like to discuss a bill in greater detail with your legislator, ask the staff person taking your opinion to relay your name and telephone number to your policy maker or a legislative assistant and ask that your call be returned.

From *APHA Legislative Advocacy Handbook: A Guide for Effective Public Health Advocacy*, p. 30, Washington, DC: Author. © American Public Health Association. Used with permission.

Highlight Values and Accomplishments

Always accentuate the positive values and vision relating to your organization's work. For example, you may ultimately be working toward improved community health, safe workplaces and streets, a clean community environment, or quality education. Everybody wants to experience these things, so it's difficult for opponents or skeptics to argue against the kind of values you promote.

- Prevent wasteful arguments or resistance by keeping public attention focused on values and principles that benefit everyone and that help move your initiative along.

- Communicate to others your group's accomplishments: the new programs, policies, and practices it helped bring about.

FYI 12.8   **Tips for Visiting Policy Makers**

Making a personal visit to a policy maker can have a powerful influence. The following tips from the APHA *Legislative Advocacy Handbook* will guide you in arranging and conducting a meeting with your policy maker.

Tips for Arranging a Meeting with Your Policy Maker

- **Send a letter, a fax, or call to request an appointment.** If you want to meet with your legislator in the district, send the request to the district office. If you will be visiting the capitol, send the letter to that office.

- **Be sure to identify yourself as a constituent** and address the letter to the legislator and to the attention of the appointment scheduler. Include information about who you are, the nature of your visit (identify what you want to discuss), when you would like to meet, and the names of any friends or colleagues who may accompany you.

- **Call the policy maker's office after a few days to follow up the letter.** Ask to speak with the appointment scheduler or the administrative assistant who handles appointments. Explain who you are and why you are calling, and refer to the letter you sent to the office. If the legislator is unavailable at that time or will not be in the area on the date you would like to meet, the appointment scheduler may offer you another date/time or provide you the opportunity to meet with the legislative staff member who handles the issue you want to discuss.

- **Send a letter or make a phone call confirming the appointment.**

Tips for Conducting a Meeting with Your Policy Maker or Staff

- **Arrive on time.** If meeting with a staff member, be sure you have the correct contact name. Do not underestimate the power of the staff person in helping to shape the policy maker's opinions and positions on issues or a particular piece of legislation.

- **Bring two or three colleagues with you.** Prior to the meeting, you should agree on what points will be made and which points each of you will discussion.

- **Try to deliver your message in three minutes.** Be sure to introduce yourself and your colleagues and explain why you are concerned with the issue and your expertise regarding the issue. Be concise, polite, and professional.

- **Be prepared to answer questions.** Clearly explain your interests and issues.

- **Be a resource for the policy maker and his/her staff.** Offer your time and assistance if he/she wants to talk about your areas of interest and expertise in the future.

- **Provide material to support your position.** Leave behind a business card and a one-page fact sheet summarizing your position.

- **Follow up with a thank-you letter.** Be sure to include any additional information you may be promised or that may be relevant to the issue.

From *APHA Legislative Advocacy Handbook: A Guide for Effective Public Health Advocacy*, pp. 30–31, Washington, DC: Author. © American Public Health Association. Used with permission.

Measure Success Each Step of the Way

Sometimes people can get discouraged if it seems like months have gone by without any significant gains. If members of your group aren't able to see any progress after dedicating a lot of time and effort to your mission, their interest and motivation won't last very long. People like to see results, no matter how small. Sometimes, significant progress on a particular community issue is slow to show itself. To break up the time that passes without major breakthroughs occurring, develop a plan of action that has some shorter term or intermediate objectives. For example, let's say that your organization has an outcome objective to provide necessary immunizations to at least 98% of all children ages two or younger within your county within three years. You need those three years to establish the program and get community support; however, you need to measure success throughout this time period as well. To do so, you can plan a number of activities that will allow you to determine whether you are moving toward your goal. Referring to the example above, you may host some educational workshops in the community for mothers with children two years or younger. Measure attendance and change in knowledge and attitudes about immunization at these outreach activities to determine if your program is getting closer to achieving its goals. Do the mothers feel more compelled to have their children immunized? Is the attendance at these events high? Is your marketing working effectively? Celebrations along the way to "the big win" will build the confidence and reputation of your group.

Frame the Issues

If opponents to your program put forth criticisms, don't respond in the terms set forward by your opponents. Instead, shift support away from their perspective by framing the issue in your own voice. Here is a great example provided by the Community Toolbox (KU Work Group, 2007d):

> There is a growing group of individuals who claim that mothers on welfare take advantage of "the system" by having more babies to get "free money" from the government. This sentiment is in direct opposition to your agency, which seeks to help mothers who have uninsured children get the care they need. Rather than attack or take an aggressive stance, responding to their criticism by underscoring that no woman could possibly profit from the small amount of extra money a month per child the state pays, you choose to reframe the issue by focusing on what contributes to mothers being on welfare in the first place: lack of employment opportunities, lack of education or training, inadequate day care, etc. (chap. 30, sect. 2, para. 4)

Develop a Public Identity

If you are too closely linked with a larger and better-known organization, the public may transfer its positive and negative image of the larger organization to your small group. Therefore, it's important to carve out your own identity and let the public know you are unique. For example, there are many breast health organizations in the U.S. that are funded by the Susan G. Komen for the Cure breast cancer foundation. In fact, it is possible to see at least two or three breast health organizations in the same community funded by this one foundation. Being affiliated with a big foundation such as this can have benefits, but also can have drawbacks. If your mission and objectives are not uniquely your own, people may have a hard time remembering your agency or assume it offers the same services as the funding source. Not only is it important to carve out your own niche, it will make you more effective in reaching your intended clientele. For example, perhaps your mission is similar to other breast health organizations in the area (i.e., to save lives), but what makes you distinct from others is that you serve primarily Latina women and offer events at local churches. Or, perhaps you are the only agency that provides prosthetics and wigs, while another agency provides mobile mammography. You're all similar enough to be working together toward your mission of saving lives, but unique in the services you offer and strategies you use to achieve this goal.

Know Your Facts

Understand your organization's issues and actions inside and out. This involves being able to quote a source of information or point to reliable statistics for claims you make publicly. Facts should guide your actions and public statements. If you are caught with inaccurate information or documentation, you could seriously damage your organization's reputation, embarrass yourself, and take attention away from important issues.

Keep It Simple

Small successes help build morale and sustain commitment to the issues. They don't always happen as a result of complex, super-involved actions. Offer simpler, short-term solutions that move toward a bigger solution: in other words, gradually build toward a greater complexity. For example, if a goal of your organization or program is to help orphans in Sierra Leone secure a better future, you could become paralyzed by all of the factors that impede this goal. Instead, begin with a needs assessment, identifying areas of priority. For example, what can your organization do in terms of providing some of the most basic needs for these children—such as shelter, food, medical care, or education? Perhaps your program can only focus on one of these based on your resources, or perhaps quite a few. Whether your budget is ample or lean, it is always important to develop simple, realistic, and measurable objectives that will help you chart your course.

Be Passionate and Persistent

As we mentioned earlier, advocacy is not for the faint of heart. However, persistence and passion are two tools that will help you fight the uphill battle. Solutions must be supported by the community, not just a few, and having passion and persistence will help others see the value of your work and become invested in your mission. Creativity, persistence, and passion fuel health advocacy, so it's important that you engage yourself and others in activities that will allow you to experience internal as well as external rewards so you have the momentum to proceed.

Be Prepared to Compromise

Building healthy communities sometimes calls for compromise with groups whose goals may not be identical to your own. Although you want to stay true to your vision, be open to alternative plans of action or compromises that, although not ideal, may get you closer to your goals. Here is another great example provided by the Community Toolbox (KU Work Group, 2007d):

> Tobacco control advocates in San Francisco wanted to include bars in a policy to ban smoking in public places. The advocates realized a ban on smoking in bars was considered too extreme by the general public, and including bars in the list of targeted establishments would greatly decrease support for the ban. The advocates decided to drop bars from their list of places to target. This was perceived as a reasonable compromise by the public, and the ordinance passed. (chap. 30, sect. 2, para. 5)

Capitalize on Opportunity

Look for opportunities to promote your goals and seize them when they come along. This may involve lying in wait for an appropriate, "natural" time when you can capitalize on some event related to your objectives. For example, February, a time associated with love for others, may be the perfect time to spread the message of breast health with mothers, aunts, sisters, girlfriends, and other loved ones. Or perhaps a well-known celebrity recently announced she has been diagnosed with breast cancer—now that the media has captured people's attention, perhaps it's a great time to flood your community with messages about mammography, survival, and hope.

Stay the Course

Advocates have successfully gone head-to-head with some pretty powerful people, including politicians, CEOs of well-known businesses, and national lobbying organizations like the National Rifle Association. Facing such influential opponents can be daunting, especially when they have greater name recognition and more resources to oppose you. As an advocate for your community, you will have some credibility with the public—after all, you're fighting for their well-being, whether that means safer streets, decent jobs, cleaner air, or better access to medical care. The public will recognize this! The bottom line is this: If you are intimidated into inaction, your opponents will automatically win and nothing will change.

Look for the Good in Others

When you encounter members from groups that disagree with your goals or viewpoint, don't assume they are "out to get you" or ready to pick a fight. If an opponent criticizes your organization, begin by assuming the person doesn't have the same understanding that you do and is speaking out of a lack of information. Educate the opponent and the public about how they may be misinformed.

Keep Focused on the Goal

Opponents may try to distract you from your advocacy activities by attacking you personally. By responding to their name-calling, you waste precious energy and lessen your chances for future cooperation or compromise with these people. Also, your public image may suffer if the general public sees you involved in mudslinging. Instead of giving in to the temptation to fight back, stay focused on the really important issues at hand. Sometimes it may be necessary to respond to their attacks in order to maintain your credibility in the eyes of the public. When you do, make sure your defense or counter attack is well documented with facts and data to back you up.

Make Issues Local and Relevant

When you bring your issues to the local level, you increase your chances for public support. Issues become relevant to community members when they are close to home. For example, Mothers Against Drunk Driving (MADD) has been successful in many communities because many people know someone who has lost a child to an alcohol-related accident. Some ways to really bring issues home to people in your area include using local statistics for the issue, capitalizing on local role models like business people or volunteers, or presenting the issues in a certain way to help community members understand how they will be affected. The Community Toolbox (KU Work Group, 2007d) offers yet another perfect example:

> Imagine that your organization works to build self-esteem and create life options for local teenage mothers. Invite local business people to speak to your organization on how they are working to create more part-time employment for teens and suggest what kind of skills the employers would like future employees to obtain. Perhaps you can create a mentoring pool where professionals from your community would work with these young mothers to help them develop career goals. (chap. 30, sect. 2, para. 7)

Find Common Ground and Generate a Large Support Base

Sometimes it may seem as if becoming part of an advocacy movement automatically puts you in opposition to state and federal policies, politicians, community leaders, and private organizations. Even though there may be some differences between your group and key segments of the community, you may all be more or less working toward the same broad goals of promoting healthier communities. It's important to include people from "inside the system" in your advocacy efforts. This helps you not only widen your perspective on the issues, but it helps you identify "ins" with key agencies and people who can provide valuable support and clout to your efforts.

Tie Your Advocacy Group's Efforts to Related Events

Watch for events that might be relevant to your group's objectives or tactics. Linking to such events helps publicize your cause and strengthen your position in the community. For example, advocates wanting to increase public assistance to individuals who cannot pay for their electric bill could link their cause to the recent death of a local man who died of heat exhaustion when he couldn't afford to fix his air conditioner.

In Conclusion

Community health workers must unite and advocate for important health issues. The power of many voices can make a difference in health outcomes. Advocacy is not a single activity. Knowledge, coalitions and partnerships, lobbying, grassroots activities, media, and legislative activism are excellent advocacy tools. Be sure to employ the tips and guidelines for advocacy that other advocates have found to be useful.

REVIEW QUESTIONS

1. List and define the advocacy terms presented in this chapter.

2. Compare and contrast four advocacy tools.

3. Describe topics you feel are important to cover in a training session for people who wish to visit a policy maker.

4. Select two health issues that you believe warrant advocacy. Write a few paragraphs giving important facts about your issues.

5. Prepare a phone script related to a health issue of your choice that you would use to contact your legislator's office. Deliver your message and reflect on whether or not your efforts were effective.

6. Identify a health issue that is not presented in the chapter but that you consider an important advocacy topic. Justify your choice.

FOR YOUR APPLICATION

Preparing for Advocacy

Select a health issue that you think warrants further advocacy in your state.

1. Collect some information about the issue.

2. Create a one-page fact sheet that you could give to other health educators who would be willing to join you in advocating for the issue.

3. Ask some of your classmates to comment on or make additions to your fact sheet.

Putting Advocacy into Practice

Select a health issue that warrants further advocacy or use the one that you selected in the previous activity.

1. Write a letter to one of your state legislators (preferably the individual from your home district) about your selected issue.

2. Use the tips provided in this chapter.

3. Ask your instructor to read your letter and provide feedback.

4. Revise your letter and send it to your legislator.

5. Put a copy in the Resource Section of your portfolio.

Making an Advocacy Resource List

Create an advocacy resource list that includes the names, titles, and contact numbers of individuals within your community who can publicize and garner support for certain health issues.

thirteen

Resource Access and Management

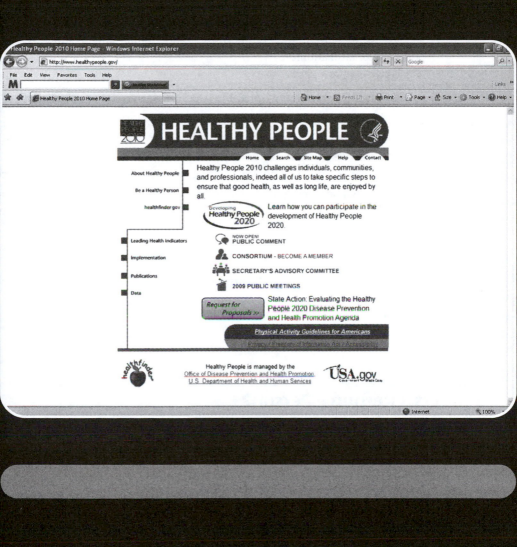

As a community health professional, you will likely act as a resource person. But what does that mean? Do you need to know everything there is to know about health? Do you need to know every important person in health care and be well versed in every computer program as well as the Internet? The good news is, absolutely not! If you are capable of all this, you are special indeed; but let's face it—no one can know everything. What is important for you to know is how to access information and where to go for help.

CHAPTER OBJECTIVES

1. Describe what it means to be a resource person in a community health setting.
2. Review different health occupations and discuss how various occupations can work together to improve community health.
3. Discuss the importance of recruiting and maintaining volunteers within health organizations.
4. Define networking.
5. Describe how community health professionals may act as consultants.
6. Analyze parameters of effective consultative relationships.
7. Discuss networking as a necessary skill to develop and maintain consultative relationships.
8. Provide an overview of government agencies that serve as health resources.
9. Distinguish between government-provided insurance such as Medicare and Medicaid versus private insurance options such as HMOs, PPOs, and fee-for-service plans.
10. Locate online sources of information using the Internet, library databases, and online journals.
11. Evaluate the credibility of health information sources.
12. List health care agencies that might be resources for the community.

What Is a Resource Person?

Regardless of the health setting (i.e., school, hospital, state agency, nonprofit, or corporate), one of your responsibilities as a community health professional will be to know (a) how to get information, (b) where to find available services, and (c) who will be able to help in a given situation. A good resource person doesn't have to know everything but, rather, knows where to find information and services. In this chapter we discuss several types of resources, including people, computers, and organizations.

People as Resources

People are the world's most valuable resources. The wisdom, knowledge, and skills that a diverse group of individuals can bring to a project are considerable. We encourage you to appreciate the wealth of available human resources.

Health and Allied Health Professionals

Health professionals are an obvious source of knowledge and skills to benefit your health education programs. Although not all health professionals have related experiences or outlooks, there is a common goal across all health disciplines—to improve the quality of life and health for all individuals. The following occupational descriptions from the U.S. Department of Labor (2008) will give you a better idea of the range of potential resources from the health professions.

Dental Hygienists and Dentists

Hygienists help people keep their teeth clean, and they conduct an initial assessment of the integrity of the teeth and gums. Most importantly, the hygienist teaches people how to care for their teeth and prevent problems. The dentist diagnoses and treats problems that occur with teeth and gums. Among the specialty areas in dentistry are endodontics (treatment of roots of teeth) and oral surgery.

Health Educators

"Health educators are professionals who design, conduct, and evaluate activities that help improve the health of all people. These activities can take place in a variety of settings that include schools, communities, health care facilities, businesses, universities, and government agencies" (NCHEC, n.d.). A **Certified Health Education Specialist (CHES)** is someone who has successfully passed the national credentialing exam (CHES exam) and has demonstrated competency with regard to the responsibilities delineated by the NCHEC.

Nurses

Most of us understand the basic responsibilities of nurses. We have seen them in a variety of settings, ranging from schools to hospitals. They observe, assess, and record signs and symptoms; administer medications and treatments; and provide patient instruction. You are probably most familiar with registered nurses, who have either a two-year diploma or a bachelor's degree in nursing. Licensed practical or vocational nurses train in one year. They have fewer responsibilities regarding treatment and must be supervised by a registered nurse.

Nurse Practitioners

These are registered nurses who are qualified through advanced training to assume some of the duties and responsibilities formerly assumed only by a physician. For example, some nurse practitioners work in clinics without doctor supervision, and others work with doctors as a health care team. Their scope of practice and authority depends on state laws. For example, some states allow nurse practitioners to write prescriptions, while other states do not. The term "nurse practitioner" encompasses the adult nurse practitioner, advanced practice nurse, certified nurse midwife, certified nurse practitioner, certified registered nurse anesthetist, clinical nurse specialist, clinical specialist in mental health nursing, family nurse practitioner, gerontological nurse practitioner, neonatal nurse practitioner, pediatric nurse practitioner, and school nurse practitioner.

Nutritionists

These professionals, also called dieticians, are trained to blend the science of nutrition with the planning and preparation of meals. They work in many settings, such as hospitals and schools, and may counsel groups of people or work one-on-one with individuals. As you can see, education is a large part of their job.

Occupational Therapists

The goal for the occupational therapist is to help individuals develop and maintain daily living skills. The people with whom they work may be mentally, physically, developmentally, or emotionally challenged. Occupational therapists may work in a client's home or in a health care facility.

Physical Therapists

Physical therapists, like occupational therapists, help individuals restore function. A primary difference is that physical therapists generally work with individuals who have experienced normal functioning in the past and have had an injury that impairs their ability to function. Physical therapists work less with daily living skills and more on the functioning of a joint or limb.

Physicians

We assume that all of you have seen a physician at some time in your life. They are involved primarily in the treatment of disease but are beginning more frequently to address prevention. They use a wide variety of equipment and practice primarily in private offices and health care facilities. The term *physicians* refers to medical doctors (M.D.) and doctors of osteopathy (D.O.). Osteopaths use traditional forms of treatment, including medicines and surgery, but they place special emphasis on the musculoskeletal system. Many M.D. and D.O. specialty areas exist; perhaps you can name a few.

Physician's Assistant (PA)

This is a mid-level health practitioner with special training to provide basic medical care, acting under the supervision of a physician. A physician's assistant may perform such duties as conducting medical examinations, taking medical histories, ordering laboratory tests, interpreting the test results, and performing minor surgical procedures.

Respiratory Therapists

These therapists are literally concerned with the breath of life. They might be involved in diagnosis, treatment, or maintenance of respiratory function. They use a variety of equipment and may treat patients at home or in a health care facility. They educate patients about their respiratory status and how to improve it.

Other Therapists

Other types of therapy include art therapy, dance therapy, recreational therapy, music therapy, pet therapy, and horticulture therapy. The primary goal of each is to help people attain and maintain independence. The wide variety of therapy types allows therapists to combine their interest in health with other interests, and allows patients to use the medium of choice to improve their functional capacity.

Ultrasound, X-Ray, and Imaging Technicians

Technological advancements have expanded employment for imaging technicians. An increasing number of imaging techniques, like ultrasound and magnetic resonance scans, do not use X-rays. Each type of imaging requires specific knowledge and skills.

A Few Examples

We were reminded of the value of health professionals as resources recently when we sought specific information on the dollar value of lives saved through early detection of breast cancer. We searched the online databases and the Web but could not find the specific information we needed. We mentioned the problem to one of our students, an X-ray technician. She had the information we needed within five minutes. What an incredible resource we had without realizing it!

Another example we offer relates to grant writing. In developing a community grant-funded program to increase breast cancer screening and follow-up care for uninsured or low-income Hispanic/Latina and African American women in Denton County, TX, it was necessary for the health educator to collaborate with a clinic or medical practice that would serve as the health care provider and interpret the screening results for the women participating in the free and reduced cost mammogram services. Otherwise, the funding source would not award the grant. Ethically, it would not be responsible for an organization to offer free or low cost mammograms without having a physician or other medical specialist review the results with the client and refer her to the appropriate treatment if needed. One could also argue that providing screening without access to treatment is also inhumane.

The health educator in this example contacted the director of a local nonprofit health clinic, which was funded by multiple grants and provided a number of medical services to low-income and uninsured persons in the county. The clinic's existing funding did not provide for culturally relevant breast health education services that would encourage more women in the community, especially those from ethnic minority backgrounds, to participate in early detection. It seemed like both sides could benefit from a partnership.

Consequently, the collaboration between the health educator and the director of the clinic was advantageous for all involved: the clinic director could connect patients to breast health education and mammography services offered through the health educator's grant-funded program; the health educator could offer women without a primary care physician an opportunity to receive the results and any follow-up referrals through the clinic; and uninsured or low-income minority women in the community would have access to a more comprehensive breast health program and potentially life-saving service (i.e., screening, follow up, and treatment). To be effective in your role as a community health professional, you must be resourceful enough to not only access general health information but to recognize other health professionals who might serve as allies in locating specific information or coordinating services. The old saying is true: Together, everyone achieves more!

Volunteers

Almost any health-related agency for which you will work will depend on volunteers. As Penner and Finkelstein (1998) explain, "If the trend toward fewer government services for disadvantaged and ill individuals continues, the need for unpaid volunteers will increase" (p. 525).

In fact, "Lack of money to purchase health care coupled with societal forces and sociodemographic factors limit the ability of poor families to achieve and maintain adequate health status" (Beardain & Grantham, 1993, p. 2). Volunteers, both health professionals and lay individuals, help increase the volume of health-related services provided by community programs (Penner & Finkelstein, 1998). Moreover, they may be the only hope for some agencies to make a difference in the health status of people in their community.

There are many reasons beyond financial savings to utilize volunteers. The more connected to a community people feel, the more likely they are to take responsibility for the community and engage themselves in its growth and overall health. Mobilizing community resources and expanding capacity through volunteers may also enhance an organization's general profile, which can attract more volunteers, participants, and funding.

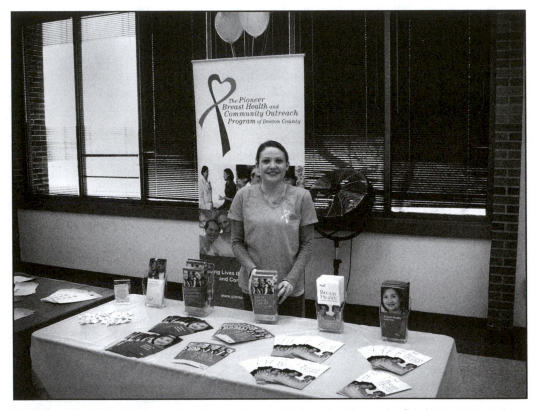

Virtually all health-related agencies rely on volunteers to broaden the reach of their programs and enhance their ability to respond to community needs. (Photo by Jody Oomen-Early)

As noted in *Successful Strategies for Recruiting, Training, and Utilizing Volunteers*, a manual compiled by the U.S. Department of Health and Human Services (2004b), other potential benefits of using volunteers include the following:

- An increased ability to serve clients and respond to the needs of the community (e.g., increased services, expanded hours of operation, shorter wait times)
- Greater staff diversity (e.g., age, race, social background, income, education)
- Increased skill set (volunteers have a diverse array of talents)
- Expanded community support
- Networking that may lead to greater resources and cost savings for the organization

Sometimes the magnitude of dismal news in the media gives the impression that few people choose to be helpful and giving. However, volunteerism is alive and well in this country. According to a recent report from the U.S. Bureau of Labor Statistics (BLS, 2007b), between 2005 and 2006, nearly 3 out of 10 people in the civilian, noninstitutional population age 16 and older did volunteer work. This number was slightly lower than in 2003 and 2004, but higher than in 2002.

You will need to know something about *who* volunteers and *why* they do so in order to recruit and retain the people you need. People who volunteer often have more education and higher incomes than those who do not. Married people, especially married women, volunteer more frequently (BLS, 2007b; Zweigenhaft, Armstrong, Quintis, & Riddick, 1996). However, the number of men who volunteer is increasing, as is the percentage of older Americans who volunteer (BLS, 2007b; Chambre, 1993). As a whole, volunteers donate a median of 50 hours of service a year; however, this number increases with age, with the largest amount of volunteer time belonging to those 65 years and older.

People volunteer for various reasons (Snyder, 1993), and are influenced by a number of factors. Some of the reasons people give for choosing to volunteer include personal satisfaction, professional responsibility, perceived community need, desire to help others (BLS, 2007b; Ward, 1998); commitment to service, business networking, career development (Ellis, 1993); recreation, a desire to make friends (Glascoff, Baker, & Glascoff, 1997); and recognition. Other notable characteristics of volunteers in America are listed in FYI 13.1 on the following page.

As the Bureau of Labor Statistics (2007b) reports, volunteers perform a myriad of important tasks, but the main activities reported were fund-raising (10.9%) and tutoring or teaching (10.8%). Men and women tend to engage in different activities. Men who volunteer are most likely to engage in general labor (13.5%) or to coach, referee, or supervise sports teams (10.2%), while women volunteers are most likely to fund-raise (12.5%), or tutor or teach (12.5%).

If in the future you need volunteers in your work, we encourage you to tailor recruitment and retention efforts for specific types of individuals. Creating an environment where volunteers can make a difference in health status requires more than just providing an opportunity to volunteer. A comprehensive understanding of why people volunteer, what barriers prevent them from volunteering, and what keeps them motivated to continue to volunteer may improve the volunteer experience and have a powerful impact on the effectiveness of volunteer services. Volunteers will also need

FYI **13.1   Who Volunteers in America?**

- About 61.2 million people in the U.S. volunteer annually (that's over a quarter of the U.S. population).

- The value of volunteer time, on average, is $17.19 an hour.

- Volunteers donate an average of 52 hours of time a year.

- About 30.1% of women volunteer compared to 23% of men.

- People 35 to 54 years old are most likely to volunteer.

- Individuals ages 20–24 have the lowest volunteer rates.

- More married persons (32.2%) volunteer compared to those nonmarried (20.3%) and those with other marital status (21.3%).

- Volunteers are most likely to work with religious groups, education, or youth.

- The most common volunteer activities performed are fund-raising, teaching, mentoring, or coaching.

Source: *Successful Strategies for Recruiting, Training, and Utilizing Volunteers: A Guide for Faith- and Community-Based Service Providers* [online manual]. U.S. Department of Health and Human Services, 2004.

training and development opportunities. We hope you will accept the challenge of maximizing your volunteer resources through a respectful understanding of them as individuals. Some helpful tips for recruiting and working with volunteers are listed in FYIs 13.2 and 13.3 (p. 316).

Consultants

Consultants, people you hire to assist with a specific project or program, can offer a combination of five abilities: expertise, perspective, authenticity, friendship, and accomplishment (Bellman, 1990). Let's discuss these abilities in a little more detail.

Expertise

This ability pertains to a special knowledge or skill. You might, for example, want to hire a consultant to help you evaluate a specific program. According to Bellman (1990, p. 129), you may want to use a consultant's expertise for one or more reasons:

1. You may not have the knowledge and skills yourself.

2. You may have the knowledge and skills but not the time.

3. You may not be in the right position to do the work.

4. You may not want to do the work yourself.

Be honest with consultants about why you are hiring them. If you happen to be serving as a consultant yourself, be sure to find out why you are being hired.

FYI **13.2   Strategies for Recruiting Volunteers**

- Contact your local volunteer center.
- Use current volunteers—they are convincing salespeople because they are dedicated to your cause and believe in your organization.
- Use the mass media (e.g., television, radio, the Internet, newspapers, billboards), as well as neighborhood newspapers, newsletters, and organizational bulletins.
- Make announcements at services, educational sessions, meetings, and social gatherings of your congregation or organization.
- Post volunteer opportunities on appropriate Web sites.
- Make personal appearances at schools, senior centers, career fairs, and community events.
- Generate personal interest stories based on volunteer experiences.
- Staff booths and exhibits at special events.
- Use mass mailings or personalized, handwritten notes.
- Get referrals from staff, ministers, friends, and lay leaders.
- Register with volunteer referral organizations.
- Volunteer in other organizations' projects.
- Collaborate with schools that require community service hours for graduation.
- Ask people to volunteer; most people volunteer because they are asked.
- Create print materials such as flyers and brochures about your organization and include descriptions of the volunteer opportunities available.

Source: *Successful Strategies for Recruiting, Training, and Utilizing Volunteers: A Guide for Faith- and Community-Based Service Providers* [online manual]. U.S. Department of Health and Human Services, 2004.

Perspective

This ability involves seeing the world in a new way, or bringing a fresh perspective to a situation. Sometimes an organization or program isn't running smoothly because an individual or individuals are not performing as they should. For example, your authors were helping public health personnel access information and found that they rarely used the Internet as a tool. We made the assumption that they lacked the skills to use the Internet. According to Bellman (1990, p. 131), however, the lack of performance isn't usually lack of skills, as normally perceived by supervisors, but instead faulty perceptions about the use of skills. For example, such people

- see the situation in a way that precludes using the skills that would be appropriate to the situation.
- don't understand that the skills might be necessary.
- are scared to use the skills they have because of perceived consequences.
- don't want to use their skills because they think it would be inappropriate.

- don't know when to use their skills because no one has indicated that the skills are needed.
- suffer in some way when they use their skills.

FYI **13.3   How to Write a Volunteer Position Statement**

If your agency, company, or organization depends largely upon volunteers, you may be asked to recruit them. As part of this task, you may need to develop descriptions of the volunteer position. Some things to consider when developing a written description are outlined below:

1. **Position Title**
   A specific, descriptive title provides the volunteer with a sense of identity and ensures that salaried staff and other volunteers understand this particular role. Steer away from descriptions that have to do with the presence of lack of pay. For example, why call the receptionist a "volunteer" receptionist? You don't say "paid" receptionist for a staff member.

2. **Work Location**
   Where will the individual be working? Can the work be done at home or only on site, or at a particular site? Make sure that there is public transportation near your work site so you can recruit people who might not have their own transportation.

3. **Purpose of the Position**
   How will the volunteer's work affect the project's outcome, clients, or mission? It is important to identify the expected impact for both direct service and administrative assignments so that volunteers will understand how important their work is.

4. **Responsibilities and Duties**
   Specifically identify the volunteer position's responsibilities and duties. Define what is expected from the volunteer.

5. **Qualifications**
   It pays to be clear and concrete in listing qualifications for any volunteer position. Include education, personal characteristics, skills, abilities and/or experience required.

6. **Commitment Expected**
   What do you expect of the volunteer? Include length of service, hours per week, hours per day. Include any special requirements such as weekend work.

7. **Training**
   List what training the volunteer will receive. Include general training that all positions receive plus any position-specific training for this assignment.

8. **Other**
   Include the date the description was written or the date that it was updated. List the volunteer supervisor's name and his/her contact information. Include information about how to get more information and who to call if interested. You might want to include signature lines for the volunteer manager and the site supervisor if appropriate.

Source: *Successful Strategies for Recruiting, Training, and Utilizing Volunteers: A Guide for Faith- and Community-Based Service Providers* [online manual]. U.S. Department of Health and Human Services, 2004.

In our case, the individuals with whom we were working mistakenly believed that they were not allowed to use the Internet. Whether your organization needs a new perspective or requires help in pinpointing a lack of training, a consultant can assist.

Authenticity

A consultant can help people in an agency recognize the true nature of the organization. The previous section talked about seeing the world in a new way, but authenticity is "seeing" reality. The consultant must be personally authentic (know and understand self) in order to add this dimension to the consulting process.

Friendship

Bellman (1990) notes that characteristics we expect from our friends are the same characteristics we should expect in a consulting relationship:

- We want friends to be honest.
- We expect our friends to allow us to take responsible risks.
- We want to be able to talk about what is important to us with our friends and to be taken seriously.
- We want to accomplish things, reach goals shoulder to shoulder, and enjoy our accomplishments with our friends.
- We want be able to talk with friends about concerns, knowing that they will be supportive.

Although friendship might seem out of place in a business relationship, the elements of friendship we have listed are necessary to honest appraisal and true teamwork.

Accomplishment

The normal expectation from a consulting relationship is that results will be achieved. Obviously, results are the bottom line for hiring a consultant. We caution you, however, to be careful in the way you define *results*. Sometimes we have personal agendas for accomplishments that are not based in reality. For example, if you hire someone to help you evaluate a program, you cannot demand that the results show the program in a completely positive light. Accomplishment in this case is gaining information that will help you improve your program. You might also want to think in terms of small successes. Give yourself and your programs credit for the process of improvement, not just the final outcome.

The costs associated with hiring a consultant need to be considered. Yet, in cases where you are "stuck" due to overwork, lack of skills, or inability to gain perspective, the benefits of hiring a consultant may far outweigh the costs. A good consultant can save a program or project.

Currently, there is very little research published about the opportunities or trends in consulting within the field of community health. However, FYI 13.4 offers some insight into consulting in health education. As the health care system continues to evolve, with increasing emphasis on prevention and on program accountability and sustainability, the opportunities for consulting should multiply.

FYI **13.4   Consulting in Health Education**

In an effort to learn more about health educators as consultants, Keating, Boham, and Ransdell (2007) surveyed health education/promotion consultants via the Health Education Directory (HEDIR) Listserv. Participants who were health education consultants (a total of 25) completed a quantitative survey that also contained a few qualitative questions. The researchers found the following:

- The majority of health education consultants participating in this survey had graduate degrees, diverse backgrounds, and more than 15 years of experience.
- CHES certification was held by 28% of the sample. Most participants held full-time jobs and participated in consulting part-time as a way to secure additional income.
- Consulting opportunities were most likely to arise due to expertise, reputation in the field, services requested, and/or networking.
- When hired as a consultant, individuals were most likely to: (a) design, implement, or evaluate programs; (b) conduct seminars or presentations; (c) write and review grants; or (d) combine multiple responsibilities, as specified in a contract designed by the entity for whom consulting is conducted.
- The majority of the consultants who participated in the study earned an annual income between $50,000 and $59,000.
- When asked how someone could become a health education consultant, participants suggested developing an area of expertise within health, providing necessary services such as grant writing or program evaluation, and networking.
- One-third of the survey participants worked as consultants on a part-time basis and had primary careers in other areas of health education such as in schools, government organizations, or corporate health.
- Program design and implementation were the most commonly reported job responsibilities assigned to health education consultants.

Source: "Consulting in Health Education/Promotion: Everything You've Always Wanted to Know but Were Afraid to Ask," by M. Keating, M. Boham, and L. Ransdell, 2007, *California Journal of Health Promotion*, vol. 5 (3), pp. 92–99.

Networking

Do you hear people talking about networking but just can't get a handle on what it means? Networking is an important tool for serving as a resource person. Look at Figure 13.1 and you will see the potential connections generated through meeting and getting to know people. For example, if you meet and share information with person A, you have the potential of gaining resources from persons A, B, C, and E. Person A knows and talks with B, C, and E; and if you ask, he or she will most likely be willing to pass along your name, needs, or skills. Networking can take you even further because each individual knows other individuals. The key to networking is that you place yourself in situations where you can meet and talk with other professionals. You

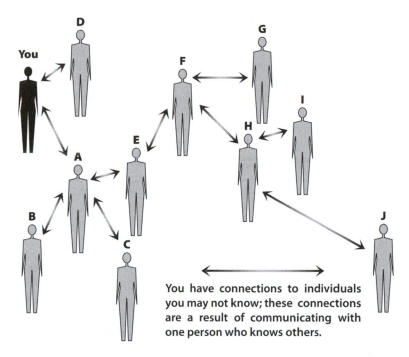

You have connections to individuals you may not know; these connections are a result of communicating with one person who knows others.

Figure 13.1   Networking.
Networking is a key factor when you are serving as a resource person and when you are seeking resources. Communicating with a couple of key individuals could be of great benefit to you and your agency.

must be willing to discuss your needs as well as those skills you are willing to share with others. Professional conferences, workshops, and other professional development activities are good places to start networking.

Computers as Resources

Technology is a powerful tool for acquiring and sharing health information. Through the click of a button, people from any side of the world can now access health information 24 hours a day, 7 days a week on the Internet. Acting as a health-related resource person requires you to possess the computer skills necessary to not only search and find health information through the World Wide Web, but to be able to determine its accuracy and credibility. Some commonly used terms and strategies for sharing and evaluating online health information are discussed next.

The World Wide Web

As you know, the World Wide Web (WWW), part of the Internet, is a network of servers that connect with links. The **links** help an individual at one computer access files at another site. A link generally goes to a **home page** (the introductory page to a Web site). The home page often acts as a table of contents or guide to the site's other pages and links to more sites (McLean, 1996). For example, if you go to the Texas Woman's University home page at http://www.twu.edu you will find options like Get info about TWU, Admissions, and Student Life. If you put the cursor on one of these phrases, you will note that it turns into a small hand, indicating a link to another page. You simply click on the link, and your Web browser will retrieve the page from where it is stored and display it on your computer.

Links between sites are made with the help of hypertext. **Hypertext** also helps users find information through key words and phrases. You know you are using hypertext to access information when you type in "http:" as part of the address. HTTP stands for hypertext transport protocol (Daniel & Balog, 1997).

Search Tools

Web Browser

A Web **browser** is software that helps you view the World Wide Web on your computer. According to Daniel and Balog (1997), "There are three basic types of Web browsers: full screen browsers (e.g., Lynx), graphical browsers (e.g., Internet Explorer or Mozilla Firefox), and line mode browsers" (p. 261). Full screen browsers display only text on the screen. The others show text and graphics and provide other services. If you want to know more about browsers, you might visit http://www.browsers.com. As a World Wide Web user, you travel from one **Uniform Resource Locator** (URL) to another. The URL is a Web address.

The Web's contribution to community health can be phenomenal: Health facts can be at your fingertips in seconds. But you need to make sure that the information you choose is indeed factual (see the discussion later in the chapter), and you can expect to get frustrated over the plethora of addresses, types of sites, and contradictory information. You probably have a favorite search tool; if not, try one of those mentioned in the following paragraphs.

Search Engines

A **search engine** is a database created by software that searches the Web for titles and phrases. In other words, when you initiate a search using a search engine, you are not searching the Web itself but, rather, the search engine database. The numerous search engines all have similarities, but they differ in size and in the types of Web pages they list. Some of the most well-known search engines are Google (http://www.google.com) and Yahoo (http://www.yahoo.com). Google currently claims to index over 3.3 billion pages, while Alltheweb.com (one of Yahoo's many search properties) claims to index over 3.1 billion (Barlow, 2004). Search engines that require site owners to pay to have their sites indexed, such as Ask.com, index fewer pages. Although they are all similar in ways, you must be the judge of which best serves your purpose. The effectiveness and utility of search engines depends largely upon the information you seek.

A **meta-search engine** allows you to enter a query and search multiple search engines and their databases of Web pages simultaneously. Within a few seconds, you get results from all the search engines. Examples of meta-search engines include Dogpile (http://www.dogpile.com), Clusty (http://www.clusty.com), and Surfwax (http://www.surfwax.com).

Directories

Although the terms *search engine* and *directory* are often used interchangeably, they are not the same thing. A **directory** is a database that usually organizes Web sites by topic and is managed by humans, unlike a search engine, which uses software (Kennedy, 1999). Web sites are categorized by subject, date, and even format. Some well-known directories are YouTube (http://www.youtube.com), Yahoo (http://www.yahoo.com), About.com (http://www.about.com), and LookSmart (http://www.looksmart.com). As of early 2006, YouTube emerged as one of the ten most popular Web sites on the Internet (Burke, Snyder, & Rager, 2009). The world's largest online video directory, YouTube gives individuals the ability to watch homemade and professionally produced video clips or upload their own video content to share on a wide range of topics. FYI 13.5 includes a listing of popular search engines and health directories. We encourage you to try them all and compare your results.

Search Agents

A **search agent** (i.e., "agents" or "intelligent agents") is a software tool that you can download to your computer that will help you find information on the Internet in less

---

FYI 13.5   Popular Internet Search Engines and Health Directories

Search Engines	Health-Related Directories
Google	Health.com
http://www.google.com	http://www.health.com
Yahoo	Intellihealth
http://www.yahoo.com	http://www.intellihealth.com
Ask	Intute
http://www.ask.com	http://www.intute.ac.uk
Aolsearch	Scirus
http://www.aolsearch.com	http://www.scirus.com
Alltheweb	Google Scholar
http://www.alltheweb.com	http://scholar.google.com
Hotbot	Health6.com
http://www.hotbot.com	http://www.health6.com
Livesearch	Just Health Sites
http://www.livesearch.com	http://www.justhealthsites.com
Altavista	Healthfinder
http://www.altavista.com	http://www.healthfinder.gov
Gigiblast	Highlight Health
http://www.gigiblast.com	http://www.highlighthealth.info
Lycos	Medlineplus
http://www.lycos.com	http://www.nlm.nih.gov/medlineplus

time (Sullivan, 2005). These "agents" will automatically do certain jobs on the Internet according to what you ask them to do. For example, a search agent will send your search question to all of the best ranked search engines simultaneously and rank the results so you quickly find what you need. There are agents that speed up your computer downloads, ones that remove ads from your computer screen or block "pop up" advertising or "spyware." There are even search agents that will scan your e-mail for "spam" or junk mail or tell you what the weather will be like! Some of the best-known search agents are Copernic, Firststop, Webseeker, and Myspiders (Sullivan, 2005). Unfortunately, search agents usually provide only a limited number of hits per site they search.

Listserv

A **Listserv** is an e-mail discussion group or mailing list that is bound by a common interest. Transcripts of a Listserv can be saved and the archives can be reviewed. An example of a Listserv relating to health is the **HEDIR** (Health Education Directory) that was developed and copyrighted by Dr. Mark J. Kittleson. In addition to sharing messages, a Listserv could be a portal for sharing health information and ideas with your peers. For example, are you interested in finding out how many health educators work in school settings versus corporations? Or, perhaps you'd like to discuss the current CHES requirements? The HEDIR Listserv could be a valuable medium for collecting this information in a short span of time. Listservs exist in every field and are an effective way to communicate with a large group.

Online Databases for Professional Literature

Don't forget about professional journals when you are seeking information. Sometimes the ease of gathering information electronically makes seeking and reading professional journals less attractive. However, as you will learn in a later section of this chapter, the information you collect must be verified through research. Because professional journals are generally the means by which research is disseminated, it is vitally important that you stay abreast of what they report.

Locating professional articles has become as simple as searching the Web. Large databases that archive articles and abstracts exist for most professions. For example, Medline is a database compiled by the U.S. National Library of Medicine that archives articles and abstracts from approximately 4,300 medical journals. Other databases that health educators might find useful include CINAHL (the Cumulative Index to Nursing and Allied Health Literature), Psychlit (psychology-related journals), and ERIC (educational journals). Most databases for professional journals can be accessed via the Web, but we suggest that you visit your university library and speak with a reference librarian to gain more information. Or, you may want to attend a library workshop on database searching or tour your library's Web pages to learn more about searching the databases available to you. There are more than you can imagine.

There are also growing numbers of online health-related professional journals; some of the most popular peer reviewed periodicals relating to community health are:

- Journal of Community Health
- American Journal of Health Education
- Journal of Family and Community Health

- American Journal of Public Health
- Health Promotion Practice
- Journal of School Health
- The International Electronic Journal of Health Education
- The Internet Journal of Allied Health Sciences and Practice

More than likely, you will have access to these journals through your university library. In fact, your library may actually have a directory of all electronic journals related to health as well as other subjects. As with hard-copy journals, electronic journals also require subscriptions, and there is a schedule for publication. Although you have the option of printing a hard copy of a journal article if necessary, you will not have to store or dispose of a pile of journals. This plays a small but important role in preserving the environment in which we live.

Web 2.0 Technology

The Internet has rapidly evolved over the last decade, making it easier for people to share information quickly and with tools that allow for more personalization. This new wave of user capabilities and creativity is often referred to as "Web 2.0." The number 2 does not denote a "second version" of the Internet but rather a perceived second generation of Internet tools and communities (O'Reilly, 2005). Blogs, wikis, podcasts, and video directories are just a few examples of Web 2.0 technology that can be sources of health information.

Blogs

As defined by *Webster's New Millennium Dictionary of English* (2007), a Web log, or **blog**, is a frequently updated online diary or personal chronological log of thoughts published on a Web page. Blogs are typically published by individuals, and their style is personal and informal. Anybody with an Internet connection can publish his or her own blog. Blogging has evolved from its origins as a medium for the online publication of personal diaries to a respected vehicle for editorials on specific topics including social, economic, and political-based issues (Oomen-Early & Burke, 2007). The quality, content, and ambition of blogs varies greatly, and they may have anywhere from a handful to tens of thousands of daily readers (Lenhart & Fox, 2006). Some blogs are explicitly or implicitly fictional, though the standard genre expectation, particularly for health and education-based sites, is nonfiction. (Educause Learning Initiative, 2005; Lenhart & Fox, 2006).

In 2006, almost 70 million American adults were reading or hosting blogs (Lenhart & Fox, 2006). About 100,000 new blogs are created each day, and the Blogosphere (total blogs tracked) doubles every five to seven months (Technocrati, 2006). These facts reflect not only the growth in blogging, but also a blog's popularity as a vehicle to provide and share information. In fact, you may already be familiar with blogging and have your own "blogspot" on such popular sites as Blogger, Blogspot, LiveJournal, MySpace, Facebook, or WordPress. In addition to providing opportunities for personal expression, blogs may be an effective strategy for delivering health information, connecting health professionals, raising social conscience, and advocating for the field and specific health issues (Oomen-Early & Burke, 2007).

Wikis

The term "Wiki" is a Hawaiian term meaning "super fast" (Tonkin, 2006). A **Wiki** is a piece of server software that allows users to freely create and edit Web page content using any Web browser. According to the original creator, Ward Cunningham, "a Wiki is the simplest online database that could possibly work" (Tonkin quoting Cunningham, 2006, p. 43). Wikis support hyperlinks and have a simple text syntax for creating new pages and crosslinks between internal pages which are user-friendly. A Wiki is unique compared to other collaborative communication mechanisms in that it allows all users to contribute and edit the content (Tonkin, 2006). Wikis can be used for such things as sharing helpful Web sites on specific topics (also called webliographies); comparing fieldwork notes; presenting and reviewing favorite articles, pictures, or papers within groups; collecting peer feedback; scheduling events or appointments; and a multitude of other tasks. Like many simple concepts, "open editing" has some profound and subtle effects on Wiki usage. "Allowing everyday users to create and edit any page in a Web site is exciting in that it encourages democratic use of the Web and promotes content composition by nontechnical users" (Herman, 2005, para. 2). The most widely used Wiki to date is **Wikipedia** (see FYI 13.6). One of the disadvantages of using Wikis to find or present health information is that you do not always know who is authoring or editing a Wiki; therefore, you cannot guarantee that the information you find is accurate or unbiased.

Podcasts

A **podcast** is an audio broadcast that has been converted to a file type called "MP3" or other audio file format for playback in a digital music player or computer. The "pod" in podcast was coined from iPod, the predominant portable, digital music player by Apple on which the podcasts can be downloaded and played. Podcasts are not just limited to MP3 players or iPods, however. You can listen to a podcast from your computer by downloading free software that can be found on popular Web sites like iTunes, Playpod, Smartfeed, and Newsfire. Although podcasts are mostly verbal, they may also contain music (PCMag.com, n.d.). A podcast is distinguished from other digital media formats by its ability to be syndicated, subscribed to, and downloaded automatically when new content is added (PCMag.com, n.d.). Podcasting is becoming a popular medium for presenting information because of its immediacy, archiving capabilities, and ability to reach a global audience. For example, the National Institutes of Health (NIH) uses podcasting to disseminate health information. Individuals can subscribe to NIH Radio and receive free podcasts on a variety of health presentations by some of the nation's leaders in health. You can browse the NIH Radio archives and listen to a variety of podcasts by visiting http://www.nih.gov/news/radio/podcast/nihpodcastarchive.htm.

Webinars and Webcasts

A **webinar** is a seminar broadcasted on the Internet that may be interactive. It can contain both audio and video elements. Webinars connect people synchronously and are superior to teleconferencing in that participants can be anywhere on the planet and participate in the presentation. Presenters have the ability to use presentation slideshows, video, or link to places on the Internet while facilitating the webinar. Wimba and Elluminate are common webinar platforms. Webinars may be archived to be viewed later, at which time they may become webcasts. **Webcasts** differ from webinars in that data is transmitted one way and does not allow interaction between the presenter and the audience. Webinars and webcasts are powerful tools for health professionals because they can connect people from all points of the globe and serve a

FYI **13.6   Wikipedia: The Online Encyclopedia**

Wikipedia is an online encyclopedia that can be edited by anyone. It was based on *Nupedia,* an earlier prototype by Jimmy Wales. Larry Sanger built upon Wales' ideas and launched Wikipedia on January 15, 2001. The concept behind Wikipedia was to establish a free, "living" encyclopedia that could quickly build upon global knowledge and perspectives (*Wikipedia: Size Comparisons*, n.d., para. 2). Information is therefore accessible and "controlled" by anyone and everyone. The innovation quickly spread. By February 12, 2001, the project surpassed 1,000 articles, exceeding 10,000 articles by September 7. In the first year of its existence, Wikipedia grew to 20,000 encyclopedia entries—a rate of more than 1,500 articles per month! On August 30, 2002, the article count reached 40,000. As of January 2008, Wikipedia has amassed over 2,153,002 articles and over 5 million registered accounts. By the time you read this, it will surely have grown even more! The combined Wikipedias in all languages together contain 1.74 billion words in 7.5 million articles in approximately 250 languages; the English Wikipedia gains a steady 1,700 articles a day, with the wikipedia.org domain name ranked at around the 10th busiest on the Internet (*Wikipedia: Size Comparisons*, n.d., para. 3.).

Wikipedia continues to garner visibility by the press and has steadily gained some acceptance as a secondary source. However, even though credibility of Wikipedia is growing as its quality assurance and fact checking improves, people should still **be cautious in using it as a sole source of information**. The fact that it is an "open source" means that it is only as credible as the authors who contribute to it. In fact, some critics of Wikipedia have called it "garbage, an incoherent hodge-podge of dubious factoids that adds up to something far less than the sum of its parts" (Orlowski, 2005). In fact, co-founder Larry Sanger, who is no longer a part of Wikipedia, has openly urged former colleague Wales to seek more "established sources of expertise" (Orlowski, 2005, para. 2).

Wikipedia also acknowledges its need for improvement on its own Web site. "Many of the articles are of poor quality and some mainstream encyclopedia topics are not covered adequately. And, the average article length is only a little over half the size of that in *Encyclopedia Britannica*. Over time the balance of the editorial effort is expected to slowly tilt toward a greater emphasis on increasing the quality, scope, classification, and interlinkage of existing articles" (*Wikipedia: Size Comparisons*, n.d., para. 5). When searching for health information, you might consider Wikipedia as a first stop or springboard to lead you to other sources or ideas on the topic. As with any source, it is always important to think critically about what is presented and be judicious in the application of this information based on its apparent credibility and accuracy.

Sources: "Wikipedia Founder Admits to Serious Quality Problems," by A. Orlowski, 2005, [Newsbrief], *The Register.* Retrieved January 4, 2008, from http://www.theregister.co.uk/2005/10/18/wikipedia_quality_problem; *Wikipedia: Size Comparisons.* (n.d.). Retrieved January 18, 2008, from http://en.wikipedia.org/wiki/Wikipedia:Size.comparisons.

multitude of purposes, including training, simulations, focus groups, meetings, lectures, and press conferences.

Analyzing Computer Resources

Think about a time when you used information from the Web for a paper or other class assignment. How did you know that the information you used was accurate, objective, and appropriate? Did the author or authors seem credible? Was the content thorough? The Internet provides massive amounts of information, but, unfortunately, some of the easiest Internet sources to access don't provide reliable, unbiased information. There are actually five categories to consider when analyzing a source of information: accuracy, authority, objectivity, currency, and coverage. FYI 13.7 provides guidelines for analyzing your computer sources of information.

FYI 13.7   Five Criteria for Evaluating Web-Based Content

Evaluation of Web documents	How to interpret the basics
1. Accuracy	
• Who wrote the page and can you contact him or her?	• Make sure the author provides e-mail or a contact address/phone number.
• What is the purpose of the document and why was it produced?	• Know the distinction between author and Webmaster.
• Is this person qualified to write this document?	
• Is the information reliable and error free?	
2. Authority	
• Is there an author listed?	• What credentials are listed for the authors?
• Who published the document and is this entity separate from the "Webmaster"?	• Where is the document published? Check URL domain.
• Check the domain of the document. What institution publishes this document?	
• Is the author qualified? An expert?	
• Does the author list his or her qualifications?	
• If the page includes neither a signature nor indicates a sponsor, *is there any other way to determine its origin?*	
+ Look for a header or footer showing affiliation.	
+ Look at the URL: http://www.fbi.gov	
+ Look at the domain: .edu, .com, .ac.uk, .org, .net	

3. **Objectivity**
   - What goals/objectives does this page meet?
   - How detailed is the information?
   - What opinions (if any) are expressed by the author?
   - Does the information show a minimum of bias?
   - Is the page designed to sway opinion?
   - Is there any advertising on the page?
   - Determine if the page is a mask for advertising; if so, information might be biased.
   - View any Web page as you would an infomercial on television. Ask yourself why was this written and for whom?

4. **Currency**
   - When was it produced? Is there a date listed?
   - When was it updated?
   - How up-to-date are the links (if any)?
   - Have some expired or moved?
   - How many dead links are on the page?
   - Are the links current or updated regularly?
   - Is the information on the page outdated?

5. **Coverage**
   - What topics are covered?
   - What does this page offer that is not found elsewhere?
   - How in-depth is the material?
   - Are the links (if any) evaluated and do they complement the documents' theme?
   - Is it all images or a balance of text and images?
   - Is the information presented cited correctly?
   - If the page requires special software to view the information, how much are you missing if you don't have the software?
   - Is it free or is there a fee to obtain the information?
   - Is there an option for text only, or frames, or a suggested browser for better viewing?

Putting it all together

Accuracy—If a Web page lists the author and institution that published the page and provides a way of contacting him/her and . . .

Authority—If the page lists the author credentials and its domain is preferred (.edu, .gov, .org, or .net), and . . .

Objectivity—If the page provides accurate information with limited advertising and it is objective in presenting the information, and . . .

Currency—If the page is current and updated regularly (as stated on the page) and the links (if any) are also up-to-date, and . . .

Coverage—If you can view the information properly—not limited to fees, browser technology, or software requirement, then . . .

Accuracy

The term **accuracy** refers to the correctness of the information. We can all agree that you need to present the most accurate information possible. If you are a member of HEDIR (the Listserv mentioned earlier), you have read discussions about **urban myths**. These myths are anecdotes and supposed facts that are widely disseminated but have no accuracy. An example of such a myth is the claim that antiperspirants cause cancer. The assertion sounds somewhat plausible. You might read that an antiperspirant can block sweat glands and, further, that a blocked sweat gland might result in cellular changes that, in turn, could possibly result in cancer. Despite the apparent plausibility of the claim, however, current research does not document a relationship between antiperspirants and cancer.

Unfortunately, much Web information is presented as fact, even though it has no empirical basis. Empirical research would involve an experimental study design. Recall from chapter 3 that an experimental design is a type of research study that uses at least two groups of subjects, one for the intervention and another for comparison. When you present information, be sure to identify the experimental studies that document what you are saying.

Sometimes research alone isn't enough to document the accuracy of information because of the presence of bias or flaws in some research designs. In cases like these, it may be wise to check the opinions of experts in the field to verify information you are presenting. To find expert opinion, check the databases for peer-reviewed journals; experts will have published articles on their area of concentration.

Authority

When evaluating online content, one must also question the authority who is sponsoring the information. For example, is the Web site produced by a pharmaceutical company? A physician? A governmental organization like the Centers for Disease Control? An angry blogger? Would your reaction to the information be different if you knew the document was written from the perspective of one of these? Knowing who is generating the information will allow you to put what you are reading into proper context and consider the bias or objectivity in delivery of the content. When examining the authority of a Web page or Web site, consider such things as its domain (.org, .edu, or .com); the credentials of the author(s); headers or footers that provide information about the sponsoring agency; and where the document or Web site is published (i.e., China, U.S., the U.K., etc. . . .).

Objectivity

The **objectivity** of information can be determined by assessing its source. If the source presents two or more different perspectives accompanied by citations, it may be more appropriate than sources offering just one perspective. You can be more confident that the information is not based on one biased viewpoint. But look for evidence of bias if the source is a for-profit organization or is funded by an organization that wishes to propound a specific viewpoint.

Currency

Currency of information is also important. You usually need the most timely information or enough background material for a historical perspective. Determine your specific needs, but make a deliberate decision about the time issue rather than accept information no matter when it was written.

Coverage

The **coverage** of information has to do with its depth. For example, the statement "Smoking causes health problems" has meaning by itself. It can be backed by research that is current and independent. It is not likely to be misconstrued even if it stands alone. Some statements need to be supported by additional information that is also accurate and appropriate in order to have meaning. For example, the statement "Herbal preparations can enhance health" does not stand alone. Many herbal preparations haven't even been studied. If you are discussing herbs, you will want to give supporting evidence. Frequently, it's difficult to determine the extent of coverage of a topic from a Web page. The page may or may not include links to other Web pages or print references that might provide the full picture of the issue. Sometimes Web information is "just for fun," a hoax, someone's personal expression that may be of interest to no one, or even outright silliness. It is up to you to make certain that the information is adequate either by itself or in combination with additional information.

Evaluating Podcasts and Blogs

As you know, Web pages are not the only sources of health information. As mentioned earlier, podcasts and blogs can be helpful in disseminating health content. Apply the same standards mentioned in FYI 13.7 in reviewing the content contained in these sources and consider questions outlined in FYI 13.8 and FYI 13.9 as well.

FYI **13.8   Questions to Ask When Evaluating Blogs**

- Does the title of the blog provide information about its content?
- Is the purpose of the blog stated on the blog page?
- Is there a link to lead you to further information about the blog creator?
- Can you determine the credentials of the creator from the blog content?
- If you conduct a search on the creator's name in a search engine or in Google Groups, can you find out what provides the creator with the authority to write about the blog topic?
- Can you tell from the comments on the blog that others treat the creator as an expert in the topic that the blog covers?
- Do many other blogs link to this one? (Conduct a URL search in a blog search engine like Google BlogSearch or Technorati.)
- When looking at the blogger's posts, can you recognize any bias?
- Is the content found in the blog written in a readable manner, with correct grammar/spelling?
- Does the content in the blog contradict information found in another source?
- Is the information on the blog updated on a regular basis?

From "Critical Evaluation of a Blog." *Kathy Schrock's Guide for Educators* [online manual], by K. Schrock, 2006. Retrieved from http://discoveryschool.com/schrockguide/. Used with permission.

FYI **13.9   Questions to Ask When Evaluating Podcasts**

- Did the podcast include content that appeared accurate? Timely? Appropriate?
- Were the technical qualities (audio, slides, etc.) acceptable in the production?
- Was a written transcript of the podcast available?
- Was the podcast linked from a site that included subject tags?
- Who was the sponsor of the podcast? Did it appear to be credible?
- Was the podcast linked from a site that included links to other resources?
- Did the podcast adhere to the copyright guidelines in its use of music, pictures, etc.?
- Was the length of the podcast appropriate for its content? (20 min. or less)
- Was the podcast part of a regularly scheduled series?
- Did the presenter in the podcast keep you interested?
- What were the presenter's credentials?
- Did the presenter seem biased?
- Did the podcast flow smoothly (introduction, content, summary)?
- Was it obvious how to add the podcast feed to your aggregator? (RSS)
- If the item was an enhanced podcast, did the use of slides enhance the content?
- If the item was an enhanced podcast, was it available in various file formats to allow viewing on various hardware devices?

From "What Makes a Good Podcast?" *Kathy Schrock's Guide for Educators* [online manual], by K. Schrock, 2006. Retrieved from http://discoveryschool.com/schrockguide/. Used with permission.

Organizations as Resources

We introduced the importance of health organizations in chapter 2. These organizations can have a powerful impact on the health of a community. It will be important to familiarize yourself with the organizations in your community and network with the professionals staffing them.

Voluntary Health Organizations

Voluntary health organizations are powerful allies for community health professionals and help to build healthier communities. Brief descriptions of a few of the many voluntary health organizations follow. Appendix A lists URLs for these and other organizations.

- *The American Cancer Society.* This organization is dedicated to helping people who face cancer through research, patient services, early detection, treatment, and education. The national office is located in Washington, D.C., but the organization has state and local affiliates.

- *The American Heart Association.* The mission of this organization is to help people build healthier lives, free of heart disease and stroke, through health education and advocacy. It is divided physically into the National Center (located in Dallas, Texas) and nine affiliate offices that cover the United States and Puerto Rico.

- *The American Lung Association.* Fighting lung disease for more than 90 years, the American Lung Association is a leader in tobacco education and regulation. It has a strong focus on the prevention of lung diseases like asthma, tuberculosis, pneumonia, and emphysema.

- *March of Dimes.* Four major problems threaten the health of America's babies: birth defects, infant mortality, low birth weight, and lack of prenatal care. The March of Dimes has adopted goals to bring us closer to the day when all babies will be born healthy. The goals include a commitment to "reduce birth defects by 10%, reduce infant mortality to 7 per 1,000 live births, reduce low birth weight to no more than 5% of all live births, and increase the number of women who get prenatal care in the first trimester of their pregnancy to 90%" (March of Dimes, 1999, p. 1).

- *Muscular Dystrophy Association.* This voluntary health agency is working to defeat 40 neuromuscular diseases through worldwide research, comprehensive services, and public health education.

- *National Kidney Foundation.* The National Kidney Foundation seeks to prevent kidney and urinary tract diseases. It also seeks to improve the health and well-being of individuals and families affected by these diseases and increase the availability of all organs for transplantation.

- *Cystic Fibrosis Foundation.* The mission of the Cystic Fibrosis Foundation is ongoing improvements in the quality of life for individuals with this disease.

- *American Red Cross.* This organization has multiple functions and services. The primary mission, however, is to help prevent, prepare for, and cope with emergencies. Approximately 30 million people are assisted each year.

- *The National Academies of Practice.* This organization is dedicated to quality health care for all. The members, nominated by individuals in their respective fields, have spent a significant portion of their careers in direct health care delivery to consumers. The NAP serves as an interdisciplinary policy forum, addressing public policy, education, research, and inquiry.

Government Agencies

We discussed the National Institutes of Health (NIH) and the Centers for Disease Control and Prevention (CDC) in chapter 2. These two agencies have a powerful influence on the health of the nation. You will find more detailed information about each in the paragraphs that follow. Keep in mind, however, that even government agencies that don't seem to be directly health-related can have an impact on health.

National Institutes of Health

The NIH mission is "to uncover new knowledge that will lead to better health for everyone" (NIH, 1999, p. 1). The NIH, housed in Bethesda, Maryland, has 20 institutes and seven centers (see Appendix E for a complete list). It is one of the eight agencies of the Public Health Service, which is part of the Department of Health and Human Services. The institutes work toward their mission by conducting research in their own laboratories; supporting research at universities, medical centers, and other institutions; and assisting in the training of research investigators.

The NIH has supported about 325,000 **principal investigators** (scientists who take the lead in a research project) and researchers in conducting health-related research. The agency employs more than 18,000 people—from research scientists to support personnel.

According to the NIH (2008), research it supported played a role in the following accomplishments:

- Infectious diseases—such as rubella, whooping cough, and pneumococcal pneumonia—that once killed and disabled millions of people are now prevented by vaccines.

- Quality of life for 19 million Americans suffering with depression has improved as a result of more effective medication and psychotherapy.

- The sequencing of the human genome set a new course for developing ways to diagnose and treat diseases like cancer, Parkinson's disease, and Alzheimer's disease, as well as rare diseases.

- In response to the anthrax attacks of 2001, the NIH launched and expanded research to prevent, detect, diagnose, and treat diseases caused by potential bioterrorism agents.

- New and improved imaging techniques let scientists painlessly look inside the body and detect disease in its earliest stages when it is often most effectively treated.

- Researchers are aggressively pursuing ways to make effective vaccines for deadly diseases like HIV/AIDS, tuberculosis, malaria, and potential agents of bioterrorism.

- Progress in understanding the immune system may lead to new ways to treat and cure diabetes, arthritis, asthma, and allergies.

- New, more precise ways to treat cancer are emerging, such as drugs that zero in on abnormal proteins in cancer cells.

- Novel research methods are being developed that can identify the causes of outbreaks, such as Severe Acute Respiratory Syndrome (SARS), in weeks rather than months or years.

Centers for Disease Control and Prevention

As you may recall from chapter 2, the CDC's mission is to "promote health and quality of life by preventing and controlling disease, injury, and disability" (CDC, 2008a, para. 1). Its main office is in Atlanta, Georgia. An organizational chart that outlines its arrangement of offices, institutes, and centers appears in Appendix E. The CDC seeks to accomplish its mission by working with partners throughout the nation and the world to:

- monitor health

- detect and investigate health problems

- conduct research to enhance prevention
- develop and advocate sound public health policies
- implement prevention strategies
- promote healthy behaviors
- foster safe and healthful environments
- provide leadership and training

The CDC employs almost 8,000 people in about 170 different occupations. The employees work in Atlanta and in 10 locations across the United States.

Organizations That Impact Health Care Delivery

Most of us are aware of the typical organizations that deliver health care: hospitals with emergency rooms, community outreach clinics or health centers, and doctors' offices. Much education is provided by these organizations. Unfortunately, health information is not always presented appropriately or in a culturally sensitive manner. Moreover, the timing of information presentation is not always beneficial to the patient. For example, providing education during a crisis in the emergency room is not generally effective. Nevertheless, these organizations can be valuable health information resources.

Even schools can serve as health-related resources. Public Law 94-142 requires that all children in the United States be provided free and appropriate public education. Because some children need health care in order for education to be meaningful, schools have implemented many health services. Among them are physical therapy, occupational therapy, counseling, speech therapy, and nursing services (Rodman et al., 1999).

Insurance Companies

Insurance companies affect health care delivery tremendously because they create and sell the plans that cover our health care expenses. There are two broad categories of insurance with which you should be familiar: private (fee for service and managed care) and government.

Private—fee for service.   Insurance is about money. In 1960 the United States spent only 5.2% of GDP on health care. By 2004 that number had risen to 16%, which is more than America spends on food (Krugman & Wells, 2006). Insurance helps people cover the cost of health care. Two basic categories of private insurance exist: payment after and payment before services are delivered. Before the 1990s, payment after the delivery of services, or **fee for service**, was the most common form of health insurance (Baker & Baker, 1999). Today, almost all insurance provides predetermined-per-person delivery of services. Each insurance company will negotiate with the health care delivery institution and physician the fee that will be paid for each service. Therefore, hospitals and physicians may receive different amounts for the same services from various insurance companies.

Private—managed care.   The concept of **managed care** refers to a "means of providing health care services within a network of health care providers" (Baker & Baker, 1999, p. 26). In the managed care model, all health care services for an individual are coordinated and provided by the network. The network consists of health care providers and agencies that agree to be members. **Health maintenance organizations**

(HMOs) are the most common type of managed care plan. Several varieties of HMOs currently exist, but they all have similarities. The insurance company pays a preset monthly fee to the health care providers who belong to the HMO. An insured individual must use the providers who are designated in the plan or pay higher fees. Health care providers employed by the insurance company review cases and play a role in the selection of health care. The insurance company may charge physicians in some way if they order services that are not suggested by the company.

Most plans cover hospital services (surgical and emergency room), long-term care services, home care, primary care physician (PCP) visits, selected lab work, radiology, and pharmaceutical needs. Unfortunately, many managed care organizations include only limited mental health services despite the fact that millions of people each year need services for mental health. Dental and eye care are often covered under separate plans.

Preferred provider organizations (PPOs) are another type of private insurance plan. Similar to HMOs, they consist of a panel of providers that range from hospitals to specialty physicians. The panel members provide utilization review or a review of the services ordered by a physician. They make recommendations about the necessity of services, and the physician is expected to follow those recommendations. Doctors may be charged in some way for services that are deemed unnecessary. People who select PPOs must use the providers who are members of the plan or pay higher fees. The types of services offered are very similar to those offered in HMO plans. See FYI 13.10 for a helpful review of managed care terms.

FYI **13.10   Managed Care Terms**

Term	Definition
Capitation rates	Predetermined upper limit for treatment cost.
Case managers	Individuals in the employ of the insurance company who oversee and manage treatment for an individual receiving health care.
Copayment fees	Predetermined fee for which the insured is responsible.
Deductibles	Predetermined amount of money that the insured will pay before insurance coverage begins.
Fee for service	Payment after the delivery of health care services.
Formularies	Descriptions of approved treatment regimes.
Managed care	A means of providing health care services within a network of health care providers.
Preventive medicine	Health care delivery before the occurrence of disease or disease progression.
Primary care physician	The physician who determines the need for and authorizes specialty health care.
Utilization review	Review and management of treatment selected by physicians who are members of the HMO or PPO.

HMOs and PPOs create problems for many underserved U.S. populations. The motivation behind HMOs is to decrease expenses, not improve health status. The rationale for the HMO or PPO model is that physicians and patients overutilize the health care system. In order to solve the problem, the physician becomes the gate-keeper to prevent unnecessary services. We know, however, that many underserved populations, working poor, and those living below poverty level, in fact, do not access health care as often as do European Americans and people from middle- or upper-income families. They also have poorer health.

When many poor individuals eventually visit their HMO, they may have a back-log of illnesses. Their course of illness is likely to be longer and more severe due to lack of adequate housing, food, and clothing. Compounding these problems is the fact that utilization review is largely based on statistical norms for European Americans. It will be important for you to understand how insurance companies impact health care delivery and find ways to help those who are hurt by our current insurance programs.

Government insurance.   In 1965, legislation established "Health Insurance for the Aged and Disabled" as part of the Social Security Act (Baker & Baker, 1999). Known as **Medicare**, this insurance program has two parts, called simply Part A and Part B. Part A covers hospital stays, and Part B covers such things as physician visits, labs, x-rays, diagnostic tests, and medical equipment such as wheelchairs or walkers. An individual chooses to purchase Part B. Anyone working in the United States pays a tax to cover Part A. Part B is charged to the individuals, generally through deductions from Social Security benefit payments.

Medicaid was also established in 1965 as part of the Social Security Act. This program was created to assist needy individuals with health care expenses. Although the federal government provides broad eligibility criteria, each state sets its own specific criteria and payment rates for services. This is the largest program to help people with low incomes pay for health care.

Other government programs include the Department of Veteran Affairs health programs, migrant health care services, mental health services, drug and alcohol services, and the Indian Health Service.

In Conclusion

Although you don't need to know everything and everyone related to health, you do need to be able to access and use health resources. You should begin by understanding your most valuable resource: people. Other health care professionals can offer knowledge and skills that you alone cannot hope to attain in one lifetime. They may serve as volunteers or form a vital resource network for you. Devoting time and attention to your relationships with other health professionals is a wise career investment.

In addition to people, technology is a vital resource. In today's world, technology enables people to find information quicker than ever before. Your ability to locate and present information depends on your mastery of current computer technology and your efforts to keep up to date with innovations.

Finally, organizational resources are abundant, whether they are voluntary health organizations, health care facilities, or government agencies. Your understanding of their missions and roles will guide your search for information and enable you to use it effectively. So, how do you manage all of this information? A resource inventory is a tool that can help community health professionals manage and locate resources expeditiously. Appendix D provides a template for you to use. Serving as a resource person is a key responsibility for those working within a community setting. People need to have accurate, credible information as well as know how to apply this information and where to go for additional help or services. Navigating people toward essential information, community agencies, organizations, or health services is key to building healthier, empowered communities.

REVIEW QUESTIONS

1. Identify three health professionals working in community health and describe how each might serve as a resource for a health educator.

2. List five reasons people might volunteer. What can you do to help maintain volunteers?

3. Describe the five abilities that a consultant might bring to a client.

4. Reflect on consulting within the field of health and list three things one might consider before beginning consulting work.

5. Define networking and discuss its importance.

6. Identify the differences between search engines, search agents, and directories.

7. Discuss five criteria for evaluating online materials.

FOR YOUR APPLICATION

Conducting an Internet Search

Select one health-related organization and search the Internet to collect information about it. Write several paragraphs describing your findings.

Recruiting and Keeping Volunteers

Imagine that you work for a voluntary health association. Select a specific agency and create a hypothetical activity in which that agency might be involved. Develop a list of methods you will use to recruit volunteers for the activity you have chosen. Make a second list of methods you will use to keep those volunteers.

Evaluating Electronic Information

Choose a health issue to explore. Locate a Web site, an online article or brochure, and a podcast or blog related to this health issue. Using the criteria included in this chapter, evaluate the reliability, credibility, and overall effectiveness of these health materials.

Subscribing to a Health Listserv or Health Blog

Learn more about health-related Listservs and blogs in your field such as the HEDIR (www.hedir.org), The HEDIR Blog (http://hedir.hpcareernetwork.com/), or HPCareer.Net. If the membership is free (like it is for the HEDIR), consider joining it for at least a week. Keep track of the kinds of discussion and information sent through this Listserv or posted on the blog. What is the quality of the discussion? Overall, do you think this is an effective way to share health information?

Creating a Resource File

Imagine that you are a college campus health educator. Using Appendix D, create a resource list of health materials and resources that could be used for planning and implementing campus-based health events.

Future Trends in the Global Community

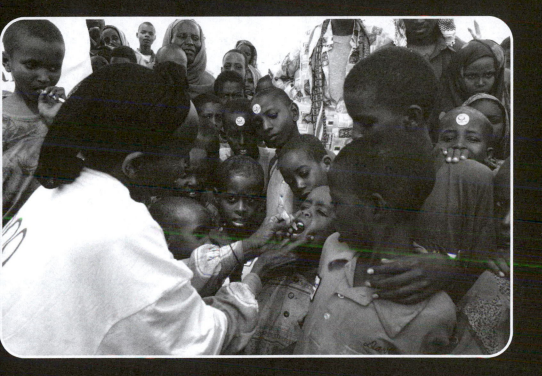

As you sit down to enjoy your favorite Thai cuisine at a local restaurant, a scrolling headline on the television screen within your view captures your attention: "Soaring cost of rice leads to social unrest and violence internationally." As you dive into your meal, you ponder how such a common staple, like the one on the plate in front of you, could be causing such mayhem worldwide. The television images of chaos, violence, and starvation in places like Haiti and Sierra Leone jump out at you and generate even more questions: What is causing this crisis? What impact does it have on communities in those countries and others around the globe? And, how does it affect you?

CHAPTER OBJECTIVES

1. Define globalization.

2. Discuss the trends and projections relating to globalization, world demographics, and health.

3. Explain how technology may serve as both a barrier and as an asset to building healthier global communities.

4. Describe predicted changes in health care systems and their potential influence on community health.

5. Describe predicted job-market growth patterns as they relate to community health.

6. Discuss the importance of promoting community empowerment at the local and global levels.

7. List strategies for career development and lifelong learning that will increase one's ability to work successfully in the field of community health.

Global Health and Quality of Life

The world is rapidly changing at a pace that makes it difficult to keep up. Globalization has become a buzzword for the 21st century to describe this change process. The World Health Organization defines **globalization** as "a comprehensive worldwide process involving the internationalization of communication, trade, and economic organization. It involves parallel rapid social, economic, and political change" (WHO, 2004). Ongoing changes in these socio-ecological factors (see chapter 1) can put the health of a community in a state of constant flux. Though globalization benefits many parts of the world, it can exacerbate disparities and significantly impact health and quality of life for poor and marginalized populations in developed and undeveloped economic regions.

Isn't that how we began this textbook—with a discussion about the meaning of health and quality of life? How fitting that we have now come full circle. Yet we dare not simply repeat what we said at the beginning of the textbook. There is so much more that you need to know to be equipped for the health professions of the future. The pace of change in the world and within these professions compels us to describe in this final chapter some future trends and recommendations for professional development. We begin this venture with brief comments about these two concepts within the context of a global future.

Global Health Concepts

Access an Internet search engine, type in the words *global health*, and an avalanche of links to information and opportunities will appear. The plethora of choices will be overwhelming, particularly if you are trying to focus on only a few key concepts. Finding a simple, concise definition that encompasses the broad spectrum that global health represents is also a challenge. Instead, we offer five characteristics of global health based on a variety of sources (Global Health Council, n.d.; Skolnik, 2008) and our own experiences. Each characteristic, in isolation, is an insufficient description of all that comprises global health. Collectively, however, these descriptive statements begin to paint the broader picture.

- *Global health is* a process through which public health and community health promotion principles are applied across national boundaries.

- *Global health is* a goal that stretches beyond the mere absence of disease and embraces the concepts of total wellness and quality of life for all.

- *Global health is* a worldview in which individual members are seen as interdependent for survival and well-being.

- *Global health is* a partnership in which "countries work together not only to understand critical health issues but also to solve them" (Skolnik, 2008, p. 7).

- *Global health is* the common ground where individuals and nations can meet from across a complex array of boundaries (geographic, political, ideological, etc.) to share a common goal.

Quality of Life on a Global Scale

Quality of life has been described as "the perception of individuals or groups that their needs are being satisfied and that they are not being denied opportunities to pursue happiness and fulfillment" (Green & Kreuter, 2005, p. 34). Quality of life comparisons on a global scale reveal enormous inequities related to satisfied needs and denied opportunities. The richest 10% of the world's population holds 54% of the world's wealth while an additional 40% of the population has access to only 5% of the global income (United Nations Development Programme [UNDP], 2005). Though quality of life improvements have been achieved in some parts of the world in recent years, "violent conflicts, insufficient resources, lack of coordination and weak policies continue to slow down development progress, particularly in Africa" (UNDP, 2007/2008, p. 4).

Contributing factors and potential solutions for these inequities in quality of life can be viewed within the context of the trends we describe in the following sections. We offer them as issues to consider as you prepare to promote global health.

Trends in the Global Community

As we pointed out earlier, our world is evolving at lightening speed. The populations, languages, cultures, economies, technology, and diseases of the 19th and 20th centuries are markedly different than those in the 21st. This continual metamorphosis will have a profound impact on the quality of life and prosperity of people in every corner of the world. Established in 1948, the World Health Organization has expanded its focus over the last six decades to include improving overall well-being rather than just survivorship. In fact, it reports that, due to socioeconomic development and technological advances, the world as a whole is moving toward a healthier, longer life span (WHO, 2008b). As you look toward and plan for the future, consider the emerging trends that will shape our global community as well as your role as a health professional.

Trend #1: World Population Continues to Grow

Though it might be hard to believe, the rapid growth of the world population is a fairly recent phenomenon. As Table 14.1 indicates, population growth in the earliest centuries was relatively slow, and the number of people in the world did not significantly expand over periods of time. For those inhabitants of early civilization, life was harsh. Living conditions were poor and death rates were high. War, famine, disease, poverty, illiteracy, and lack of technological innovation kept the population in check. Because both fertility and mortality were high, the world census changed very little in the years leading up to 1800. It is estimated that two thousand years ago, the world's population was 300 million (about as large as the population of the United States today!); ten centuries later, it may have increased only by 10 million. It rose to about 500 million by 1500, and by 1800 the population had climbed to almost 1 billion.

With the advances brought on by the Enlightenment and the Industrial Revolution, the world's population nearly doubled between 1800 and 1900. Still, that gain is modest compared to the unprecedented population boom that occurred in the 20th century. With the introduction of scientific and technological innovations such as vaccines and medications, public health and epidemiological strides to control disease, better access to food and water, and the rise of modern industry and communications, world population *nearly quadrupled*! Over the course of 100 years, the world's population grew from 1.65 billion in 1900 to 6.11 billion in 2000, an increase of 4.46 billion (UN, 2009). Even more wondrous is the fact that over half of this growth (80%) took place in the second half of the century. This incredible upward trend will continue throughout the 21st century (see Figure 14.1). The population of the world is projected to continue to increase, but at a slower pace. By 2050, world population is expected to reach 9.15 billion (see Table 14.1). Most population growth is expected to occur in developing countries, while more developed regions will either remain constant or slightly decline in numbers. India will become the world's most populous country by 2050, and China and the U.S. will also remain in the top three (Table 14.2).

In fact, the current population of the most developed regions is expected to remain relatively constant, from its present 1.23 billion to 1.27 billion by 2050. In lesser developed areas, populations will climb to 7.87 billion in 2050 and then to 8.42

billion by 2100 (UN, 2009). How will this growing census impact world resources, economies, and overall health? This is a hot topic of debate among world leaders, economists, sociologists, health scientists, and researchers across the world.

Related to the issue of increasing population is the world's rapid urbanization (WHO, 2006a). About 45% of the world's population lived in urban areas in 1995. By 2025, that proportion is expected to increase to 60%. People are flocking to cities all over the world to be closer to jobs and other resources. As more children are born in those areas, city boundaries will expand by necessity.

This growth rate gives rise to growing concerns about our ability to maintain a sustainable environment for all those people. In a **sustainable environment**, such factors as

Table 14.1 World Population Estimates and Projections, Year 1 to 2050

Year	Population in Billions
1	.30
1000	.31
1500	.50
1800	.98
1900	1.65
1925	1.96
1950	2.53
1975	4.07
2000	6.11
2025	8.01
2050	9.15

Source: *World Population Prospects: The 2008 Revision* (2009); *World Population Prospects: The 1998 Revision* (1999), United Nations, Population Division, New York: Author.

Table 14.2 The 20 Most Populous Countries by 2050

Rank	Country	Population in 2050 (in millions, medium variant)	% of world total
1	India	1,614	17.6
2	China	1,417	15.5
3	U.S.	404	4.4
4	Pakistan	335	3.7
5	Nigeria	289	3.2
6	Indonesia	288	3.1
7	Bangladesh	222	2.4
8	Brazil	219	2.4
9	Ethiopia	174	1.9
10	Dem. Republic of the Congo	148	1.6
11	Philippines	146	1.6
12	Egypt	130	1.5
13	Mexico	129	1.4
14	Russian Federation	116	1.2
15	Vietnam	112	1.3
16	United Republic of Tanzania	109	1.1
17	Japan	102	1.2
18	Turkey	97	1.0
19	Iran (Islamic Republic of)	97	1.1
20	Uganda	91	1.0

Source: Adapted with permission from *World Population Prospects: The 2008 Revision, Highlights*, Table A.3, United Nations, Population Division, 2009, New York: Author.

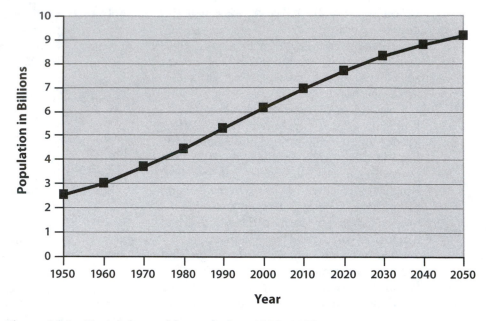

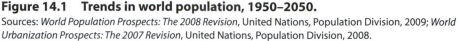

Figure 14.1   Trends in world population, 1950–2050.
Sources: *World Population Prospects: The 2008 Revision*, United Nations, Population Division, 2009; *World Urbanization Prospects: The 2007 Revision*, United Nations, Population Division, 2008.

housing, education, health and nutrition, and the use of natural resources keep adequate pace with population growth and distribution patterns (WHO, 2006a). In other words, a sustainable environment is one in which the people who live in it have access to what they need to live.

The downside of rapid urban growth is crowding and stress. Those who can afford to move out of crowded inner-city areas and into more attractive suburbs leave behind those who face poverty and marginalization. The result is often inadequate housing, poor waste disposal and sanitation systems, and stress-induced violence and accidents. It is possible that, as the urbanization phenomenon grows, so will the number of people living in this poverty gap.

Trend #2: People Are Living Longer

You probably remember from chapter 4 that the U.S. population is aging. That is also true from a global perspective. The United Nations Development Programme (UNDP, 2006) reported that in 2000, 19.5% of the world's population was over the age of 60. By 2010, that percentage will rise to 21.7; by 2015, it will be 23.5; and by 2020, nearly one in four people on the planet will be over the age of 60. As more people live longer, the primary challenge will be to help individuals develop and sustain their well-being into old age. The focus will continue to rest on healthy lifestyle behaviors such as exercise, diet, and abstinence from tobacco. Newly expanding needs will center on efforts to help the elderly remain active in their communities, maintain and develop new social contacts, and engage in intergenerational activities (UN, 2009).

Consequently, the average human life span is continuing to increase worldwide (Table 14.3). This is true for both men and women. Life expectancy for men is expected to increase from 65.4 to 73.3 by 2050, and for women, it will increase from 69.8 to 77.9 (Table 14.4 on the following page). The number of persons aged 60 years or over is expected nearly to triple, increasing from 673 million in 2005 to 2 billion by 2050 (UN, 2009). Over the same period, the share of older persons living in developing countries is expected to rise from 64% in 2005 to nearly 80% in 2050. Today, about half of the oldest-old (those 80 years and older) live in developing countries, but that share is expected to reach 71% in 2050. The **median age**, or the age that divides the population in two halves of equal size, is an indicator of population aging. At the world level, the United Nations (2009) reports that the median age is projected to increase from 28.9 to 38.4 years between 2009 and 2050. Within countries with the oldest

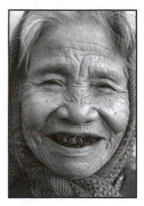

Average life spans are increasing for men and women across the globe. (© Teoman Alemdar)

populations, this will increase to 55.8 (Table 14.5 on the following page). According to the United Nations (2009), North America currently has the greatest life expectancy of 79.3 years and this will increase to 83.5 by 2050. The Central Intelligence Agency's *World Factbook* (2008) estimates the U.S. life expectancy at birth at 78.1, which ranks 50th among countries worldwide. Figure 14.2 illustrates the continuing upswing in the percentage of people aged 60 years and older. This graying of our global society will undoubtedly have an impact on not only the health care system, but other facets of society. For example, with more people living longer, active lives, the age of retirement will continue to increase, businesses and entertainment will continue to tailor services and advertising to this growing segment of the population, and our entire notion of "growing old" will evolve. Perhaps 60 will be the new 50 by 2020?

Table 14.3   Life Expectancy at Birth for the World, Major Development Groups and Major Areas, 2005–2010 and 2045–2050

Major Area	2005–2010	2045–2050
World	67.6	75.5
More developed regions	77.1	82.8
Less developed regions	65.6	74.3
Least developed countries	55.9	68.5
Other less developed countries	67.7	75.9
Africa	54.1	67.4
Asia	68.9	76.8
Europe	75.1	81.5
Latin America and the Caribbean	73.4	79.8
North America	79.3	83.5
Oceania	76.4	82.1

From *World Population Prospects: The 2008 Revision, Highlights,* Table III. 1, 2009, United Nations, Population Division, New York: Author. Used with permission.

Table 14.4 Life Expectancy by Sex for the World and Major Development Groups, 2005–2010 and 2045–2050

| | Life expectancy at birth (years) | | | |
| | 2005–2010 | | 2045–2050 | |
Major Area	Male	Female	Male	Female
World	65.4	69.8	73.3	77.9
More developed regions	73.6	80.5	79.9	85.6
Less developed regions	63.9	67.4	72.2	76.5
Least developed countries	54.7	57.2	66.7	70.4

From *World Population Prospects: The 2008 Revision, Highlights*, Table III. 2, 2009, United Nations, Population Division, New York: Author. Used with permission.

Table 14.5 Ten Countries or Areas with the Oldest and Ten Countries with the Youngest Populations, 2009 and 2050

| 2009 | | | 2050 | | |
Rank Country or Area		Median Age	Rank Country or Area		Median Age
A. Oldest Population			**A. Oldest Population**		
1.	Japan	44.4	1.	China, Macao SAR	55.8
2.	Germany	43.9	2.	Japan	55.1
3.	Italy	43.0	3.	Republic of Korea	53.7
4.	Finland	41.8	4.	Singapore	53.5
5.	Channel Islands	41.7	5.	China, Hong Kong SAR	52.7
6.	Switzerland	41.6	6.	Bosnia and Herzegovina	52.2
7.	Bulgaria	41.5	7.	Cuba	51.9
8.	Austria	41.4	8.	Germany	51.7
9.	Slovenia	41.4	9.	Netherlands Antilles	51.1
10.	China, Hong Kong SAR	41.3	10.	Poland	51.0
B. Youngest Population			**B. Youngest Population**		
1.	Niger	15.1	1.	Niger	20.2
2.	Uganda	15.5	2.	Afghanistan	23.5
3.	Dem. Republic of the Congo	16.5	3.	Somalia	23.6
4.	Burkina Faso	16.7	4.	Uganda	24.2
5.	Zambia	16.8	5.	Chad	24.5
6.	Malawi	16.8	6.	Zambia	24.7
7.	Afghanistan	16.8	7.	United Republic of Tanzania	24.8
8.	Chad	17.0	8.	Guinea-Bissau	24.8
9.	Timor-Leste	17.2	9.	Timor-Leste	25.0
10.	Angola	17.3	10.	Burkina Faso	25.1
	WORLD	28.9		WORLD	38.4

Adapted with permission from *World Population Prospects: The 2008 Revision, Highlights,* Table A.11, 2009, United Nations, Population Division, New York: Author.

Note: Only countries or areas with 100,000 persons or more in 2009 are considered.

Though the highest proportion of population expansion will be among the elderly, the world's adolescent population will continue to grow as well. The World Health Organization coined the phrase **global teenager** in 1999 to emphasize the emerging changes in how this age group, worldwide, will view and function in emerging societies (WHO, 1999). According to a United Nations report (2006), the number of young people between ages 10 and 19 has reached a peak at 1.2 billion, or nearly a sixth of the total world population. Over 90% of these teenagers live in developing countries, due to the high fertility and low death rates globally (UN, 2006). However, besides being the largest teenage population the world has seen, this group faces dangers associated with their characteristic vulnerability. Teenagers comprise the demographic most vulnerable to HIV/AIDS and the health impacts of poverty, drugs, discrimination, violence, and sexual trafficking (UN, 2006). If their health care and social needs could be met, however, teenagers could develop into the largest, most vibrant workforce ever seen when they reach adulthood.

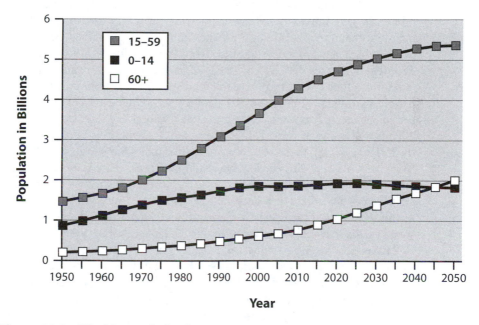

Figure 14.2   World population by age groups, 1950–2050.

From *World Population Prospects: The 2006 Revision*, Fact Sheet, Series A, March 7, 2007, United Nations, Population Division, New York: Author. Used with permission.

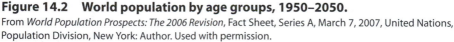

Trends in the Global Burden of Disease

As the world population grows and life expectancy increases, we will continue to battle diseases both infectious and chronic. Global surveillance, modern medicine, and health education and prevention will play important roles in battling and preventing worldwide epidemics and pandemics.

Trend #3: Infectious Diseases Are Making a Comeback

In this era of globalization, medicine, and technology, it might seem paradoxical to think that many of the infectious diseases that plagued populations in centuries past are now resurging—and with a vengeance. As described in chapter 3, an **infectious disease** is a communicable disease spread from individual to individual or from insects, animals, or other carriers to humans. Infectious diseases are sometimes called **tropical diseases** because they are endemic and epidemic infections that cause disease and disability for people living or visiting warmer climates of the world (WHO, 2008a). However, it is important to note that "tropical" diseases are not necessarily *caused* by climate or geography. They are actually due in part to poor and disenfranchised people having limited or no access to a public health infrastructure (Koop, Pearson, & Schwarz, 2002).

While epidemiologists, medical scientists, health organizations, and governments have made great strides in controlling some of history's most pestilent infectious diseases in developed countries, such as guinea worm, leprosy, onchocerciasis ("river blindness"), lymphatic filariasis, Chagas disease, and trachomal, these diseases still plague some of the world's poorest and the most marginalized populations. These diseases, which have faded in industrialized parts of the world, are deemed **Neglected Tropical Diseases** (NTDs) by the World Health Organization because they have faded from focus in terms of research and support. Even though an estimated 1 billion people worldwide (one out of six people) are affected by NTDs, less than 1% of all drugs registered between 1975 and 2007 were for these tropical diseases (WHO, 2008a). For some of these NTDs, the cost of treatment is mere pennies. According to the WHO (2008a), there are simple and affordable diagnostic tools that cost as little as four cents per test. For those who reside in more isolated areas, an NTD may prove fatal before it can be diagnosed because the currently available diagnostic tools require skilled health workers and hospital care. NTDs are now on the global health agenda as the WHO and other health organizations realize that the programs to combat such treatable diseases must be expanded and made accessible to the poor.

Likewise, attention must also be given to acute infectious diseases such as malaria, cholera, tuberculosis, HIV, Ebola, SARS (Severe Acute Respiratory Syndrome), avian flu, and dengue fever as they pose great health, economic, and security threats to modern society. HIV will remain a world killer, especially among poor countries, throughout the 21st century (see Table 14.6). Malaria, cholera, and tuberculosis were once under control in industrialized countries during the early part of the 20th century, but they are making a comeback in the 21st century as the world population becomes increasingly mobile, transcontinental travel is now commonplace, and new strains of diseases emerge as a result of antibiotic resistance. We have made great strides in vaccine development and immunization programs. However, a number of bacteria strains have become resistant to medicines, and new and reemerging microbes are still a problem. For example, tuberculosis (TB), a disease that had largely been contained by the earlier half of the 20th century, has reemerged with more aggressive strains (WHO, 2008a). Now TB kills more than 2 million people a year, and is one of the three leading infectious killers worldwide (Doctors Without Borders, n.d.).

Table 14.6   HIV Prevalence in the Countries Most Affected by the HIV/AIDS Epidemic, 2009 and 2025

Country	Prevalence (percentage) 2009	Prevalence (percentage) 2025	Country	Prevalence (percentage) 2009	Prevalence (percentage) 2025
Africa			**Europe**		
Swaziland	26.7	24.6	Ukraine	1.7	1.4
Botswana	24.7	20.1	Estonia	1.2	0.6
Lesotho	23.5	21.7	Russian Federation	1.0	0.7
South Africa	18.8	16.4	**Latin America and the Caribbean**		
Namibia	15.6	14.1	Bahamas	3.1	2.5
Zambia	15.2	13.3	Suriname	2.7	2.4
Zimbabwe	14.6	7.2	Guyana	2.5	2.0
Mozambique	12.8	10.7	Haiti	2.2	2.1
Malawi	11.9	9.9	Belize	2.1	1.9
Kenya	7.9	6.5	Jamaica	1.6	1.3
Central African Republic	6.5	5.6	Trinidad and Tobago	1.4	1.2
Gabon	6.4	5.8	Barbados	1.2	0.9
United Republic of Tanzania	6.3	5.4	Dominican Republic	1.1	0.7
Cameroon	5.4	4.1	Brazil	0.7	0.6
Uganda	5.1	2.8	Honduras	0.7	0.4
Asia			**North America**		
Thailand	1.4	1.0	United States of America	0.7	0.5
Cambodia	1.1	0.6	**Oceania**		
India	0.4	0.3	Papua New Guinea	1.8	1.9
China	0.1	0.1			

Adapted with permission from *World Population Prospects: The 2008 Revision, Highlights*, Table A.20, 2009, United Nations, Population Division, New York: Author.

Note: Prevalence relates to the population aged 15–49.

The WHO, in a report called *The Global Burden of Disease* (2008a), prepared projections of mortality and burden of disease by cause from 2004 to 2050. These projections indicated that infectious diseases, other than HIV and tuberculosis, will decline at faster rates than diseases that are more chronic in nature (i.e. heart disease, diabetes, and respiratory illnesses). They point to current efforts in antibiotic development and control technologies that, if rigorously attended to in the future, should be able to keep up with expected infectious disease emergencies. To counter increasing risks from infectious diseases, WHO (2008a) has created a number of initiatives to contain and eradicate infectious diseases and worldwide epidemics. Some of these include:

- Vaccines, molecular biology, and genetic engineering.
- Roll Back Malaria Project—a global coalition involving UNDP, UNICEF, WHO, and the World Bank to help health systems deliver cost-effective interventions like better health care, insecticide-treated bednets, and improved environmental management.

- STOP TB Initiative—a political and social movement to fight TB throughout the world by promoting the use of cost-effective Directly Observed Treatment (DOT).

- Partnerships for long-term goals—with support from public and private organizations and institutions, NGOs, and the pharmaceutical industry, the WHO has targeted seven infectious diseases—filariasis, leprosy, guinea-worm disease, tetanus, Chagas disease, measles, and polio—for eradication/elimination. This effort is focused primarily on lesser developed countries without health infrastructure that are vulnerable to outbreaks of these diseases.

- Antimicrobial Resistance Monitoring and Containment Network—a partnership of laboratories throughout the world working to decrease the speed at which antimicrobial resistance develops. These laboratories diagnose resistant infections and promote the development of policies for correct antibiotic use.

- Epidemic and Pandemic Alert Response—uses computer-generated geographical display systems to map the prevalence of infectious diseases in relation to the surrounding topography and health care infrastructure. This powerful technology helps identify health problems and enables global health workers to formulate appropriate resolutions given local resources.

- Modification of negative developments in world travel and trade as well as land use and ecology to prevent the emergence and spread of microbes.

Trend #4: Chronic Diseases Are Leading Killers across the Globe

While there is good news that life expectancy across the globe is increasing and many are enjoying socioeconomic improvements (UN, 2007a), the bad news is that, as people live longer and adopt unhealthy Western lifestyle habits (such as smoking, sedentary living, and high-fat diets), a global epidemic of chronic diseases such as heart disease, cancer, diabetes, obesity, and depression is expected (UN, 2007b). Chronic diseases are now among the leading causes of death for people in high, middle, and low-income countries (see Table 14.7). In low-income countries less than a quarter of all people reach the age of 70, and more than a third of all deaths are among children under 14 (WHO, 2008e). Although cardiovascular diseases are among the leading cause of death in these countries, the combined toll of infectious diseases (especially HIV/AIDS, lung infections, tuberculosis, diarrheal diseases, and malaria) claims more lives. In middle-income countries, nearly half of all people live to age 70 and chronic diseases are the major killers. In high-income countries, more than two thirds of all people live beyond age 70 and predominantly die of chronic diseases (WHO, 2008e). We have at our disposal the knowledge to combat the lifestyle choices that contribute to chronic disease. The exciting news is that you, as a future community health professional, are part of the potential solution!

Trends in Global Capacity

Have you ever heard the phrase, "health is wealth"? It's not just catchy—it's true. A country's economic prosperity, stability, or decline has a momentous impact on the

Table 14.7   Ten Leading Causes of Death by Broad Income Group, 2004

Low-income countries	Deaths in millions	% of deaths
Lower respiratory infections	2.94	11.2
Coronary heart disease	2.47	9.4
Diarrheal diseases	1.81	6.9
HIV/AIDS	1.51	5.7
Stroke and other cerebrovascular diseases	1.48	5.6
Chronic obstructive pulmonary disease	0.94	3.6
Tuberculosis	0.91	3.5
Neonatal infections	0.90	3.4
Malaria	0.86	3.3
Prematurity and low birth weight	0.84	3.2
Middle-income countries	**Deaths in millions**	**% of deaths**
Stroke and other cerebrovascular disease	3.47	14.2
Coronary heart disease	3.40	13.9
Chronic obstructive pulmonary disease	1.80	7.4
Lower respiratory infection	0.92	3.8
Trachea, bronchus, lung cancers	0.69	2.9
Road traffic accidents	0.67	2.8
Hypertensive heart disease	0.62	2.5
Stomach cancer	0.55	2.2
Tuberculosis	0.54	2.2
Diabetes mellitus	0.52	2.1
High-income countries	**Deaths in millions**	**% of deaths**
Coronary heart disease	1.33	16.3
Stroke and other cerebrovascular diseases	0.76	9.3
Trachea, bronchus, lung cancers	0.48	5.9
Lower respiratory infections	0.31	3.8
Chronic obstructive pulmonary disease	0.29	3.5
Alzheimer and other dementias	0.28	3.4
Colon and rectum cancers	0.27	3.3
Diabetes mellitus	0.22	2.8
Breast cancer	0.16	2.0
Stomach cancer	0.14	1.8

Source: *The Top 10 Causes of Death*, World Health Organization Fact Sheet No. 310, November 2008.

health of its citizens. Simply put, the health status of each country's citizens will impact their ability to add to their country's **gross national product (GNP)**, or the sum of all goods and services a country produces for a given year. Health is a resource that enables more individuals to work, generating productivity and economic activity. In turn, the wealth generated helps stabilize a country economically and politically and improves the standard of living or quality of life for those living there. As countries in the 21st century harness new technologies, expand their sources of industry and revenue, maximize their natural resources, educate and train those in the labor force, and respond to demands from the global economy, they will strengthen their ability to establish and maintain a stable or expanding economic environment, which is also known as **global capacity**. Conversely, those countries which lack natural resources, industry, education, political stability, internal peace, and a strong labor force will be vulnerable to widespread poverty, disease, and violence.

Trend #5: Technology Is Impacting Poverty and Disease

It seems almost absurd to think that individuals in low-income or developing countries who often have little or no access to running water much less a computer or any other technology could be "lifted from poverty" by something as ubiquitous as a cell phone. However, there are a growing number of economists who maintain that cell phones and other communication technology can restructure developing countries. The possibilities afforded by a proliferation of cell phones are potentially revolutionary. In 2008, there were more than 3.3 billion mobile-phone subscriptions worldwide, which means that there are at least another three billion people who don't own cell phones—the bulk of them in Africa and Asia. Even the smallest improvements in communication and efficiency, amplified across those additional three billion people, could raise the GNP for these countries and reshape the global economy in ways that we are just beginning to understand.

The ideal case study of this antipoverty innovation comes from Bangladesh, once the poorest country in the world. In 1990 the Grameen Bank, an unconventional enterprise that makes **microloans** to the poor, provided a loan to Grameen Telecommunications, a nonprofit organization that provides low-cost phone services in rural areas. Using the borrowed money, village entrepreneurs purchased mobile phones which they then used to sell phone services to other villagers. This led to a rise of mobile phone entrepreneurs, of which 95% were female. Villagers reaped the benefit of instant communication, and village entrepreneurs earned a steady income. Even the poorest of the poor could use the phones to communicate with family, sell their goods to others who lived out of the area, find employment elsewhere, check prices in other markets before selling their goods, and have more options during emergency situations (Corbett, 2008). This mobile phone enterprise created a "domino effect," spurring other economic activities, lifting people from poverty, and replacing feelings of fatalism with hope. Most importantly, this case study has shown that even individuals living in the most abject poverty have proven themselves to be more technologically savvy and more enterprising than people would have believed.

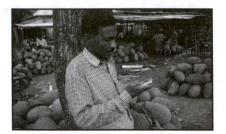

Some economists maintain that cell phones and other technology can help developing countries restructure their economies. (© Teoman Alemdar)

Trend #6: The World Is Becoming Greener

"Going Green" in the 21st century means more than leaning toward a certain hue or the fact that satellite data show plant growth has been measurably more vigorous over the last 25 years (United Nations Environmental Program, 2004). In fact, the movement represents a whole new way of living—using the earth's resources wisely and trying to improve the overall health of the planet. The World Health Organization maintains that a new approach to urbanization offers us the opportunity to develop healthy cities by pooling our concentrated resources to create positive environments. WHO refers to it as the **preferred future**:

> We create an environment in which everyone's health is promoted and pro-
> tected—whether this is in schools, workplaces, or the home. An environment in
> which the air is clear, the water safe, and where health, transport, and waste man-
> agement services are well managed and effective. An environment in which every-
> one enjoys access to social amenities such as safe play areas for children. An
> environment in which the different "players"—civilians young and old, industries
> and companies, municipal authorities, nongovernmental organizations, and public
> utilities—work together to optimize use of the resources, skills, and capacities that
> are often abundant in urban areas. In short, a healthy city that meets needs for
> work, learning, rest, and play. (WHO, 1999)

Former U.S. Vice President Al Gore, a champion against global climate change and a 2007 Nobel Peace Prize winner for his environmental advocacy, has awakened the political and social consciousness of America to the impending energy and cli-mate crisis. In a 2008 speech at a national convention, he warned that the United Sates and the rest of the world were "facing unprecedented problems, including grow-ing demand for electricity, dangerous changes in the climate driven largely by emis-sions of carbon dioxide, and political instability in regions that produce much of the world's oil" (Broder, 2008). "The survival of the United States of America as we know it is at risk," he warned, and "the future of human civilization is at stake" (Broder, 2008). Clearly, the time has come to take action to reverse this trend. As the world population grows and urbanization spreads, the earth's natural resources, habitats, and climates will be increasingly imperiled unless we can learn to balance our need to industrialize and modernize with the future sustainability of the earth. It will take everyone to make this "preferred future" a reality.

Trend #7: Poverty Is a Pivotal Factor

While the percentage of the world's poor has declined, the absolute number of people living in poverty has not. Over 2.5 billion people (40% of the global popula-tion) live on less than $2.00 a day (UNDP, 2005). A large proportion of these individ-uals are women. In many parts of the world, women are relegated to lower social status than men and, in some areas, have few legal rights or the ability to succeed financially without the assistance of a male family member. In such countries, lower levels of education are common among women and, in some cases, social and cultural restraints prevent women from seeking needed health care. These factors negatively impact the health of women at levels that are disproportionate to the health levels of men (Skolnik, 2008).

Children in particular suffer from global poverty. Nearly half the world's children, especially girls, have no guarantee of early childhood education (UNICEF, 2008b) and many female students drop out of school when they reach puberty because of poor school sanitation (UNICEF, 2008a). "In a world of unprecedented wealth, almost 2

million children die each year for want of a glass of clean water and adequate sanitation" (UNDP, 2006, para. 2), and "more than 5,000 children under five die every day
as a result of diarrheal diseases, caused in part by unsafe water, lack of access to basic
sanitation facilities and improved hygiene" (UNICEF, 2008a, para. 4). It is estimated
that worldwide over 30,000 children under the age of five die every day (Skolnik,
2008). The sad truth is that most of these deaths occur in poverty-stricken areas of the
world and, with simple, low-cost interventions in place, could have been prevented.

Trend #8: Escalating Global Violence Is Leading to Greater Rates of Death and Poverty

In chapter 2 we described Maslow's hierarchy of needs and explained that, along
with the physiological basics, a primary human need is to be safe (Maslow, 1954). Yet,
the world is a violent place, with wars and internal strife displacing large populations
of people around the globe (USAID, 2008). On September 11, 2001, a calculated terrorist attack on U.S. soil left many in shock and disbelief that a nation viewed as a safe
haven could also be vulnerable. Following the attack on 9/11, a series of anthrax
attacks incited fear about the rising threat of bioterrorism. Since then, *emergency preparedness and response* has become a commonplace component of public health efforts
to safeguard the nation's air, water, food, and medical supplies and prevent the deliberate spread of disease-causing agents (CDC, n.d., *Bioterrorism*).

Yet when we think of global violence, we must focus not only on the hazards of
war and other forms of political unrest, but also organized crime (UNDP, 2008) and
acts of random violence that plague many areas of the world. Violent practices against
women and children are even acceptable practices in some societies. For example,
because male offspring bring honor in some societies, female fetuses may be aborted
and female infants neglected in some populations (Mahbub ul Haq Human Development Centre, 2000; UNDP, 2005). Young girls can be sold or forced into prostitution
or burned by their husband's family if their bridal dowry is deemed unacceptable
(Skolnik, 2008). The reported percentages of women who are victims of sexual abuse
(including rape, molestation, incest, assault, and harassment) and domestic violence
have ranged from 10% to as high as 60% (Skolnik, 2008; UNDP, 2005). Yet in some
societies, domestic violence is considered an acceptable marital reality and sexual violence has been used as a tool of war (UNDP Azerbaijan, 2007; USAID, 2008).

In a study conducted by the United Nations Secretary General, the research team
discovered that "most violent acts against children are carried out by people they
know and should be able to trust" (2006, *Main findings*). The community can also be a
source of violence, with peer and gang violence, police brutality, sexual violence, and
even *cyber harassment* via the Internet or mobile phones becoming a growing threat.
"Violence against children includes physical violence, psychological violence such as
insults and humiliation, discrimination, neglect, and maltreatment. Although the consequences may vary according to the nature and severity of the violence inflicted, the
short- and long-term repercussions for children are very often grave and damaging"
(UN, 2006, *Main findings*).

Trends in the Global Health System

The World Health Organization (2008d) defines a health system as "all the organizations, institutions, resources, and people whose primary purpose is to improve health" (para. 1). Two trends in the global health system that might impact your future as a health professional are the global health worker shortage and the increasing emphasis on global health promotion.

Trend #9: The Health Worker Shortage Is Increasing

According to the WHO (2008d), the "global health worker shortage has reached crisis levels. In Africa alone, 1 million more health workers are urgently needed, and for the rest of the world, the shortfall is another 3.3 million" (para. 2). This shortage is driven by a number of factors that we have already described in this chapter. Populations are living longer in high-income countries, which are struggling with increasing rates of heart disease, diabetes, and other chronic conditions. At the same time, these countries are not producing or maintaining the number of health workers needed to keep up with the chronic disease epidemic.

Health workers from around the world are drawn to countries where working conditions and quality of life options are more favorable. Health worker migration tends to move "from the poorest regions to richer cities within a country and then to high-income countries." Within most countries, there is also movement from the public to the private sector, particularly if there are considerable differences in income levels (WHO, 2006a, para. 3).

The workforce shortage and migration trends are also true within the United States, where dwindling numbers of primary care providers in medicine and dentistry cannot meet the demands of a growing and aging population (Perlino, 2006). A public health workforce crisis is also looming (ASPH, 2008; Perlino, 2006; U.S. Health Resources and Services Administration [USHRSA], n.d.). According to a 2008 report from the Association of Schools of Public Health (ASPH), this workforce has decreased by over 50,000 employees since 1980, is expected to dwindle an additional 23% by 2012, and will not be able to meet the expected demand for an additional 250,000 workers by 2020.

Think for a moment about the implications of these health workforce trends. The global health workforce is flocking to private health care positions in *high*-income countries while the global population is rapidly increasing in *low*-income countries where epidemics of infectious disease and the rise of chronic health problems are already taking a heavy toll. Primary care and public health workers in the United States work on the front lines of the American health system to meet the health needs of low-income and refugee populations. They are also the U.S. professionals most likely to become part of the solution to critical global health problems (ASPH, 2008; WHO, 2006a).

Consequences of these worker shortages are already beginning to reverberate in the U.S. and around the world (ASPH, 2008; WHO, 2006a). However, we encourage you to think of the global health challenge as an opportunity for you to use your training in community health to make a significant impact. The key to becoming part of the global health solution is to think beyond what can be seen at the moment. BigPic-tureSmallWorld, Inc. (www.BigPictureSmallWorld.com) creates Web movies for the United Nations Environmental Programme and other organizations that inspire and challenge the world to think creatively. A quote from their Web movie, *America America* (Gabel, 2006), reminds us that:

> What you do matters.
> Every person is a suggestion of what they should be.
> Every country is the seed of what it could be.
> We walk as prophesies of the next age. (frames 12–13)

Trend #10: Global Health Promotion Is the New Horizon

In 2000, at the beginning of the new millennium, global leaders signed the **United Nations Millennium Declaration**, a commitment "to combat poverty, hunger, disease, illiteracy, environmental degradation, and discrimination against women" (WHO, 2008b, para. 1). These leaders developed eight **Millennium Development Goals** (MDGs) to guide these efforts:

- **Goal 1:** Eradicate extreme hunger and poverty. Halve the proportion of people living on less than $1 a day and halve malnutrition.

- **Goal 2:** Achieve universal primary education. Ensure that all children are able to complete primary education.

- **Goal 3:** Promote gender equality and empower women. Eliminate gender disparity in primary and secondary schooling, preferably by 2005 and no later than 2015.

- **Goal 4:** Reduce child mortality. Cut the under-five death rate by two-thirds.

- **Goal 5:** Improve maternal health. Reduce the maternal mortality rate by three-quarters.

- **Goal 6:** Combat HIV/AIDS, malaria and other diseases. Halt and begin to reverse HIV/AIDS and other diseases.

- **Goal 7:** Ensure environmental stability. Cut by half the proportion of people without sustainable access to safe drinking water and sanitation.

- **Goal 8:** Develop a global partnership for development. Reform aid and trade policies with special treatment for the poorest countries. (UNDP, 2005, p. 15)

Most of these goals were targeted for achievement by 2015, a challenge that led to "a new trend in international assistance, with the emergence of a variety of actors that have become known as Global Health Initiatives (GHIs)" (WHO, 2008c, p. 1). Over 80 GHIs, most of them based on public-private partnerships, focus on specific diseases or populations in need. "Some of the largest and best known of the GHIs include the Global Fund to Fight AIDS, Tuberculosis and Malaria (the Global Fund); the Global Alliance for Vaccines and Immunization (GAVI); and the U.S. President's Emergency Plan for AIDS Relief (PEPFAR)" (2008c, p. 1).

In 2008 the WHO issued its "Report on the Expert Consultation on Positive Synergies between Health Systems and Global Health Initiatives" (2008c). In it, global leaders made a number of recommendations for promoting global health that mirrored much of what we have discussed in this textbook as important principles when developing healthy communities (chapter 2). For instance, the leaders touched on elements of the ecological approach in their recommended focus on primary health within the context of "social and environmental determinants of health" (p. 2). They also emphasized the importance of "country-driven processes" (p. 7) for developing trust and strong partnerships.

It would be too simplistic for us to imply that everything we have covered in this textbook will work in all global health situations. In fact, whether you apply this textbook content in a country that differs from your own or in your local community, adaptation to population interests, needs, cultures, and unique situations is always warranted. Nevertheless, leaders of the International Union for Health Promotion and Education (IUHPE, 2007) have pointed out that the general principles and framework of health education and health promotion are embedded in the millennium development goals, and health promotion is already a recognized professional paradigm in many countries of the world. The IUHPE recommends that future workers in the global health arena possess tools for "developing the knowledge and skills for advocacy and mediation with politicians and the private sector, assessing the impact of policies on health and its determinants, accessing and using available information and evidence, and evaluating interventions" (2007, p. 5) in global health settings.

Healthy People in a Healthy World is one of the CDC's six overarching health protection goals for the 21st century (CDC, 2007b). One of the sub-goals relates directly to global health promotion: "Global health will improve by sharing knowledge, tools, and other resources with people and partners around the world" (p. 7). To this end we offer some advice in FYI 14.1 that may seem contradictory at a glance but really isn't. The first paired set of recommendations in that FYI, "Think globally. Act locally," can truly be accomplished simultaneously if you master the art of addressing local com-

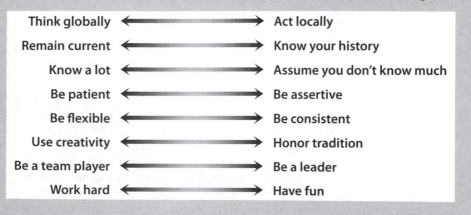

FYI 14. 1   **Insights and Approaches for Future Success**

These insights and approaches are not as contradictory as they may seem at first glance.

Think globally	Act locally
Remain current	Know your history
Know a lot	Assume you don't know much
Be patient	Be assertive
Be flexible	Be consistent
Use creativity	Honor tradition
Be a team player	Be a leader
Work hard	Have fun

munities within the context of global perspectives. Furthermore, FYI 14.2 and Appendix A list important health organizations and resources that will be valuable guides as you seek to learn more and expand your view of the global landscape.

FYI 14.2   **Global Health Organizations and Resources**

Centers for Disease Control and Prevention (CDC) Coordinating Office for Global Health	www.cdc.gov/cogh
The Clinton Global Initiative	www.clintonglobalinitiative.org
Department of Commerce—U.S. Census Bureau	www.census.gov
Food and Drug Administration (FDA) Office of International Programs	www.fda.gov/oia/homepage.htm
Bill and Melinda Gates Foundation	www.gatesfoundation.org
The Global Fund to Fight AIDS, Tuberculosis, and Malaria	www.theglobalfund.org
Global Health Council	www.globalhealth.org
Global Health Education Consortium	www.globalhealthedu.org
Global Partnerships	www.globalpartnerships.org
One Campaign	www.one.org
Pan-American Health Organization (PAHO)	www.paho.org
Partners in Health (PIH)	www.pih.org
UNICEF	www.unicef.org
United Nations	www.un.org
U.S. Agency for International Development (USAID)	www.usaid.gov
U.S. State Department	www.state.gov
World Health Organization	www.who.org

In Conclusion

As discussed in this chapter and throughout this text, we live in a rapidly evolving society in which change is the only true constant. Staying abreast of global trends and needed information and skills will require an ongoing commitment on your part, particularly after you graduate. Some health professionals who are working in the field find it difficult to carve out of their busy schedules the time needed for professional development. In light of the rapid pace at which our profession and the world are changing, we urge you to view continual renewal as a necessity rather than a luxury. To be adequately equipped for success in the field of community health, we encourage you to:

- Reach beyond the confines of course expectations and grade incentives, and view learning as the lifeline to your professional future.
- Adopt and implement a plan for professional development beyond graduation.
- Develop a deep-rooted understanding of community health within the context of global social structures and quality of life.
- Pay close attention to predicted trends, and embrace new ideas and technologies as they develop.
- Assume that there is always more to learn, and take the frequent initiative to do so. Establish a regular period (at least one day a month) in which you read professional literature and visit reliable Internet sources.
- Broaden your community perspective; visit and revisit community organizations and information sources, attend community events, remain actively involved in the community, and listen to its members.
- Be patient when working toward community goals since wide-sweeping change, especially at the policy level, can take time. When necessary, initiate small tasks with reachable objectives at the beginning of each community effort.
- Be willing to try something new if you think it will appeal to targeted members of a community, but be sure to always consider and respect the culture and unique characteristics of your community.
- Remember that it really does "take a village." Community health is about working together and empowering people to help themselves. It is not a didactic process where professionals, who claim to know what is best, reign over those who are most in need. Everyone plays an important role in improving quality of life on a global scale. We challenge you to adopt this mind-set, and as you work with others toward this common goal, lead in the spirit of unity:

Tao of Leadership
Go to the people
Live with them
Love them
Learn from them
Start with what they have
Build on what they know.

But of the best leaders
When their task is accomplished
Their work is done
The people will all remark
We have done it ourselves.

—Lao Tzu, from *The Tao of Leadership* (ancient Chinese text)

REVIEW QUESTIONS

1. Analyze the concept of quality of life from a global perspective.
2. Discuss the health needs that may arise in the future as a result of what is happening in the world and in U.S. communities today.

3. Describe predicted changes in world demographics, health care systems, and their potential influence on community health education opportunities.

4. Explain how chronic diseases have overtaken infectious diseases as the world's leading killers.

5. Discuss why many infectious diseases, such as TB, are making a comeback.

6. Explain the role technology plays in reversing the poverty cycle in a country.

7. Describe predicted job-market growth patterns as they relate to community health.

8. Provide suggestions for lifelong learning and career development in community health.

☞ FOR YOUR APPLICATION

Addressing Quality-of-Life Issues

Interview three people whose age, culture, and lifestyle differ from one another. Ask each to describe his or her personal definition of quality of life and the specific health issues that affect it. Use the results to:

- compare responses across interviews and identify similarities and differences
- identify at least two professional disciplines outside of your own that could help enhance the quality of life of your interviewees
- brainstorm efforts that could involve representatives of these disciplines in a collaborative effort.

Global Impact of Disease

Research a chronic or infectious disease that is a major concern for the 21st century. Explain the historical trend of the disease globally as well as the projected impact of the disease in geographic, economic, social, and political terms. Highlight the role community health professionals can play in reducing the impact of the disease worldwide.

Polishing Your Portfolio

Review the narrative of your philosophy of health (chapter 1, "For Your Application"). Critique it in light of what you have learned from this textbook, particularly from this chapter, about quality of life for our global community and future trends. Revise the narrative to more accurately reflect your current perspectives about health, health education, and your role as a future health educator. Ask two health professionals who are working in your targeted employment area to review your entire portfolio (see Appendix C) and suggest format and content changes. Continue to add portfolio content as you progress through your degree program. Don't wait until graduation to seek out profession-related work and volunteer experiences. Carve time from your busy schedule to prepare yourself for the job market of the future.

Web Resources

Professional Development Resources

Professional Development and the Job Market (*Selected Sites*)

- **Bureau of Health Professions** (under HRSA) http://bhpr.hrsa.gov/
- **National Center for Health Workforce Information & Analysis** (Bureau of Health Professions, HRSA) http://bhpr.hrsa.gov/healthworkforce/
- **National Commission for Health Education Credentialing** http://www.nchec.org
- **National Implementation Task Force for Accreditation in Health Education** www.healthedaccred.org/
- **United States Bureau of Labor Statistics** *Occupational Outlook Handbook* (See *health educators*, Code: 21-1091). http://www.bls.gov/oco/
- **What Is Public Health?** http://www.whatispublichealth.org/resources/ index.html

Professional Associations (*Selected Sites*)

- **American Association for Health Education** http://www.aahperd.org/AAHE/
- **American Medical Association** http://www.ama-assn.org
- **American Psychological Association** http://www.apa.org
- **American Public Health Association** http://www.apha.org
- **American School Health Association** http://www.ashaweb.org
- **National Wellness Institute** http://www.nationalwellness.org
- **Society for Public Health Education** http://www.sophe.org

U.S. Health Agencies and Organizations

U.S. Department of Health and Human Services (USDHHS)
http://www.hhs.gov

- **Administration for Children and Families (ACF)** http://www.acf.hhs.gov/
- **Administration on Aging (AOA)** http://www.aoa.dhhs.gov
- **Agency for Healthcare Research and Quality (AHRQ)** http://www.ahcpr.gov
- **Agency for Toxic Substances and Disease Registry (ATSDR)** http://www.atsdr.cdc.gov
- **Centers for Disease Control and Prevention (CDC)** http://www.cdc.gov
- **Centers for Medicare & Medicaid Services** http://www.cms.hhs.gov/
- **Food and Drug Administration (FDA)** http://www.fda.gov
- **Health Resources and Services Administration (HRSA)** http://www.hrsa.gov/
- **Indian Health Service (IHS)** http://www.ihs.gov
- **National Institutes of Health (NIH)** http://www.nih.gov
- **Program Support Center (PSC)** http://www.psc.gov
- **Substance Abuse and Mental Health Services Administration (SAMHSA)** http://www.samhsa.gov

Centers for Disease Control and Prevention (CDC, under USDHHS)
http://www.cdc.gov

- **Office of Minority Health & Health Disparities (OMHD)** http://www.cdc.gov/omhd/
- **Epidemiology Program Office** http://www.cdc.gov/epo
- **National Center for Chronic Disease Prevention and Health Promotion** http://www.cdc.gov/nccdphp
- **National Center for Environmental Health** http://www.cdc.gov/nceh
- **National Center for Health Statistics** http://www.cdc.gov/nchs
- **National Center for HIV, STD, Viral Hepatitis, and TB Prevention** http://www.cdc.gov/nchstp/od
- **National Center for Injury Prevention and Control** http://www.cdc.gov/ncipc
- **National Immunization Program** http://www.cdc.gov/vaccines/
- **National Institute for Occupational Safety and Health** http://www.cdc.gov/niosh
- **National Vaccine Program Office** http://www.hhs.gov/nvpo/
- **CDC Media Relations** http://www.cdc.gov/media/
- **National Office of Public Health Genomics** http://www.cdc.gov/genetics

- **Office of Global Health** http://www.cdc.gov/ogh
- **Office of Health and Safety (OHS)** http://www.cdc.gov/od/ohs
- **Office of Women's Health** http://www.cdc.gov/women/

Health Resources and Services Administration (HRSA)
http://www.hrsa.gov/

- **Bureau of Health Professions** http://bhpr.hrsa.gov/
- **Bureau of Primary Health Care** http://www.bphc.hrsa.gov
- **Center for Public Health Practice** http://bhpr.hrsa.gov/publichealth/index.htm
- **HIV/AIDS Bureau** http://hab.hrsa.gov/
- **Maternal and Child Health Bureau** http://www.mchb.hrsa.gov
- **Office for the Advancement of Telehealth** http://telehealth.hrsa.gov
- **Office of Minority Health** http://www.omhrc.gov/
- **Office of Rural Health Policy** http://ruralhealth.hrsa.gov/

National Institutes of Health (NIH, under USDHHS)
http://www.nih.gov

- **National Cancer Institute** http://www.nci.nih.gov
- **National Eye Institute** http://www.nei.nih.gov
- **National Heart, Lung, and Blood Institute** http://www.nhlbi.nih.gov
- **National Human Genome Research Institute** http://www.nhgri.nih.gov
- **National Institute of Allergy and Infectious Diseases** http://www.niaid.nih.gov
- **National Institute of Arthritis and Musculoskeletal and Skin Diseases** http://www.nih.gov/niams
- **National Institute of Child Health and Human Development** http://www.nichd.nih.gov
- **National Institute of Deafness and Other Communication Disorders** http://www.nidcd.nih.gov/
- **National Institute of Dental and Craniofacial Research** http://www.nidr.nih.gov
- **National Institute of Diabetes and Digestive and Kidney Diseases** http://www.niddk.nih.gov
- **National Institute of Environmental Health Sciences** http://www.niehs.nih.gov
- **National Institute of General Medical Sciences** http://www.nih.gov/nigms
- **National Institute of Mental Health** http://www.nimh.nih.gov
- **National Institute of Neurological Disorders and Stroke** http://www.ninds.nih.gov
- **National Institute of Nursing Research** http://www.nih.gov/ninr
- **National Institute on Aging** http://www.nih.gov/nia

- **National Institute on Alcohol Abuse and Alcoholism** http://www.niaaa.nih.gov
- **National Institute on Drug Abuse** http://www.nida.nih.gov

Office of Public Health and Science (OPHS, under USDHHS)
http://www.hhs.gov/ophs/

- **Office of Disease Prevention and Health Promotion**
  http://odphp.osophs.dhhs.gov
- **National Disaster Medical System (NDMS)**
  http://www.hhs.gov/aspr/opeo/ndms/index.html
- **Office of HIV/AIDS Policy** http://www.hhs.gov/ophs/ohap/
- **Office of Global Health Affairs** http://www.globalhealth.gov/
- **Office of Minority Health Resource Center** http://www.omhrc.gov
- **Office of Population Affairs** http://www.hhs.gov/opa/
- **Office of Research Integrity** http://ori.dhhs.gov
- **Office of the Surgeon General** http://www.surgeongeneral.gov
- **Office on Women's Health** http://www.4woman.gov/owh
- **President's Council on Physical Fitness and Sports** http://www.fitness.gov/

Other U.S. Government Agencies

- **Environmental Protection Agency (EPA)** http://www.epa.gov
- **Occupational Safety and Health Administration (OSHA, under Department of Labor)** http://www.osha.gov

Voluntary Health Organizations and Foundations (*Selected Sites*)

- **Alzheimer's Association** http://www.alz.org
- **American Cancer Society** http://www.cancer.org
- **American Diabetes Association** http://www.diabetes.org
- **American Heart Association** http://www.americanheart.org
- **American Lung Association** http://www.lungusa.org
- **American Red Cross** http://www.redcross.org
- **Arthritis Foundation** http://www.arthritis.org
- **Council on Foundations** http://www.cof.org
- **Cystic Fibrosis Foundation** http://www.cff.org
- **Epileptic Foundation of America** http://www.efa.org
- **Foundation Center of New York** http://www.foundationcenter.org
- **Leukemia Society of America** http://www.leukemia.org
- **Lupus Foundation of America** http://www.lupus.org
- **March of Dimes for Birth Defects** http://www.modimes.org

- **Muscular Dystrophy Association** http://www.mdausa.org
- **National Kidney Foundation** http://www.kidney.org
- **National Osteoporosis Foundation** http://www.nof.org
- **National Safety Council** http://www.nsc.org/
- **Planned Parenthood Federation of America**
  http://www.plannedparenthood.org
- **Public Health Foundation** http://www.phf.org/chsi/index.htm
- **Robert Wood Johnson Foundation** http://www.rwjf.org

U.S. Health-Related Information and Data Sources

General Health-Related Information and Data Sources

- **CDC Wonder** (Centers for Disease Control) http://wonder.cdc.gov
- **Fastats** (Centers for Disease Control) http://www.cdc.gov/nchs/fastats
- **Health Finder** (U.S. Department of Health and Human Services)
  http://www.healthfinder.gov
- **HealthierUS.gov** (U.S. Department of Health and Human Services)
  http://www.healthierus.gov/index.html
- **National Center for Health Statistics** http://www.cdc.gov/nchs/
- **Health Topics A to Z** (Centers for Disease Control)
  http://www.cdc.gov/az/a.htmL
- **MedlinePlus** (U.S. National Library of Medicine)
  http://www.nlm.nih.gov/medlineplus/
- **National Bureau of Labor Statistics** http://stats.bls.gov
- **National Center for Health Statistics** http://www.cdc.gov/nchs
- **National Center for Policy Analysis** http://www.ncpa.org
- **National Center for Public Policy** http://www.public-policy.org
- **National Health Information Center** http://www.health.gov/NHIC/
- **U.S. Census Bureau** http://www.census.gov

Age- and Gender-Specific Information Resources

Maternal and Infant Health

- **March of Dimes for Birth Defects Foundation** http://www.modimes.org
- **Maternal and Child Health Bureau** http://www.mchb.hrsa.gov
- **Pregnancy Risk Assessment Monitoring System (PRAMS)**
  http://www.cdc.gov/PRAMS/
- **National Healthy Mothers, Healthy Babies Coalition** http://www.hmhb.org

- **Office of Adolescent Pregnancy Programs (Office of Population Affairs, USDHHS)** http://www.hhs.gov/opa/index.html
- **Mothers and Infants (under CDC)** http://www.cdc.govinccdphp/mothers.htm
- **Infants and Toddlers (CDC *LifeStages*)**
  http://www.cdc.gov/LifeStages/infants_toddlers.html
- **Pregnancy (CDC *LifeStages*)**
  http://www.cdc.gov/ncbddd/pregnancy_gateway/default.htm
- **Women Infants and Children (WIC)** http://www.fns.usda.gov/wic/

[See also *Women's Health*]

Child Health

- **Administration for Children and Families (ACF)** http://www.acf.hhs.gov/
- **American Academy of Child and Adolescent Psychiatry** http://www.aacap.org
- **Childstats.gov** (*Federal Interagency Forum on Child and Family Statistics*)
  http://www.childstats.gov/index.asp
- **Children (CDC *LifeStages*)** http://www.cdc.gov/LifeStages/children.html
- **Healthy Youth (CDC)** http://www.cdc.gov/HealthyYouth/index.htm
- **Kids Health** (Nemours Foundation) http://kidshealth.org/
- **National Institute of Child Health and Human Development**
  http://www.nichd.nih.gov
- **National Resource Center for Health and Safety in Child Care** (under Maternal and Child Health Bureau, HRSA) http://nrc.uchsc.edu

Adolescent and Young Adult Health

- **Adolescents (CDC *LifeStages*)** http://www.cdc.gov/HealthyYouth/az/index.htm
- **Adolescent Health "On-Line"** (American Medical Association)
  http://www.ama-assn.org/ama/pub/category/1947.html
- **Healthy Youth (CDC)** http://www.cdc.gov/HealthyYouth/index.htm
- **National Adolescent Health Information Center** http://nahic.ucsf.edu/
- **Texas Youth Commission Office of Prevention** http://www.tyc.state.tx.us/
- **Youth Risk Behavior Surveillance System** (under CDC)
  http://www.cdc.gov/nccdphp/dash/yrbs

Middle-Aged Adult Health

- **Health Conditions of the Americas** (under PAHO)
  http://www.paho.org/english/country.htm

[See also disease/health issue-specific organizations, CDC, NIH, and OPHS]

Older Adult Health

- **Administration on Aging** (under USDHHS) http://www.aoa.dhhs.gov
- **American Association of Retired Persons (AARP)** http://www.aarp.org

- **National Institute on Aging** (under NIH) http://www.nih.gov/nia
- **Healthy Aging for Older Adults** http://www.cdc.gov/aging/

Women's Health

- **Women (CDC *LifeStages*)** http://www.cdc.gov/women/
- **Women's Health.gov** (under USDHHS) http://www.womenshealth.gov/
- **Office of Women's Health** http://www.fda.gov/womens/default.htm

[See also *Maternal and Infant Health*]

Men's Health

- **Men's Health** (under CDC) http://www.cdc.gov/men/

Ethnic and Minority Information Resources

General Information Sources

- **Diversity Rx** http://www.diversityrx.org
- **Ethnomed** http://ethnomed.org/
- **Healthy People 2010** http://www.health.gov/healthypeople
- **Office of Minority Health & Health Disparities** http://www.cdc.gov/omhd/About/about.htm
- **Minority and Ethnic Groups (CDC)** http://www.cdc.gov/std/stats/minorities.htm
- **Minority Health Network** http://www.pitt.edu/~ejb4/min/
- **Minority Health Professional Foundation** http://www.minorityhealth.org
- **National Center for Health Statistics: Faststats AtoZ** *(Click on "Health of . . ." various special populations)* http://www.cdc.gov/nchs/fastats/Default.htm
- **Office of Minority Health** http://www.omhrc.gov
- **U.S. Census Bureau Reports (ethnicity- and poverty-specific)** http://www.census.gov/hhes/www/poverty/poverty.html

African American Health Issues

- **African American Program** (American Diabetes Association) http://www.diabetes.org/communityprograms-and-localevents/africanamericans.jsp
- **Black Health Net** http://blackhealthnet.com

American Indian /Native American Health Resources

- **Association of American Indian Physicians** http://www.aaip.org/
- **American Indian Research and Education Center** http://airec.unlv.edu/index.htm
- **Code Talk (Office of Native American Programs, HUD)** http://www.hud.gov/offices/pih/ih/codetalk/
- **Indian Health Service (IHS)** http://www.ihs.gov

Asian and Pacific Islander Health Information Resources

- **Asian and Pacific Islander American Health Forum** http://www.apiahf.org/
- **Association of Asian Pacific Community Health Organizations** http://www.aapcho.org

Hispanic American/Latino Health Resources

- **Chicano/Latino Net Health** http://latino.sscnet.ucla.edu/
- **Latino Cardiovascular Health Resources** (National Heart, Lung, and Blood Institute) http://www.nhlbi.nih.gov/health/prof/heart/latino
- **Midwest Latino Health, Research, Training, and Policy Center** (University of Illinois at Chicago): http://www.uic.edu/jaddams/mlhrc/mlhrc.html
- **The National Alliance for Hispanic Health** http://www.hispanichealth.org
- **National Hispanic Medical Association** http://home.earthlink.net/~nhma

Global Health Information Resources

International Organizations/Information Resources

- **Child Family Health International** www.cfhi.org
- **Christian Connections for International Health** www.ccih.org
- **Essential Health Links** (Center for Health Information and Technology) http://www.healthnet.org/essential-links/index.html
- **Global Health Council** http://www.globalhealth.org/
- **Global Health Education Consortium** http://globalhealthedu.org/pages/default.aspx
- **International Clinical Epidemiology Network (INCLEN)** www.inclen.org
- **International Red Cross** http://www.icrc.ch/eng
- **Lifewind International** http://www.lifewind.org/
- **Pan American Health Organization** http://www.paho.org
- **Project Hope** http://www.projecthope.org/
- **Students Partnership Worldwide** http://www.spw.org/
- **UNICEF** http://www.unicef.org/index.php
- **World Bank** http://www.worldbank.org/
- **World Health Organization** http://www.who.int/en/

Global Health Information Sources in the United States

- **EthnoMed** http://ethnomed.org/
- **Gap Minder** http://www.gapminder.org/
- **Globemed** http://www.globemed.org/

- **Office of Global Health** (under CDC) http://www.cdc.gov/ogh
- **Office of Global Health Affairs, U.S. Dept. of Health & Human Services** http://www.globalhealth.gov/index.html
- **University Coalitions for Global Health** http://www.ucgh.org/
- **USAID Global Health (United States Agency for International Development)** http://www.usaid.gov/our_work/global_health/

U.S. Refugee and Immigrant Populations

- **National Center for Farmworker Health** (Buda, Texas) http://www.ncfh.org/
- **Texas Office of Border Health (Texas Department of State Health Services)** http://www.dshs.state.tx.us/borderhealth/default.shtm
- **Refugee Health Program (Texas Department of State Health Services)** http://www.dshs.state.tx.us/idcu/health/refugee_health/
- **Refugee Support Center** (Dallas, Texas) http://www.refugeesupportcenter.com/
- **The International Rescue Committee** http://www.theIRC.org
- **Refugee Health Information Network** http://www.rhin.org/
- **Women's Commission for Refugee Women and Children** http://www.womenscommission.org/
- **Homeland Security: Division of Immigration Health Services** http://www.inshealth.org/

Community Health Education Techniques (*Selected Sites*)

General Information Sources

- **CDC's Steps Program** http://www.cdc.gov/steps/
- **Community Toolbox** http://ctb.ku.edu/en/
- **Diversity Rx** http://www.diversityrx.org
- **Guide to Community Preventive Services** (under OPHS) http://www.thecommunityguide.org/
- **The Community Guide** (CDC) http://thecommunityguide.org/

Grant Funding Information and Tips *(see also specific organizations and foundations)*

- **CDC Grants: General information** http://www.cdc.gov/od/pgo/funding/grants/grantmain.shtm
- **Community Toolbox** http://ctb.ku.edu/en/ *Writing a Grant Application for Funding*
- **Foundation Center** http://foundationcenter.org/

- **Grants.gov** http://www.grants.gov/
- **National Institutes of Health Office of Extramural Funding** http://grants1.nih.gov/grants/grant_basics.htm

Online Journals

Journals (*Selected Sites*)

- *American Journal of Epidemiology* http://aje.oxfordjournals.org/
- *American Journal of Health Behavior* http://www.ajhb.org
- *International Electronic Journal of Health Education* http://www.aahperd.org/iejhe/
- *Journal of Health Communication* http://www.gwu.edu/~cih/journal/

Health-Related Internship and Job Search Sources

Internship Links

- **American Schools of Public Health** *Internship and Fellowship Programs* http://www.asph.org/document.cfm?page=752
- **Partners in Health** http://www.pih.org/home.html (See *What You Can Do*)
- **University Coalitions for Global Health** http://www.ucgh.org/
- **USAID Global Health Fellows** http://www.ghfp.net/index.fsp

Job Search Links

- **Global Health Career Network** http://www.globalhealth.org/jobs/index.php3?offset=0
- **International Jobs Center** http://www.internationaljobs.org/
- **Partners in Health** http://www.pih.org/home.html (See *What You Can Do*)

Community Assessment Project Guide

PART I

1. **Describe the makeup and history of the community to provide a context within which to collect data on its current concerns.** (Community Description)

   a. Comment on the type of information that best describes the community (e.g., demographic, historical, political, civic participation, key leaders, past concerns, geographic, assets).

   b. Describe the sources of information used (e.g., public records, local people, internet, maps, phone book, library, newspaper).

   c. Include pictures of the community to provide evidence of both resources and barriers to quality of life.

2. **Seek out community "gatekeepers" for perceptions on community health issues.**

   a. Identify at least two community gatekeepers.

   b. Interview the gatekeepers.

   c. Describe who you listened to and why.

   d. Describe how you arranged to listen to community leaders and members.

   e. Describe the methods (e.g., listening sessions, public forums, interviews, concerns surveys, focus groups) you used to listen to the community.

   f. Address whether the problems identified by the gatekeepers match epidemiological data and research information relating to the community.

   g. Describe the issues of concern to people in the community (i.e., do they care about safety, education, housing, access to health care, etc.).

   h. Discuss how important these issues are to the community.

   i. Discuss how satisfied community members are with past and current efforts to address the issues.

   j. List priority concerns based on issues of high importance and low satisfaction.

PART II

3. **Describe the health problem identified and the methods (e.g., public forums, listening sessions, focus groups, interviews, surveys, observation) used to collect descriptive information from the community.**

   a. Describe the community-level indicators—the incidence (new cases) or prevalence (existing cases) of disease, and the social indicators related to the disease (i.e., rate of poverty in the community, unemployment, etc.).

   b. Report how frequently the problem (or related behavior) occurs (i.e., current statistics).

   c. Describe how many people are affected by the problem and the severity of its effects.

   d. Conduct a PRECEDE analysis of the identified health issue (predisposing, enabling, and reinforcing factors).

   e. Explain how feasible it is to address the issue.

   f. Discuss the possible impact and/or consequences of solving it.

   g. Indicate the target populations and subgroups identified by stakeholders as particularly likely to benefit from the effort.

   h. Identify the method used to collect data from the identified target group.

   i. Describe any existing health assessment surveys available to use in data collection with the target group.

   j. Select the instrument (i.e. survey) used to collect the information.

   k. Describe the instrument in detail (authors, purpose, how it was developed). Include entire survey in an appendix.

   l. Explain how you selected the target group to take the survey.

   m. Describe your procedures (e.g., surveys, interviews) to gather information.

   n. If using a focus group or community forum in lieu of or in addition to a survey, list the question you used as well as the characteristics of the group you're interviewing (i.e. role in community, age, ethnicity, occupation, etc.).

PART III

4. **Compile and describe the evidence suggesting that identified issues should be a priority.**

   a. Analyze data collected.

   b. Explain methods used to analyze data.

   c. Present findings (use descriptive statistics, charts, and graphs).

   d. Describe the barriers and resources for addressing the identified issue(s) and achieving the goal (e.g., denial, discounting the problem). Describe how they can be minimized (e.g., reframing the issue).

5. Provide suggestions for health education program developers.

a. Address how health education can address the predisposing, enabling, and reinforcing factors related to the health issue.

b. Recommend a health education theory that can be used as a foundation for program planners.

c. Indicate what resources and assets are available and where.

d. Identify the community leaders. Describe the individuals and organizations with influence in the community who might support (or oppose) efforts to address this issue.

e. Describe the community projects currently in progress. Identify strengths and weaknesses of these sources and propose how these efforts might be supported with future health education efforts based on this community health assessment.

Table B.1　Components to Include in a Formal Community Needs Assessment Report

Title Page	Title of your assessment project, name of author/s, and date.
Executive Summary or Abstract	A brief (250 words or less) summary of the purpose of the assessment, methods used, and findings.
Table of Contents	List all of the paper content sections with appropriate first page number.
Introduction and Community Description	Overview of the community (history, demographics, geographic boundaries, etc.). Provide facts collected through secondary data.
Data-Collection Methods	Discuss the data collection strategy/ies used along with the step-by-step protocol.
Data Analysis	Explain how the data collected was analyzed.
Findings	Illustrate and discuss results from the data analyses. Include graphs and charts to display your findings.
Community Assets	Identify community assets that would be helpful in program development, coordination, implementation, evaluation, and maintenance.
Implications for Health Education and Program Development	Discuss the implications of what you found, explain emergent health priorities, segment health needs by group, provide suggestions for health education and health interventions, and suggest guiding theoretical frameworks.
Conclusion	Provide a few summary statements and offer some of the limitations of the needs assessment. Explain how the results of the study will help plan or assist programs within the community.
References	Be sure to list all references in a format such as APA and provide parenthetical reference citations throughout.
Appendixes	You may want to include copies of the surveys or questions you used for data collection, articles or handouts relating to the community, and any miscellaneous documents you feel enrich the community assessment.

Community Health Professional Portfolio Guide
(E-portfolios and Hard Copy)

Content Area/Competency	Artifacts
Assessing Community Needs and Assets	• Community needs assessment report • Community description • PRECEDE analysis • Community health survey/s • Community asset inventories • Focus group questions and summaries • Community gatekeeper interviews (written transcripts and summaries or audio/video) • Photovoice application • Videos (E-portfolios) • Web pages (linked on E-portfolio or printed)
Communicating Health Information	• Press Release • Brochure • PowerPoints • Blog/newspaper/journal article • Literature reviews • Web page (linked on E-portfolio or printed example) • Podcast (E-portfolio) • Wiki/s (links on E-portfolio or printed examples) • Vodcast (E-portfolio) • Public service announcement • Event flyers and handouts • Posters • Examples of media evaluations and peer critiques • Materials created for those with lower literacy • Training manuals

Planning for Evidence-Based Programs	• Formal program plan; written critiques of program plans • Examples of health education strategies • Application of a planning model • Written mission statement, goals, and objectives • Evaluation plan • Research grant proposals • Related presentations and handouts
Implementing and Coordinating Community Health Programs	• Evidence of public presentations or teaching (text, photos, audio, video, Web page) • Lesson/presentation plans; presentation critiques • Case studies • Evidence and photos of volunteer experience or service learning • Related presentations and handout • Supervisor, instructor, or preceptor critiques • Thank-you letters or certificates of appreciation
Resource Access and Management	• Community resource directory • Asset map/inventories • Webliography and/or wikis • Spotlights on professional organizations and agencies • Case studies • Related presentations and handouts
Evaluation and Research	• Formal program evaluation report • Examples of program evaluation strategies and objectives • Literature reviews • Research proposals/reports • Published research articles/abstracts • Market research • Evaluation surveys/instrumentation • Presentation of data (graphs, charts, tables) • Peer and self-critiques • Self-constructed exams or rubrics • Photos • Pod or vodcast (E-portfolio)
Health Advocacy	• Letters to the editor, Congress, or community leaders • Op-ed pieces • Media advocacy plan • Local media contact directory • Public service announcement • Pod or vodcast (E-portfolio) • Blog/s (E-portfolio or printed from blogs site) • Examples of community forums attended or facilitated

Resources for creating E-portfolios

McKenzie, J., Cleary, M.J., McKenzie, B., & Stephen, C.S. (2002). E-portfolios: Their creation and use by pre-service health educators. *International Electronic Journal of Health Education*, 4: 79–83.

http://www.eduscapes.com

http://www.electronicportfolios.org

Creating a Resource Inventory for Community Health

No matter what setting you work in as a health professional (i.e., clinical, school, community, corporate, nonprofit) it is likely you will need to collect resources to help you develop effective health education programs. Use this worksheet as a guide to help you compile these resources.

Topic Area: _____   Date: _____

List helpful Web sites on your topic. (Remember to consider the accuracy, authority, currency, objectivity, and coverage of each Web site.)

List phone numbers for clearinghouses or "help" or "information" lines relating to the topic.

Identify community agencies or nonprofit organizations that may have information on the topic. (Provide name, address, phone number, and email.)

List individuals who may serve as guest speakers on this topic. (Be sure you can justify their authority on this topic.)

Locate and list professional journal articles or books. (Include complete reference information, including the database you used.)

Search for podcasts or blogs that might provide helpful information. List these below. (Remember to apply the same evaluation criteria as other Web-based resources.)

Organizational Charts

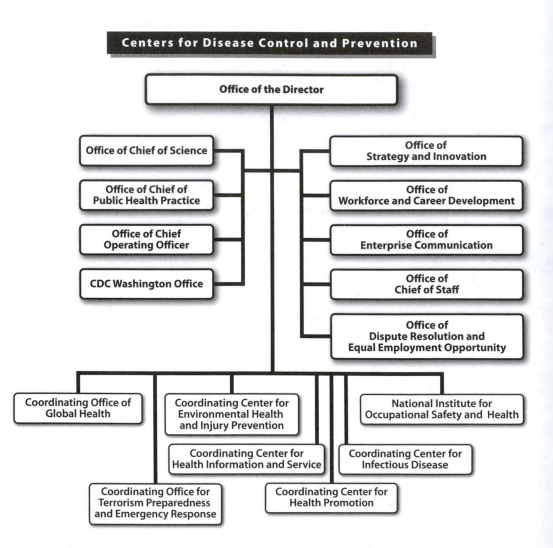

Centers for Disease Control and Prevention

Office of the Director

Office of Chief of Science

Office of Chief of Public Health Practice

Office of Chief Operating Officer

CDC Washington Office

Office of Strategy and Innovation

Office of Workforce and Career Development

Office of Enterprise Communication

Office of Chief of Staff

Office of Dispute Resolution and Equal Employment Opportunity

Coordinating Office of Global Health

Coordinating Center for Environmental Health and Injury Prevention

National Institute for Occupational Safety and Health

Coordinating Center for Health Information and Service

Coordinating Center for Infectious Disease

Coordinating Office for Terrorism Preparedness and Emergency Response

Coordinating Center for Health Promotion

U.S. Department of Health and Human Services

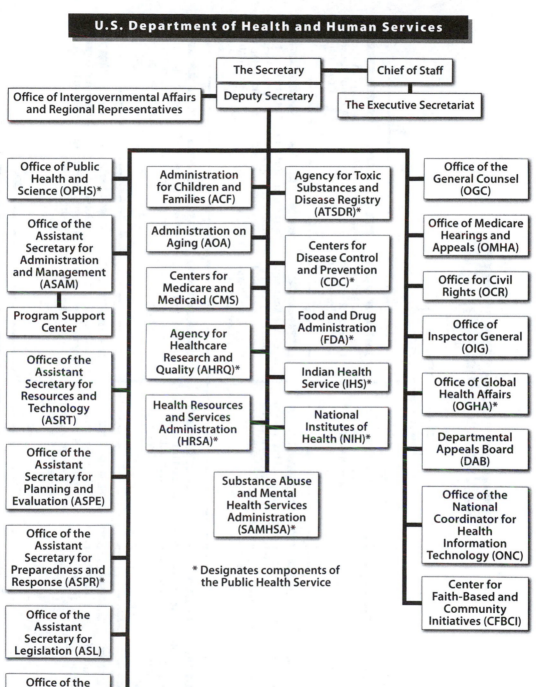

The Secretary

Chief of Staff

Office of Intergovernmental Affairs and Regional Representatives

Deputy Secretary

The Executive Secretariat

Office of Public Health and Science (OPHS)*

Administration for Children and Families (ACF)

Agency for Toxic Substances and Disease Registry (ATSDR)*

Office of the General Counsel (OGC)

Office of the Assistant Secretary for Administration and Management (ASAM)

Administration on Aging (AOA)

Centers for Disease Control and Prevention (CDC)*

Office of Medicare Hearings and Appeals (OMHA)

Program Support Center

Centers for Medicare and Medicaid (CMS)

Office for Civil Rights (OCR)

Office of the Assistant Secretary for Resources and Technology (ASRT)

Agency for Healthcare Research and Quality (AHRQ)*

Food and Drug Administration (FDA)*

Office of Inspector General (OIG)

Indian Health Service (IHS)*

Office of Global Health Affairs (OGHA)*

Office of the Assistant Secretary for Planning and Evaluation (ASPE)

Health Resources and Services Administration (HRSA)*

National Institutes of Health (NIH)*

Departmental Appeals Board (DAB)

Office of the Assistant Secretary for Preparedness and Response (ASPR)*

Substance Abuse and Mental Health Services Administration (SAMHSA)*

Office of the National Coordinator for Health Information Technology (ONC)

* Designates components of the Public Health Service

Office of the Assistant Secretary for Legislation (ASL)

Center for Faith-Based and Community Initiatives (CFBCI)

Office of the Assistant Secretary for Public Affairs (ASPA)

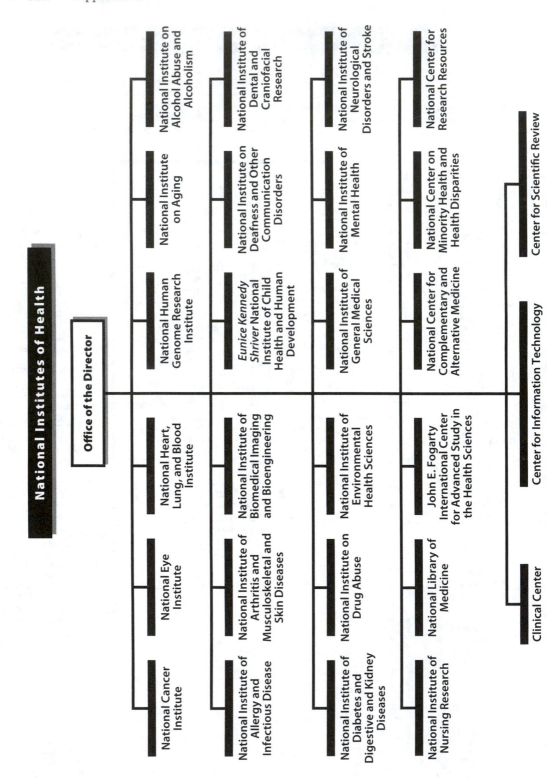

National Institutes of Health

Office of the Director

National Cancer Institute

National Eye Institute

National Heart, Lung, and Blood Institute

National Human Genome Research Institute

National Institute on Aging

National Institute on Alcohol Abuse and Alcoholism

National Institute of Allergy and Infectious Disease

National Institute of Arthritis and Musculoskeletal and Skin Diseases

National Institute of Biomedical Imaging and Bioengineering

Eunice Kennedy Shriver National Institute of Child Health and Human Development

National Institute on Deafness and Other Communication Disorders

National Institute of Dental and Craniofacial Research

National Institute of Diabetes and Digestive and Kidney Diseases

National Institute on Drug Abuse

National Institute of Environmental Health Sciences

National Institute of General Medical Sciences

National Institute of Mental Health

National Institute of Neurological Disorders and Stroke

National Institute of Nursing Research

National Library of Medicine

John E. Fogarty International Center for Advanced Study in the Health Sciences

National Center for Complementary and Alternative Medicine

National Center on Minority Health and Health Disparities

National Center for Research Resources

Clinical Center

Center for Information Technology

Center for Scientific Review

NIH Institutes

- **National Cancer Institute** (NCI)—Est. 1937
  NCI leads a national effort to eliminate the suffering and death due to cancer.

- **National Eye Institute** (NEI)—Est. 1968
  NEI conducts and supports research that helps prevent and treat eye diseases and other disorders of vision.

- **National Heart, Lung, and Blood Institute** (NHLBI)—Est. 1948
  NHLBI provides leadership for a national program in diseases of the heart, blood vessels, lung, and blood; blood resources; and sleep disorders.

- **National Human Genome Research Institute** (NHGRI)—Est. 1989
  NHGRI supports the NIH component of the Human Genome Project, a worldwide research effort designed to analyze the structure of human DNA and determine the location of the estimated 30,000 to 40,000 human genes.

- **National Institute on Aging** (NIA)—Est. 1974
  NIA leads a national program of research on the biomedical, social, and behavioral aspects of the aging process; the prevention of age-related diseases and disabilities; and the promotion of a better quality of life for all older Americans.

- **National Institute on Alcohol Abuse and Alcoholism** (NIAAA)—Est. 1970
  NIAAA conducts research focused on improving the treatment and prevention of alcoholism and alcohol-related problems to reduce the enormous health, social, and economic consequences of this disease.

- **National Institute of Allergy and Infectious Diseases** (NIAID)—Est. 1948
  NIAID research strives to understand, treat, and ultimately prevent the myriad infectious, immunologic, and allergic diseases that threaten millions of human lives.

- **National Institute of Arthritis and Musculoskeletal and Skin Diseases** (NIAMS)—Est. 1986
  NIAMS supports research into the causes, treatment, and prevention of arthritis and musculoskeletal and skin diseases, the training of basic and clinical scientists to carry out this research, and the dissemination of information on research progress in these diseases.

- **National Institute of Biomedical Imaging and Bioengineering** (NIBIB)—Est. 2000
  NIBIB improves health by promoting fundamental discoveries, design and development, and translation and assessment of technological capabilities in biomedical imaging and bioengineering, enabled by relevant areas of information science, physics, chemistry, mathematics, materials science, and computer sciences.

- **National Institute of Child Health and Human Development** (NICHD)—Est. 1962
  NICHD research on fertility, pregnancy, growth, development, and medical rehabilitation strives to ensure that every child is born healthy and wanted and grows up free from disease and disabilities.

- **National Institute on Deafness & Other Communication Disorders** (NIDCD)—Est. 1988
  NIDCD conducts and supports biomedical research and research training on normal mechanisms as well as diseases and disorders of hearing, balance, smell, taste, voice, speech, and language that affect 46 million Americans.

- **National Institute of Dental and Craniofacial Research** (NIDCR)—Est. 1948
  NIDCR provides leadership for a national research program designed to understand, treat, and ultimately prevent the infectious and inherited craniofacial-oral-dental diseases and disorders that compromise millions of human lives.

- **National Institute of Diabetes and Digestive and Kidney Diseases** (NIDDK)—Est. 1948
  NIDDK conducts and supports basic and applied research and provides leadership for a national program in diabetes, endocrinology, and metabolic diseases; digestive diseases and nutrition; and kidney, urologic, and hematologic diseases.

- **National Institute on Drug Abuse** (NIDA)—Est. 1973
  NIDA leads the nation in bringing the power of science to bear on drug abuse and addiction through support and conduct of research across a broad range of disciplines and rapid and effective dissemination of results of that research to improve drug abuse and addiction prevention, treatment, and policy.

- **National Institute of Environmental Health Sciences** (NIEHS)—Est. 1969
  NIEHS reduces the burden of human illness and dysfunction from environmental causes by defining how environmental exposures, genetic susceptibility, and age interact to affect an individual's health.

- **National Institute of General Medical Sciences** (NIGMS)—Est. 1962
  NIGMS supports basic biomedical research that is not targeted to specific diseases. NIGMS funds studies on genes, proteins, and cells, as well as on fundamental processes like communication within and between cells, how our bodies use energy, and how we respond to medicines.

- **National Institute of Mental Health** (NIMH)—Est. 1949
  NIMH provides national leadership dedicated to understanding, treating, and preventing mental illnesses through basic research on the brain and behavior, and through clinical, epidemiological, and services research.

- **National Institute of Neurological Disorders and Stroke** (NINDS)—Est. 1950
  The mission of the NINDS is to reduce the burden of neurological diseases.

- **National Institute of Nursing Research** (NINR)—Est. 1986
  NINR supports clinical and basic research to establish a scientific basis for the care of individuals across the life span—from the management of patients during illness and recovery to the reduction of risks for disease and disability; the promotion of healthy lifestyles; the promotion of quality of life in those with chronic illness; and the care for individuals at the end of life.

- **National Library of Medicine** (NLM)—Est. 1956
  NLM collects, organizes, and makes available biomedical science information to scientists, health professionals, and the public.

Source: *NIH Institutes, Centers, and Offices.* Retrieved January 4, 2008, from http://www.nihigov/welcome/ihnew.html.

NIH Centers

- **Center for Information Technology** (CIT)— Est. 1964
  CIT incorporates the power of modern computers into the biomedical programs and administrative procedures of the NIH by focusing on three primary activities: conducting computational biosciences research, developing computer systems, and providing computer facilities.

- **Center for Scientific Review** (CSR)—Est. 1946
  CSR is the focal point at NIH for the conduct of initial peer review, the foundation of the NIH grant and award process. The Center carries out peer review of the majority of research and research training applications submitted to the NIH. In addition, the Center serves as the central receipt point for all such Public Health Service (PHS) applications and makes referrals to scientific review groups for scientific and technical merit review of applications and to funding components for potential award.

- **John E. Fogarty International Center for Advanced Study in the Health Sciences** (FIC)—Est. 1968
  FIC promotes and supports scientific research and training internationally to reduce disparities in global health.

- **National Center for Complementary and Alternative Medicine** (NCCAM)—Est. 1999
  NCCAM is dedicated to exploring complementary and alternative medical (CAM) practices in the context of rigorous science; training CAM researchers and disseminating authoritative information.

- **National Center on Minority Health and Health Disparities** (NCMHD)—Est. 1993
  The mission of NCMHD is to promote minority health and to lead, coordinate, support, and assess the NIH effort to reduce and ultimately eliminate health disparities.

- **National Center for Research Resources** (NCRR)—Est. 1962
  NCRR provides laboratory scientists and clinical researchers with the environments and tools they need to understand, detect, treat, and prevent a wide range of diseases. With this support, scientists make biomedical discoveries, translate these findings to animal-based studies, and then apply them to patient-oriented research.

- **NIH Clinical Center** (CC)—Est. 1953
  CC is the clinical research facility of the National Institutes of Health. As a national resource, it provides the patient care, services, and environment needed to initiate and support the highest quality conduct of and training in clinical research.

Source: *NIH Institutes, Centers, and Offices*. Retrieved January 4, 2008, from
http://www.nihigov/welcome/ihnew.html.

Code of Ethics for the Health Education Profession

Preamble

The Health Education profession is dedicated to excellence in the practice of promoting individual, family, organizational, and community health. Guided by common ideals, Health Educators are responsible for upholding the integrity and ethics of the profession as they face the daily challenges of making decisions. By acknowledging the value of diversity in society and embracing a cross-cultural approach, Health Educators support the worth, dignity, potential, and uniqueness of all people.

The Code of Ethics provides a framework of shared values within which Health Education is practiced. The Code of Ethics is grounded in fundamental ethical principles that underlie all health care services: respect for autonomy, promotion of social justice, active promotion of good, and avoidance of harm. The responsibility of each health educator is to aspire to the highest possible standards of conduct and to encourage the ethical behavior of all those with whom they work.

Regardless of job title, professional affiliation, work setting, or population served, Health Educators abide by these guidelines when making professional decisions.

Article I: Responsibility to the Public

A Health Educator's ultimate responsibility is to educate people for the purpose of promoting, maintaining, and improving individual, family, and community health. When a conflict of issues arises among individuals, groups, organizations, agencies, or institutions, health educators must consider all issues and give priority to those that promote wellness and quality of living through principles of self-determination and freedom of choice for the individual.

Section 1: Health Educators support the right of individuals to make informed decisions regarding health, as long as such decisions pose no threat to the health of others.

Section 2: Health Educators encourage actions and social policies that support and facilitate the best balance of benefits over harm for all affected parties.

Section 3: Health Educators accurately communicate the potential benefits and consequences of the services and programs with which they are associated.

Section 4: Health Educators accept the responsibility to act on issues that can adversely affect the health of individuals, families, and communities.

Section 5: Health Educators are truthful about their qualifications and the limitations of their expertise and provide services consistent with their competencies.

Section 6: Health Educators protect the privacy and dignity of individuals.

Section 7: Health Educators actively involve individuals, groups, and communities in the entire educational process so that all aspects of the process are clearly understood by those who may be affected.

Section 8: Health Educators respect and acknowledge the rights of others to hold diverse values, attitudes, and opinions.

Section 9: Health Educators provide services equitably to all people.

Article II: Responsibility to the Profession

Health Educators are responsible for their professional behavior, for the reputation of their profession, and for promoting ethical conduct among their colleagues.

Section 1: Health Educators maintain, improve, and expand their professional competence through continued study and education; membership, participation, and leadership in professional organizations; and involvement in issues related to the health of the public.

Section 2: Health Educators model and encourage nondiscriminatory standards of behavior in their interactions with others.

Section 3: Health Educators encourage and accept responsible critical discourse to protect and enhance the profession.

Section 4: Health Educators contribute to the development of the profession by sharing the processes and outcomes of their work.

Section 5: Health Educators are aware of possible professional conflicts of interest, exercise integrity in conflict situations, and do not manipulate or violate the rights of others.

Section 6: Health Educators give appropriate recognition to others for their professional contributions and achievements

Article III: Responsibility to Employers

Health Educators recognize the boundaries of their professional competence and are accountable for their professional activities and actions.

Section 1: Health Educators accurately represent their qualifications and the qualifications of others whom they recommend.

Section 2: Health Educators use appropriate standards, theories, and guidelines as criteria when carrying out their professional responsibilities.

Section 3: Health Educators accurately represent potential service and program outcomes to employers.

Section 4: Health Educators anticipate and disclose competing commitments, conflicts of interest, and endorsement of products.

Section 5: Health Educators openly communicate to employers, expectations of job-related assignments that conflict with their professional ethics.

Section 6: Health Educators maintain competence in their areas of professional practice.

Article IV: Responsibility in the Delivery of Health Education

Health Educators promote integrity in the delivery of health education. They respect the rights, dignity, confidentiality, and worth of all people by adapting strategies and methods to the needs of diverse populations and communities.

Section 1: Health Educators are sensitive to social and cultural diversity and are in accord with the law, when planning and implementing programs.

Section 2: Health Educators are informed of the latest advances in theory, research, and practice, and use strategies and methods that are grounded in and contribute to development of professional standards, theories, guidelines, statistics, and experience.

Section 3: Health Educators are committed to rigorous evaluation of both program effectiveness and the methods used to achieve results.

Section 4: Health Educators empower individuals to adopt healthy lifestyles through informed choice rather than by coercion or intimidation.

Section 5: Health Educators communicate the potential outcomes of proposed services, strategies, and pending decisions to all individuals who will be affected.

Article V: Responsibility in Research and Evaluation

Health Educators contribute to the health of the population and to the profession through research and evaluation activities. When planning and conducting research or evaluation, health educators do so in accordance with federal and state laws and regulations, organizational and institutional policies, and professional standards.

Section 1: Health Educators support principles and practices of research and evaluation that do no harm to individuals, groups, society, or the environment.

Section 2: Health Educators ensure that participation in research is voluntary and is based upon the informed consent of the participants.

Section 3: Health Educators respect the privacy, rights, and dignity of research participants, and honor commitments made to those participants.

Section 4: Health Educators treat all information obtained from participants as confidential unless otherwise required by law.

Section 5: Health Educators take credit, including authorship, only for work they have actually performed and give credit to the contributions of others.

Section 6: Health Educators who serve as research or evaluation consultants discuss their results only with those to whom they are providing service, unless maintaining such confidentiality would jeopardize the health or safety of others.

Section 7: Health Educators report the results of their research and evaluation objectively, accurately, and in a timely fashion.

Article VI: Responsibility in Professional Preparation

Those involved in the preparation and training of Health Educators have an obligation to accord learners the same respect and treatment given other groups by providing quality education that benefits the profession and the public.

Section 1: Health Educators select students for professional preparation programs based upon equal opportunity for all, and the individual's academic performance, abilities, and potential contribution to the profession and the public's health.

Section 2: Health Educators strive to make the educational environment and culture conducive to the health of all involved, and free from sexual harassment and all forms of discrimination.

Section 3: Health Educators involved in professional preparation and professional development engage in careful preparation; present material that is accurate, up-to-date, and timely; provide reasonable and timely feedback; state clear and reasonable expectations; and conduct fair assessments and evaluations of learners.

Section 4: Health Educators provide objective and accurate counseling to learners about career opportunities, development, and advancement, and assist learners secure professional employment.

Section 5: Health Educators provide adequate supervision and meaningful opportunities for the professional development of learners.

Coalition of National Health Education Organizations (CNHEO). *Code of Ethics for the Health Education Profession*. Approved November 8, 1999, Chicago, IL. www.cnheo.org. Reprinted with permission.

References

Abramson, H. J. (1980). Religion. In S. Thernstrom (Ed.), *Harvard encyclopedia of American ethnic groups*. Cambridge, MA: Harvard University Press.

Agency for Healthcare Research and Quality. (n.d.). *Introduction to state health policy: A seminar for new state legislators*. Retrieved August 8, 2008, from http://www.ahrq.gov/news/ulpix.htm

Airhihenbuwa, C. O. (1990). A conceptual model for cultural appropriate health education programs in developing countries. *International Quarterly of Community Health Education, 11,* 53–62.

Ajzen, I. (1991). The theory of planned behavior. *Organizational Behavior and Human Decision Processes, 50,* 179–211.

Ajzen, I., & Fishbein, M. (1977). Attitude-behavior relations: A theoretical analysis and review of empirical research. *Psychological Bulletin, 84,* 888–918.

Alexander, E. A. (2000). *Famous fried eggs: Students debate effectiveness, accuracy, of well-known anti-drug commercial*. CNN Student Bureau. Retrieved April 13, 2008, from http://www.mediacampaign.org/newsletter/spring98/update-04.html

Alliance for the Healthiest Nation. (2008). *Our initiative for a healthier nation*. Retrieved August 14, 2008, from http://www.healthiestnation.org/

Alward, R. R., & Camunas, C. (1991). *The nurse's guide to marketing*. Boston: Delmar.

American Academy of Pediatrics. (2003). Prevention of pediatric overweight and obesity. *Pediatrics, 112*(2), 424–430.

American Cancer Society. (2007). *Lung cancer*. Retrieved April 4, 2008, from http://www.cancer.org/downloads/PRO/LungCancer.pdf

American College Health Association. (2002). *Healthy campus 2010: Making it happen*. Baltimore, MD: Author.

American Heart Association. (2008). *Heart disease and stoke statistics*. Retrieved April 5, 2008, from http://www.americanheart.org/downloadable/heart/1200082005246HS_Stats%202008.final.pdf

American Speech-Language-Hearing Association. (1999). *Language skill disorders*. Retrieved September 22, 1999, from http://www.healthtouch.com/levl/leaflets/aslha058.htm.

Ammerman, A. S., Evenson, K. R., Keyserling, T. C., Rosamond, W. D., Tawney, K. W., Jacobs, A. D., Garcia, B. A., & Aycock, N. W. (n.d.). *WISEWOMAN in a broader context: Integrating cardiovascular disease prevention into existing health services*. Chapel Hill: Center for Health Promotion and Disease Prevention, The University of North Carolina at Chapel Hill. Retrieved July 19, 2008, from http://www.hpdp.unc.edu/WISEWOMAN/manual.htm

Anderson, J. A., & Adams, M. N. (1992). Acknowledging the learning styles of diverse student populations: Implications for instructional design. In L. L. B. Border and N. Van Note Chism (Eds.), *Teaching for diversity* (pp. 19–33). San Francisco: Jossey-Bass.

Anderson, L. W., & Krathwohl, D. R. (Eds.). (2001). *A taxonomy for learning, teaching and assessing: A revision of Bloom's taxonomy of educational objectives: Complete edition.* New York: Longman.

Armstrong, T. (1994). *Multiple intelligences.* Alexandria, VA: Association for Supervision and Curriculum Development.

Association for Worksite Health Promotion. (1999). *1999 National worksite health promotion survey.* Northbrook, IL: Author.

Association of Schools of Public Health. (n.d.). *What is public health?* Retrieved August 15, 2008, from http://www.whatispublichealth.org/

Association of Schools of Public Health. (2001). *Core areas of public health.* Retrieved July 25, 2008, from http://www.asph.org/document.cfm?page=301

Association of Schools of Public Health. (2008, February). *Confronting the public health workforce crisis: ASPH statement on the public health workforce.* Washington, DC: Author. Retrieved May 26, 2008, from http://www.asph.org/UserFiles/PHWFShortage0208.pdf

Association of State and Territorial Health Officials. (2007, April). *Innovations in public health: Understanding state public health.* Washington, DC: Author. Retrieved August 10, 2008, from http://www.astho.org/pubs/UnderstandingPHASTHO.pdf

Baker, J. J., & Baker, R. W. (1999). *Health care finance: Basic tools for nonfinancial managers.* Gaithersburg, MD: Aspen.

Baker, T. A., & Wang, C. C. (2006). Photovoice: Use of a participatory action research method to explore chronic pain experience in older adults. *Qualitative Health Research, 16*(10), 1405–1413.

Bandura, A. (1977). *Social learning theory.* Englewood Cliffs, NJ: Prentice-Hall.

Barlow, L. (2004). How to use Web search engines. *The Spider's Apprentice.* Retrieved April 21, 2009, from http://www.monash.com/spidap2.html

Bartholomew, L. K., Parcel, G. S., Kok, G., & Gottlieb, N. H. (2006). *Planning health promotion programs: An intervention mapping approach* (2nd ed.). San Francisco: John Wiley & Sons.

Bauer, R. A. (1967). *Social indicators.* Cambridge: MIT Press.

Bean, J. C. (1996). *Engaging ideas: The professor's guide to integrating writing, critical thinking, and active learning in the classroom.* San Francisco: Jossey-Bass.

Beardain, R. P., & Grantham, J. B. (1993). The use of volunteerism in indigent health care. *Journal of Health and Social Policy, 5*(1), 1–7.

Beck, S. (1997). Evaluation criteria. *The good, the bad & the ugly: Or, why it's a good idea to evaluate web sources* [Online presentation]. Retrieved January 8, 2008, from http://www.lib.nmsu.edu/instruction/evalcrit.html

Bellman, G. M. (1990). *The consultant's calling: Bringing who you are to what you do.* San Francisco: Jossey-Bass.

Bernhardt, J. (2006, July). *Health marketing musings.* Retrieved April 15, 2008, from http://www.cdc.gov/print.do?url=http://www.cdc.gov/healthmarketing/blog_071306.htm#

Bloom, B., & Cohen, R. A. (2007). Summary health statistics for U.S. children: National health interview survey, 2006. *Vital Health Statistics, 10*(234). National Center for Health Statistics.

Bloom, B. S., Englehart, M., Furst, E., Hill, W., & Krathwohl, D. R. (1956). *Taxonomy of educational objectives: The classification of educational goals. Handbook 1: Cognitive domain.* New York: Longmans.

Bornstein, D. (1996). *The blind men and the elephant: A Hindu fable by John Godfrey Saxe.* Retrieved July 31, 1999, from http://www.milk.com/random-humor/elephant_fable.html

Breckon, D. J. (1997). *Managing health promotion programs: Leadership skills for the 21st century.* Gaithersburg, MD: Aspen.

Brislin, R. W. (1986). The wording and translation of research instruments. In W. J. Lonner & J. W. Berry (Eds.), *Field methods in cross-cultural research* (pp. 137–164). Beverly Hills, CA: Sage.

Broder, J. M. (2008, July 18). Gore urges change to dodge an energy crisis. *New York Times.* Retrieved August 12, 2008, from http://www.nytimes.com/2008/07/18/washington/ 18gore.html?_r=1&oref=slogin

Bryman, A. (1996). Leadership in organizations. In S. R. Clegg, C. Hardy, & W. R. Nord (Eds.), *Handbook of organizational studies* (pp. 276–292). Newbury Park, CA: Sage.

Bullough, B., & Bullough, V. L. (1972). *Poverty, ethnic identity, and health care.* New York: Appleton-Century-Crofts.

Bureau of Labor Statistics. (2001, October). Health educators. Retrieved August 15, 2008, from http://www.bls.gov/soc/soc_f1j1.htm

Bureau of Labor Statistics. (2007a, April). Health educators. *Occupational outlook handbook, 2008–09 edition.* Washington, DC: Author. Retrieved July 20, 2008, from http://www.bls.gov/ oco/ocos063.htm

Bureau of Labor Statistics. (2007b). *Volunteering in the United States, 2007.* Retrieved January 8, 2008, from http://www.bls.gov/news.release/volun.nr0.htm

Burk, M., Wieser, P., & Keegan, L. (1995). Cultural beliefs and health behaviors of pregnant Mexican-American women: Implications for primary care. *Advances in Nursing Science, 17*(4), 37–52.

Burke, S., Snyder, S., & Rager, R. (2009). An assessment of faculty usage of YouTube as a resource. *The Internet Journal of Allied Health Sciences and Practices, 7*(1). Retrieved March 17, 2009, from http://www.ijahsp.nova.edu/articles/Vol7Num1/burke.htm

Burman, R., & Evans, A. J. (2008). Target zero: A culture of safety. *Defense Aviation Safety Centre Journal, 2008,* 22–27. Retrieved from http://www.mod.uk/NR/rdonlyres/ 849892B2-D6D2-4DFD-B5BD-9A4F288A9B18/0/DASCJournal2008.pdf

California Center for Applied Linguistics. (2008). *Dialects: African American English.* Retrieved September 4, 2008, from http://www.cal.org/topics/dialects/aae.html

Campinha-Bacote, J. (1998). African-Americans. In L. D. Purnell & B. J. Paulanka (Eds.), *Transcultural health care: A culturally competent approach* (pp. 53–73). Philadelphia: F. A. Davis.

Carnevale, A. P., Gainer, L. L., & Meltzer, A. S. (1990). *Workplace basics.* San Francisco: Jossey-Bass.

CDCSynergy. (n.d.). *Social marketing.* Retrieved August 27, 2008, from http://www.cdc.gov/ dhdsp/CDCynergy_training/Content/activeinformation/example-social.htm

Centers for Disease Control and Prevention. (n.d.). *About CDC.* Retrieved August 10, 2008, from http://www.cdc.gov/about/

Centers for Disease Control and Prevention. (n.d.). *Bioterrorism.* Retrieved August 21, 2008, from http://www.emergency.cdc.gov/bioterrorism/

Centers for Disease Control and Prevention. (n.d.). *Healthy people in a healthy world.* Retrieved August 15, 2008, from http://www.cdc.gov/osi/goals/global.html

Centers for Disease Control and Prevention. (1999). Trends in HIV-related sexual risk behaviors among high school students—Selected U.S. cities, 1991–1997. *Journal of School Health, 69*(7), 255–257.

Centers for Disease Control and Prevention. (2006a). *Advancing the nation's health: A guide to public health research needs, 2006–2015.* Washington, DC: U.S. Department of Health and Human Services.

Centers for Disease Control and Prevention. (2006b). *Bridging CDC to Congress and Washington-based partners.* Retrieved August 8, 2008, from http://www.cdc.gov/washington/

Centers for Disease Control and Prevention. (2006c, July 16). *Vision, mission, core values, and pledge. About CDC.* Retrieved August 10, 2008, from http://www.cdc.gov/about/organization/mission.htm

Centers for Disease Control and Prevention. (2007a, November 27). *About REACH across the U.S. (2007 to present).* Retrieved August 10, 2008, from http://www.cdc.gov/reach/about.htm

Centers for Disease Control and Prevention. (2007b, March). *CDC achieving greater health impact: Goals for the 21st century.* Retrieved August 15, 2008, from http://www.cdc.gov/osi/goals/Objectives0307.pdf

Centers for Disease Control and Prevention. (2007c, February 6). *CDC organization. About CDC.* Retrieved August 10, 2008, from http://www.cdc.gov/about/organization/cio.htm

Centers for Disease Control and Prevention. (2007d). *Deaths, percent of total deaths, and death rates for the 15 leading causes of death: United States and each state, 1999–2004.* Retrieved April 12, 2008, from http://www.cdc.gov/nchs/data/dvs/LCWK92004.pdf

Centers for Disease Control and Prevention. (2007e). *General considerations regarding health education and risk reduction activities.* Retrieved August 27, 2008, from http://www.cdc.gov/hiv/resources/guidelines/herrg/gen-con_intro.htm

Centers for Disease Control and Prevention. (2007f, April 9). *Health information for older adults. Healthy aging.* Retrieved September 4, 2008, from http://www.cdc.gov/aging/info.htm

Centers for Disease Control and Prevention. (2007g, March). *Health protection goals and objectives.* Retrieved August 22, 2008, from http://www.cdc.gov/osi/goals/Objectives0307.pdf

Centers for Disease Control and Prevention. (2007h, February 8). *What are some of CDC's key findings related to adult health-related quality of life?* Retrieved August 23, 2008, from http://www.cdc.gov/hrqol/findings.htm

Centers for Disease Control and Prevention. (2008a). *About us.* Retrieved January 9, 2008, from http://www.cdc.gov/about

Centers for Disease Control and Prevention. (2008b). *Behavioral risk factor surveillance system.* Retrieved March 5, 2008, from http://www.cdc.gov/brfss/about.htm

Centers for Disease Control and Prevention. (2008c, August 20). *Childhood obesity. Healthy youth.* Retrieved September 1, 2008, from http://www.cdc.gov/HealthyYouth/obesity/index.htm

Centers for Disease Control and Prevention. (2008d, April 17). *The community health promotion handbook: Action guides to improve community health.* Retrieved August 14, 2008, from http://www.cdc.gov/steps/actionguides/

Centers for Disease Control and Prevention. (2008e). *National health care surveys.* Retrieved March 30, 2008, from http://www.cdc.gov/nchs/nhcs.htm

Centers for Disease Control and Prevention. (2008f). *National notifiable diseases surveillance system.* Retrieved April 10, 2008, from http://www.cdc.gov/ncphi/disss/nndss/nndsshis.htm

Centers for Disease Control and Prevention. (2008g). *Obesity.* Retrieved August 26, 2008, from http://www.cdc.gov/nccdphp/dnpa

Centers for Disease Control and Prevention. (2008h). *Overweight and obesity.* Retrieved August 26, 2008, from http://www.cdc.gov/nccdphp/dnpa/obesity/contributing-factors

Centers for Disease Control and Prevention. (2008i, February 5). *Providers of health care services. The community guide.* Retrieved August 8, 2008, from http://www.thecommunityguide.org/providers.html

Centers for Disease Control and Prevention. (2008j). *State program evaluation guides: Writing SMART objectives.* CDC Division for Heart Disease and Stroke Prevention. Retrieved January 22, 2009, from http://www.cdc.gov/dhdsp/state_program/evaluation_guides/pdfs/smart_objectives.pdf

Centers for Disease Control and Prevention. (2008k). *The steps program in action: Success stories on community initiatives to prevent chronic diseases.* Retrieved August 1, 2008, from http://www.cdc.gov/steps/success_stories/pdf/SuccessStories.pdf

Centers for Disease Control and Prevention. (2008l, June 6). Youth risk behavior surveillance—United States, 2007. *Morbidity and Mortality Weekly Report, 57*(SS-4). Retrieved February 5, 2009, from http://www.cdc.gov/HealthyYouth/yrbs/pdf/yrbss07_mmwr.pdf

Centers for Disease Control and Prevention. (2009a, February). *The community guide: Preventive services.* Retrieved August 8, 2008, from http://www.thecommunityguide.org/index.html

Centers for Disease Control and Prevention. (2009b). *Fact sheet: HIV testing among adolescents.* Retrieved May 4, 2009, from http://www.cdc.gov/healthyyouth/sexualbehaviors/pdf/hivtesting_adolescents.pdf

Central Intelligence Agency (CIA). (2008). *The world factbook.* Retrieved April 21, 2009, from https://www.cia.gov/library/publications/the-world-factbook/rankorder/2102rank.html

Chambre, S. M. (1993). Volunteerism by elders: Past trends and future prospects. *The Gerontologist, 33*(2), 221–228.

Chaskin, R. J., Brown, P., Venkatesh, S., & Vidal, A. (2001). *Community capacity and capacity building.* Hawthorne, NY: Aldine.

Cohen, D., de la Vega, R., & Watson, G. (2001). *Advocacy for social justice: A global action and reflection guide.* Bloomfield, CT: Kumarian Press.

Commonwealth Fund Commission on a High Performance Health System. (2008, July). *Why not the best? Results from the national scorecard on U.S. health system performance, 2008.* New York: The Commonwealth Fund. Retrieved August 14, 2008, from http://www.commonwealthfund.org/publications/publications_show.htm?doc_id=692682

Connecticut Association of Non-Profits Advocacy. (2003). *Advocacy and lobbying toolkit.* Retrieved on August 23, 2008, from http://www.ctnonprofits.org/Pages/NonProfitResources/Advocacy_Lobbying_Toolkit_WordVersions.asp

Coque, T. M., Novais, A., Carattoli, A., Poirel, L., Pitout, J., Peixe, L., Baquero, F., Cantón, R., & Nordmann, P. (2008, February). Dissemination of clonally related *Escherichia coli* strains expressing extended-spectrum β-Lactamase CTX-M-15. *Emerging Infectious Diseases 14*(2). Retrieved February 26, 2008, from http://www.cdc.gov/EID/content/14/2/195.htm

Corbett, S. (2008, April). Can the cell phone help end global poverty? *New York Times.* Retrieved August 20, 2008, from http://www.nytimes.com/2004/04/13/magazine/13anthropology-html

Council on Education for Public Health. (2008, July). *Schools of public health and public health programs accredited by the Council on Education for Public Health.* Retrieved July 8, 2008, from http://www.ceph.org/i4a/pages/index.cfm?pageid=3344

Council on Linkages between Academia and Public Health Practice. (2008, May). *Core competencies for public health professionals.* Washington, DC: Author. Retrieved August 16, 2008, from http://www.phf.org/link/corecompetenciesdraft.pdf

Curran, J. (2006). Infectious disease control. In B. A. DeBuono (Ed.), *Milestones in public health: Accomplishments in public health over the last 100 years* (pp. 59–82). New York: Pfizer Global Pharmaceuticals.

Cushner, K. (1994). Preparing teachers for an intercultural context. In R. W. Brislin & T. Yoshida (Eds.), *Improving intercultural interactions: Modules for cross-cultural training programs* (pp. 109–128). Thousand Oaks, CA: Sage.

D'Souza, G., Kreimer, A. R., Viscidi, R., Pawlita, M., Fakhry, C., Koch, W. M., Westra, W. H., & Gillison, M. L. (2007). Case-control study of human papillomavirus and oropharyngeal cancer. *New England Journal of Medicine, 356*(19), 1944–1956. Retrieved June 12, 2008, from http://www.content.nejm.org/cgi/content/full/356/19/1944

Daniel, E. L., & Balog, J. I. (1997). Utilization of the World Wide Web in education. *The Journal of School Health, 28*(5), 260–267.

DeBuono, B. A. (Ed.). (2006). *Milestones in public health: Accomplishments in public health over the last 100 years.* New York: Pfizer Global Pharmaceuticals.

Detmar, S. B., Muller, M. J., Schornagel, J. H., Wever, L. D. V., & Aaronson, N. K. (2002). Health-related quality-of-life assessments and patient-physician communication: A randomized controlled trial. *Journal of the American Medication Association, 288*(23), 3027–3034.

Díaz, H. L. (2007). Community capacity and micro-economic development: A study from Peru. *International Journal of Social Welfare, 16*(4), 339–348.

Dinger, M. K., & Parsons, N. (1999). Sexual activity among college students living in residence halls and fraternity or sorority housing. *Journal of Health Education, 30*(4), 242–246, 260.

Doctors without Borders. (n.d.). *Tuberculosis patients still waiting for new diagnostic tools and treatment.* Retrieved August 22, 2008, from http://www.doctorswithoutborders.org/news/issue_print.cfm?id=2404

Doll, R. C. (1992). *Curriculum improvement: Decision making and process* (8th ed.). Boston: Allyn & Bacon.

Doyle, E. I. (2008). Toward a culturally competent health education work force. In M. A. Perez & R. Luquis (Eds.), *Cultural competence in health education and health promotion* (pp. 163–181). San Francisco: Jossey-Bass.

Dudwick, N., Kuehnast, K., Nyhan Jones, V., & Woolcock, M. (2006). *Analyzing social capital in context: A guide to using qualitative methods and data.* Washington, DC: World Bank Institute. Retrieved from http://www.siteresources.worldbank.org/WBI/Resources/Analyzing_Social_Capital_in_Context-FINAL.pdf

Eck, D. I. (2001). *A new religious America: How a "Christian country" has become the world's most religious diverse nation.* San Francisco: Harper.

Educational Testing Service. (2008). *Adult literacy.* Retrieved August 20, 2008, from http://www.ets.org/portal/site/ets/menuitem.d4640d54cfbd7becda20bc47c3921509/?vgnextoid=66f87862687da010VgnVCM10000022f95190RCRD

Educause Learning Initiative. (2005). *7 things you should know about blogs.* Retrieved January 3, 2008, from http://www.educause.edu/ir/library/pdf/ELI7006.pdf

Elliott, J., Seals, B., & Jacobson, M. (2007). Use of the Precaution Adoption Process Model to examine predictors of osteoprotective behavior in epilepsy. *Seizure, 16*(5), 424–437.

Ellis, S. J. (1993). Volunteerism as an enhancement to career development. *Journal of Employment Counseling, 30*(3), 127–132.

Federal Interagency Forum on Child and Family Statistics. (2008, July). *America's children in brief: Key national indicators of well-being, 2008.* Retrieved September 1, 2008, from http://www.childstats.gov/americaschildren/health.asp

Force Health Protection and Readiness. (2008). *The millennium cohort study offers the first comprehensive review of career-span military health.* Retrieved June 12, 2008, from http://www.deploymentlink.osd.mil/new.jsp?newsID=35

Fors, S. W., Crepaz, N., & Hayes, D. M. (1999). Key factors that protect against health risks in youth: Further evidence. *American Journal of Health Behavior, 23*(5), 368–380.

Fowler, F. J. (2002). *Survey research methods* (3rd ed.). Thousand Oaks, CA: Sage.

Friedson, E. (1988). *Profession of medicine: A study of the sociology of applied knowledge* (2nd ed.). Chicago: The University of Chicago Press.

Friis, R. H., & Sellers, T. A. (1999). *Epidemiology for public health practice* (2nd ed.). Gaithersburg, MD: Aspen.

Frohmann, L. (2005). The framing safety project: Photographs and narratives by battered women. *Violence Against Women, 11*(11), 1396–1419.

Gabel, M. (2006). *America, America.* Media, PA: BigPictureSmallWorld, Inc. Retrieved August 22, 2008, from http://www.bigpicturesmallworld.com/index.shtml

Gardner, H. (1993). *Multiple intelligences: The theory in practice* (pp. 13–34). New York: Basic Books.

Gardner, H. (2003). *Multiple intelligences after twenty years.* Retrieved August 18, 2008, from http://www.pzweb.harvard.edu/PIs/HG_MI_after_20_years.pdf

Garrand, J. (1999). *Health sciences literature review made easy: The matrix method.* Gaithersburg, MD: Aspen.

Gilmore, G. D., & Campbell, M. D. (2005). *Needs and capacity assessment strategies for health education and health promotion* (3rd ed.). Boston: Jones & Bartlett.

Glanz, K., Lewis, F. M., & Rimer, B. K. (Eds.). (1997). *Health behavior and health education: Theory, research, and practice.* San Francisco: Jossey-Bass.

Glanz, K., Rimer, B. K., & Lewis, F. M. (Eds.). (2002). *Health behavior and health education: Theory, research, and practice* (3rd ed.). San Francisco: Jossey-Bass.

Glanz, K., Rimer, B. K., &. Viswanath, K. (Eds.). (2008). *Health behavior and health education: Theory, research, and practice* (4th ed.). San Francisco: Jossey-Bass.

Glascoff, M. A., Baker, J. B., & Glascoff, D. W. (1997). Successfully promoting volunteerism by offering extrinsic rewards in a personal health course: A pilot study. *Journal of School Health Education, 28*(4), 219–223.

Global Health Council. (n.d.). *Why does global health matter?* Retrieved August 20, 2008, from http://www.globalhealth.org/images/pdf/gh_message_box.pdf

Godwin, M., Ruhland, L., Casson, I., MacDonald, S., Delva, D., Birthwhistle, R., Lam, M., & Seguin, R. (2003). Pragmatic controlled clinical trials in primary care: The struggle between external and internal validity. *BMC Medical Research Methodology, 3*(28). Retrieved from www.biomedicalcentral.com11471–12288/3/28

Gold, R. S., & Miner, K. R. (2002, January). Report of the 2000 joint committee on health education and promotion terminology. *Journal of School Health, 72*(1), 3–7.

Goodman, R. M., Speers, M. A., McLeroy, K., Fawcett, S., Kegler, M., Parker, E., Smith, S. R., Sterling, T. D., & Wallerstein, N. (1999). Identifying and defining the dimensions of community capacity to provide a basis for measurement. *Health Education and Behavior, 25*(3), 258–278.

Green, L. W., & Kreuter, M. W. (1999). *Health promotion planning: An educational and ecological approach* (3rd ed.). Mountain View, CA: Mayfield.

Green, L. W., & Kreuter, M. W. (2005). *Health program planning: An educational and ecological approach* (4th ed.). Boston: McGraw-Hill.

Greenberg, J. S. (2003). *Health education: Learner-centered instructional strategies* (5th ed.). New York: McGraw-Hill.

Gronfeldt, S., & Strother, J. B. (2006). *Service leadership: The quest for the competitive advantage.* Newbury Park, CA: Sage.

Grootaert, C., Narayan, D., Nyhan Jones, V., & Woolcock, M. (2004). *Measuring social capital: An integrated questionnaire.* Retrieved from http://www.povlibrary.worldbank.org/files/11998_WP18-Web.pdf

Hamilton, B. E., Martin, J. S., & Ventura, S. J. (2007, December). Births: Preliminary data for 2006. *National Vital Statistics Reports, 56*(7). Retrieved August 23, 2008, from http://www.cdc.gov/nchs/data/nvsr/nvsr56/nvsr56_07.pdf

Hardcastle, D. A., Powers, P. R., & Wenocur, S. (2004). *Community practice: Theories and skills for social workers* (2nd ed.). New York: Oxford University Press.

Harvard School of Public Health. (n.d.). *Center for health communication.* Retrieved April 13, 2008, from http://www.hsph.harvard.edu/chc

Health Resources and Services Administration. (n.d.). *What we do.* Retrieved August 8, 2008, from http://www.hrsa.gov/about/default.htm

Henderson, D. A. (2006). Vaccines and the eradication of smallpox. In B. A. DeBuono (Ed.), *Milestones in public health: Accomplishments in public health over the last 100 years* (pp. 5–20). New York: Pfizer Global Pharmaceuticals.

Henry, J., & Ward, S. E. (1999). The art and science of health education. Unpublished paper.

Herman, M. (2005). *How to use Wiki.* Retrieved January 4, 2008, from http://www.openspaceworld.org/cgi/netwiki.cgi?HowToUseWiki

Heron, M. P., Hoyert, D. L., Murphy, S. L., Xu, J., Kochanek, K. D., & Tejada-Vera, B. (2009, April). Deaths: Final data for 2006. *National Vital Statistics Reports, 57*(14). Retrieved May 1, 2009, from http://www.cdc.gov/nchs/data/nvsr/nvsr57/nvsr57_14.pdf

Heron, M. P., Hoyert, D. L., Xu, J., Scott, C., & Tejada-Vera, B. (2008a, June). Deaths: Preliminary data for 2006. *National Vital Statistics Reports, 56*(16). Retrieved September 4, 2008, from http://www.cdc.gov/nchs/data/nvsr/nvsr56/nvsr56_16.pdf

Heron, M. P., Hoyert, D. L., Xu, J., Scott, C., & Tejada-Vera, B. (2008b, April). U.S. Mortality drops sharply in 2006, Latest data show. *National Vital Statistics Reports, 56*(16). Retrieved August 23, 2008, from http://www.cdc.gov/nchs/data/nvsr/nvsr56/nvsr56_16.pdf

Hill, S. C., & Drolet, J. C. (1999). School-related violence among high school students in the United States, 1993–1995. *Journal of School Health, 69*(7), 264–272.

Hochbaum, G. M. (1958). *Public participation in medical screening programs: A sociopsychological study.* PHS Publication No. 572. Washington, DC: U.S. Government Printing Office.

Hofstede, G. (2001). *Culture's consequences: Comparing values, behaviors, institutions and organizations across nations* (2nd ed.). Thousand Oaks, CA: Sage.

Hogben, M. (1998). Factors moderating the effect of television aggression on viewer behavior. *Communication Research, 25*, 220–247.

Holland J. (2003). *Applying complexity science to health and healthcare.* Minneapolis: Center for the Study of Health Care Management, University of Minnesota.

Ibrahim, M. A. (1985). *Epidemiology and health policy.* Rockville, MD: Aspen.

Infed Search. (2008). *Naturalistic intelligence.* Retrieved August 25, 2008, from http://www.edwebproject.org/edref.mi.th8.html

Insel, P. M., & Roth, W. T. (1994, 2000). *Core concepts in health.* Mountain View, CA: Mayfield.

Institute of Medicine. (2000). *Promoting health: Intervention strategies from social and behavioral research.* B. D. Smedley & S. L. Syme (Eds.). Washington, DC: National Academies Press.

Institute of Medicine. (2002). *The future of the public's health in the 21st century.* Washington, DC: National Academies Press.

Institute of Medicine. (2003). *Who will keep the public healthy? Educating public health professionals for the 21st century.* Washington, DC: National Academies Press.

Institute of Medicine. (2007, June). *Training physicians for public health careers* [Report brief]. Retrieved August 16, 2008, from http://www.iom.edu/Object.File/Master/43/416/Training%20physicians%20report%20brief.pdf

International Union for Health Promotion and Education. (2007). *Shaping the future of health promotion: Priorities for action.* Retrieved August 22, 2008, from http://www.iuhpe.org/upload/File/Shaping.pdf

Ireland, J. D. (1999, June). *Udana VI.4, Tittha Sutta, various sectarians (1).* Buddhist publication society. Retrieved July 31, 1999, from http://www.world.std.com/~metta/canon/khuddaka/udana/ud6-4.html

Jack, L., Harrison, I. E., & Airhihenbuwa, C. O. (1994). Ethnicity and health belief systems. In A. C. Matiella (Ed.), *The multicultural challenge in health education* (pp. 51–72). Santa Cruz, CA: ETR Associates.

Jackson, C. (1997). Behavior science theory and principles in health education. *Health Education, 12*(1), 143–150.

Johnston, L. D., O'Malley, P. M., Bachman, J. G., & Schulenberg, J. E. (2008). *Monitoring the future national results on drug use, 1975–2007. Volume 1: Secondary school students.* NIH Publication No. 08-6418A. Bethesda, MD: National Institute on Drug Abuse.

Joint Committee on Terminology. (2001). Report of the 2000 joint committee on health education and promotion terminology. *American Journal of Health Education, 32*(2), 89–103.

Jones, C. P. (2004). Levels of racism: A theoretic framework and a gardener's tale. *American Journal of Public Health, 90*(8), 1212–1215.

Jones, P. S., Lee, J. W., Phillips, L. R., Zhang, X. E., & Jaceldo, K. B. (2001). An adaptation of Brislin's translation model for cross-cultural research. *Nursing Research, 50*(5), 300–304.

Kaiser Family Foundation. (2004). *Health insurance coverage in America, 2003 data update.* Retrieved August 18, 2008, from http://www.kff.org/uninsured/7153.cfm

Keating, M., Boham, M., & Ransdell, L. (2007). Consulting in health education/promotion: Everything you've always wanted to know but were afraid to ask. *California Journal of Health Promotion, 5*(3), 92–99.

Keck, C. W. (2006). U.S. public health infrastructure. In B. A. DeBuono (Ed.), *Milestones in public health: Accomplishments in public health over the last 100 years* (pp. 213–226). New York: Pfizer Global Pharmaceuticals.

Kegler, M. C., Norton, B. L., & Aronson, R. (2008, March 21). Achieving organizational change: Findings from case studies of 20 California healthy cities and communities coalitions. *Health Promotion International, 23*(2), 109–118.

Keller, C., Fleury, J., Perez, A., Ainsworth, B., & Vaughn, L. (2008). Using visual methods to uncover context. *Qualitative Health Research, 18*(3), 428–436.

Kelly, J. G. (1986). Context and process: An ecological view of the interdependence of practice and research. *American Journal of Community Psychology, 14*(6), 581–589.

Kennedy, A. J. (1999). *The Internet: The Rough Guide 2000.* New York: Rough Guide.

Kieffer, E. C., & Rieschmann, J. (2004). *Contributions of community building to achieving improved public health outcomes, final report.* Retrieved September 4, 2008, from http://www.aspeninstitute.org/atf/cf/%7BDEB6F227-659B-4EC8-8F84-8DF23CA704F5%7D/rcckiefferfinalreport.pdf

Kilbourne, J. (2003). *Deadly persuasion: The advertising of alcohol and tobacco* [video recording]. Sut Jhally (Director). Media Education Foundation HF5831.D434.

Kitano, M. K. (1997). A rationale and framework for course change. In A. I. Morey & M. K. Kitano (Eds.), *Multicultural course transformation in higher education: A broader truth* (pp. 1–17). Boston: Allyn & Bacon.

Komro, K. A., Perry, C. L., Veblen-Mortenson, S., Williams, C. L., & Roel, J. P. (1999). Peer leadership in school and community alcohol use prevention activities. *Journal of Health Education, 30*(4), 202–208.

Koop, C. E., Pearson, C. E., & Schwarz, M. R. (2002). *Critical issues in global health.* San Francisco: Jossey-Bass.

Kotler, P., & Zaltman, G. (1971). Social marketing: An approach to social change. *Journal of Marketing, 35*(3), 3–12.

Krugman, P., & Wells, R. (2006). The health care crisis and what to do about it. *The New York Review of Books, 53*(5). Retrieved April 21, 2009, from http://www.nybooks.com/articles/18802

KU Work Group for Community Health and Development. (2007a). *Assessing community needs and resources* (chap. 3). Lawrence: University of Kansas. Retrieved August 12, 2008, from http://www.ctb.ku.edu/en/tablecontents/chapter_1003.htm

KU Work Group for Community Health and Development. (2007b). *Coalition building I: Starting a coalition* (chap. 5, sect. 5). Lawrence: University of Kansas. Retrieved January 18, 2009, from http://www.ctb.ku.edu/en/tablecontents/section_1057.htm

KU Work Group for Community Health and Development. (2007c). *An overview of strategic planning or "VMOSA"* (chap. 8, sect. 1). Lawrence: University of Kansas. Retrieved January 16, 2009, from http://www.ctb.ku.edu/en/tablecontents/section_1085.htm

KU Work Group for Community Health and Development. (2007d). *Principles of advocacy* (chap. 30). Lawrence: University of Kansas. Retrieved July 20, 2009, from http://www.ctb.ku.edu/tools

KU Work Group for Community Health and Development. (2007e). *SWOT analysis: Strengths, weaknesses, opportunities, threats* (chap. 3, sect. 14). Lawrence: University of Kansas. Retrieved January 18, 2009, from http://www.ctb.ku.edu/en/tablecontents/section_1049.htm

KU Work Group for Community Health and Development. (2007f). *Promoting interest in community issues* (chap. 6, sect. 1). Lawrence: University of Kansas. Retrieved August 20, 2008, from http://www.ctb.ku.edu/tools/sub_section_main_1069.htm

Kung, H. C., Hoyert, D. L., Xu, J., & Murphy, S. L. (2008, April). *Deaths: Final data for 2005.* Retrieved September 5, 2008, from http://www.cdc.gov/nchs/data/nvsr/nvsr56/nvsr56_10.pdf

Lalonde, M. (1974). *A new perspective on the health of Canadians: A working document.* Ottawa, Canada: Minister of Health.

Landrum-Brown, J. (2000). *Black English.* Retrieved May 8, 2000, from http://www.staff.uiuc.edu/~jlandrum/BlkEng.html

Lashley, F. R., & Durham, J. D. (Eds.). (2007). *Emerging infectious diseases: Trends and issues* (2nd ed.). New York: Springer Publishing Company.

Lenhart, A., & Fox, S. (2006). *Bloggers: A portrait of the internet's new storyteller* [Special Report]. Washington, DC: Pew Internet and American Life Project. Retrieved January 3, 2008, from http://www.pewinternet.org/PPF/r/186/report_display.asp

Liburd, L. C., & Sniezek, J. E. (2007). Changing times: New possibilities for community health and well-being. *Preventing Chronic Disease, 4*(3), 1–5. Retrieved June 28, 2008, from http://www.cdc.gov/pcd/issues/2007/jul/07_0048.htm

Linnan L., Bowling M., Lindsay G., Blakey, C., Pronk, S., Wieker, S., & Royall, P. (2007). Results of the 2004 national worksite health promotion survey. *American Journal of Public Health, 98*(8), 1503–1509.

Longtin, J., Bastien, M., Gilca, R., Leblanc, E., de Serres, G., Bergeron, M. G., & Boivin, G. (2008, February). Human bocavirus infections in hospitalized children and adults. *Emerging Infectious Diseases, 14*(2), 217. Retrieved February 26, 2008, from http://www.cdc.gov/EID/content/14/2/217.htm

Lopez, E. D., Eng, E., Randall-David, E., & Robinson, N. (2005). Quality of life concerns of African American breast cancer survivors within rural North Carolina: Blending the techniques of Photovoice and grounded theory. *Qualitative Health Research, 15*(1), 99–115.

Mahbub ul Haq Human Development Centre. (2000). *Human development in South Asia 2000: The gender question.* Oxford: Oxford University Press. Retrieved August 21, 2008, from http://www.mhhdc.org/html/ahdr.htm

Maibach, E. (2003). *Social marketing: Can we really use communication and marketing to improve the health of populations and prevent climate change?* Retrieved from http://www.cdc.gov/healthmarketing/NCHCMM2007/Presentations/Edward_Maibach%20.pdf

March of Dimes. (1999). *March of Dimes.* Retrieved December 13, 1999, from http://www.marchofdimes.org

March of Dimes. (2008, July 29). *Preterm birth contributes to growing number of infant deaths.* Retrieved August 30, 2008, from http://www.marchofdimes.com/aboutus/22684_31074.asp

Marmot, M., & Wilkinson, R. G. (2006). *Social determinants of health.* Oxford: Oxford University Press.

Maslow, A. (1954). *Motivation and personality.* New York: Harper & Row.

Maternal and Child Health Bureau. (2007). *Women's health USA 2007.* Rockville, MD: U.S. Department of Health and Human Services. Retrieved September 5, 2008, from http://www.mchb.hrsa.gov/whusa_07/popchar/0204wp.htm

Matocha, L. K. (1998). Chinese-Americans. In L. D. Purnell and B. J. Paulanka (Eds.), *Transcultural health care: A culturally competent approach* (pp. 163–188). Philadelphia: F. A. Davis.

Mayo Clinic. (2008, January 15). *Eating disorders. Tools for healthier lives.* Retrieved August 1, 2008, from http://www.mayoclinic.com/health/eating-disorders/DS00294/DSECTION=symptoms

McDermott, R. J., & Sarvella, P. D. (1999). *Health education evaluation and measurement: A practitioner's perspective* (2nd ed.). Boston: McGraw-Hill.

McKenzie, J. F., Neiger, B. L., & Smeltzer, J. L. (2005). *Planning, implementing, and evaluating health promotion programs: A primer* (4th ed.). San Francisco: Pearson.

McKenzie, J. F., Neiger, B. L., & Thackeray, R. (2009). *Planning, implementing, and evaluating health promotion programs: A primer* (5th ed.). San Francisco: Pearson Benjamin Cummings.

McLaughlin, G. (1969). SMOG grading—A new readability formula. *Journal of Reading, 12*(May), 639–646.

McLean, D. D. (1996). *Use of computer-based technology in health, physical education, recreation, and dance.* Washington, DC: ERIC Clearinghouse on Teaching and Technical Education (ERIC Document Reproductions Service H. ED 390 874).

McLeroy, K. R., Bibeau, D., Steckler, A., & Glanz, K. (1988). An ecological perspective on health promotion programs. *Health Education and Behavior, 15*(4), 351–377.

MedTech Insight. (2003). *News.* Retrieved April 9, 2008, from http://www.medtechinsight.com/newsroom/news121203.html

Merriam-Webster, Inc. (2003). *Merriam-Webster's collegiate dictionary* (11th ed.). Springfield, MA: Author.

Merriam-Webster's Online. (2008). *Merriam-Webster's online dictionary.* Retrieved August 16, 2008, from http://www.merriam-webster.com/dictionary/cooperation

Merson, M. H., Black, R. E., & Mills, A. J. (2006). *International public health.* Sudsbury, MA: Jones and Bartlett.

Metzler, M. M., Higgins, D. L., Beeker, C. G., Freudenberg, N., Lantz, P. M., Senturia, K. D., Eisinger, A. A., Viruell-Fuentes, E. A., Gheisar, B., Palermo, A. G., & Softley, D. (2003). Abstract: Addressing urban health in Detroit, New York City, and Seattle through community-based participatory research partnerships. *American Journal of Public Health, 93*(5), 803–811. Retrieved July 6, 2008, from http://www.ajph.org/cgi/content/abstract/93/5/803

Ministry of Social Development. (2007a). *Physical environment: Desired outcomes. The social report 2007.* Wellington, New Zealand: Author. Retrieved July 26, 2008, from http://www.socialreport.msd.govt.nz/physical-environment/index.html

Ministry of Social Development. (2007b). *Social connectedness: Desired outcomes. The social report 2007.* Wellington, New Zealand: Author. Retrieved July 26, 2008, from http://www.socialreport.msd.govt.nz/social-connectedness/index.html

Minkler, M. (2004). Ethical challenges for the "outside" researcher in community-based participatory research. *Health Education & Behavior, 31*(6), 684–697.

Minkler, M. (Ed.). (2005). *Community organizing and community building for health* (2nd ed.). New Brunswick, NJ: Rutgers University Press.

Minkler, M., Blackwell, A. G., Thompson, M., & Tamir, H. (2003). Community-based participatory research: Implications for public health funding. *American Journal of Public Health, 93*(8), 1210–1213. Retrieved June 18, 2008, from http://www.ajph.org/cgi/reprint/93/8/1210.pdf

Minkler, M., & Wallerstein, N. (2005). Improving health through community organization and community building: A health education perspective. In M. Minkler (Ed.), *Community organizing and community building for health* (2nd ed., pp. 26–50). New Brunswick, NJ: Rutgers University Press.

Minkler, M., Wallerstein, N., & Wilson, N. (2008). Improving health through community organization and community building. In K. Glanz, B. K. Rimer, and K. Viswanath (Eds.), *Health behavior and health education: Theory, research and practice* (4th ed., pp. 287–312). San Francisco: Jossey-Bass.

Miranda, B. F., McBride, M. R., & Spangler, Z. (1998). Filipino-Americans. In L. D. Purnell and B. J. Paulanka (Eds.), *Transcultural health care: A culturally competent approach* (pp. 245–272). Philadelphia: F. A. Davis.

Morris, J. N. (1975). *Uses of epidemiology* (3rd ed.). Edinburgh: Churchill Livingstone.

Murray J. L., Lopez, A. D., Mathers, C. D., & Stein, C. (2001). *The global burden of disease: 2000 project aims, methods, and data sources* [Global programme on evidence for health policy discussion paper no. 36]. Geneva, Switzerland: World Health Organization.

Nardi, D. A., & Petr, J. M. (2003). *Community health and wellness needs assessment: A step by step guide*. Thomson: New York.

National Adolescent Health Information Center. (2006). *Fact sheet on mortality: Adolescents and young adults*. San Francisco: Author. Retrieved August 30, 2008, from http://www.nahic.ucsf.edu//downloads/Mortality.pdf

National Adolescent Health Information Center. (2007a). *Fact sheet on substance use: Adolescents and young adults*. San Francisco: Author. Retrieved August 30, 2008, from http://www.nahic.ucsf.edu//downloads/SubstanceUse2007.pdf

National Adolescent Health Information Center. (2007b). *Fact sheet on violence: Adolescents and young adults*. San Francisco: Author. Retrieved August 30, 2008, from http://www.nahic.ucsf.edu//downloads/Violence.pdf

National Adolescent Health Information Center. (2008). *Fact sheet on demographics: Adolescents and young adults*. San Francisco: Author. Retrieved August 30, 2008, from http://www.nahic.ucsf.edu//downloads/Demographics08.pdf

National Association of County and City Health Officials. (2006, July). *2005 national profile of local health departments*. Washington, DC: Author. Retrieved August 9, 2008, from http://www.naccho.org/topics/infrastructure/profile/upload/NACCHO_report_final_000.pdf

National Association of County and City Health Officials. (2008). *Mobilizing for action through planning and partnerships (MAPP)*. Retrieved December 26, 2008, from http://www.naccho.org/topics/infrastructure/MAPP/index.cfm

National Board of Public Health Examiners. (n.d.). *Get certified in public health!* Retrieved August 16, 2008, from http://www.publichealthexam.org/

National Cancer Institutes. (1999). How the public perceives health messages. *Health communication processes that work*. Retrieved April 11, 2008, from http://www.rex.nci.nih.gov/NCI_Pub_Interface/HCPW/Home/htm

National Cancer Institutes. (2008). *Common cancer types*. Retrieved April 10, 2008, from http://www.cancer.gov/cancertopics/commoncancers

National Center for Chronic Disease Prevention and Health Promotion. (2007, October). *Health-related quality of life*. Retrieved February 28, 2008, from http://www.cdc.gov/hrqol/

National Center for Environmental Health. (2008, June). *Healthy community design*. Retrieved August 10, 2008, from http://www.cdc.gov/healthyplaces/docs/Healthy%20Community%20Design.pdf

National Center for Health Statistics. (1996). *Health, United States, 1995*. Hyattsville, MD: Public Health Service.

National Center for Health Statistics. (2007a, November). *Health, United States, 2007: With chartbook on trends in the health of Americans*. Hyattsville, MD: Author. Retrieved September 1, 2008, from http://www.cdc.gov/nchs/data/hus/hus07.pdf#032

National Center for Health Statistics. (2007b). *U.S. life expectancy hits new high of nearly 78 years*. Retrieved March 10, 2008, from http://www.cdc.gov/nchs/pressroom/07newsreleases/lifeexpectancy.htm

National Center for Health Statistics. (2008a, July 30). *Health data for all ages*. Retrieved August 30, 2008, from http://www.cdc.gov/nchs/health_data_for_all_ages.htm

National Center for Health Statistics. (2008b, July10). *What's new? Health data for all ages*. Retrieved August 31, 2008, from http://www.209.217.72.34/HDAA/tableviewer/document.aspx?FileId=249

National Commission for Health Education Credentialing. (n.d.). *What is a health educator?* Retrieved March 15, 2009, from http://www.nchec.org

National Commission for Health Education Credentialing, Society for Public Health Education, and American Association for Health Education. (2006). *A competency-based framework for health educators—2006.* Whitehall, PA: National Commission for Health Education Credentialing.

National Institutes of Health. (1999). *NIH overview.* Retrieved December 13, 1999, from http://www.nih.gov/welcome/nihnew.htm

National Institutes of Health. (2002). *Making health communication programs work: A planner's guide.* Atlanta: U.S. Department of Health and Human Services. Retrieved August 28, 2008, from http://www.cancer.gov/pinkbook

National Institutes of Health. (2008). *NIH institutes, centers, and offices.* Retrieved January 4, 2008, from http://www.nihigov/welcome/nihnew.html

National Library of Medicine. (n.d.). *Quick guide to health literacy: Fact sheet.* Retrieved August 20, 2008, from http://www.health.gov/communication/literacy/quickguide/factsbasic.htm

National Library of Medicine and National Institutes of Health. (2006). Panel 2. *NLM health information for underserved and diverse populations in the 21st century.* Retrieved August 18, 2008, from http://www.nlm.nih.gov/pubs/plan/lrp06/panel2report.doc

National Library of Medicine and National Institutes of Health. (2007). *Director's comments transcript: Health literacy 3/30/07.* Retrieved August 20, 2008, from http://www.nlm.nih.gov/medlineplus/podcast/transcript033007.html

National Science Foundation. (1997). *User friendly handbook for missed method evaluation.* Retrieved February 7, 1999, from http://www.her.nsf.gov/HER/REC/pubs/NSF97–1531/start/htm

Naval Health Research Center. (n.d.). *Department 164 deployment: The millennium cohort study.* Retrieved June 12, 2008, from http://www.nhrc.navy.mil/department164/program.html#milco

Navarro, A. M., Voetsch, K. P., Liburd, L. C., Giles, H. W., & Collins, J. L. (2007, July). Charting the future of community health promotion: Recommendations from the National Expert Panel on Community Health Promotion. *Prevention of Chronic Disease [A].* Retrieved July 20, 2008, from http://www.cdc.gov/pcd/issues/2007/jul/07_0013.htm

New York Times. (2007). Leading causes of cancer death. Retrieved April 7, 2008, from http://www.nytimes.com/imagepages/2007/07/29/health/29cancer.graph.web.html

Nieuwenhuijsen, E. R., Zemper, E., Miner, K. R., & Epstein, M. (2006). Health behavior change models and theories: Contributions to rehabilitation. *Disability & Rehabilitation, 28*(5), 245–256.

O'Reilly, T. (2005). *What is Web 2.0?* O'Reilly Media, Inc. Retrieved January 3, 2007, from http://www.oreillynet.com/lpt/a/6228

Office of Disease Prevention and Health Promotion. (1988). *Disease prevention/health promotion: The facts.* Palo Alto, CA: Bull.

Office of Minority Health. (2001). *National standards for culturally and linguistically appropriate services in health care.* Washington, DC: U.S. Department of Health and Human Services.

Office of Minority Health. (2009, January 1). *American Indian/Alaska native profile.* Retrieved February 5, 2009, from http://www.omhrc.gov/templates/browse.aspx?lvl=2&lvlid=52

Office of Women's Health. (2008, January). *BodyWorks: A tool kit for healthy girls and strong women.* Retrieved January 27, 2009, from http://www.womenshealth.gov/bodyworks/

Oliffe, J. L., & Bottorff, J. L. (2007). Further than the eye can see? Photo elicitation and research with men. *Qualitative Health Research, 17*(6), 850–858.

Online NewsHour. (1999, July–December). *Patients' Bill of Rights: A health spotlight report.* Retrieved June 12, 2009, from http://www.pbs.org/newshour/health/patientsrights/index.html

Oomen-Early, J., & Burke, S. (2007). Entering the Blogosphere: Blogs as teaching and learning tools in health education. *The International Electronic Journal of Health Education*, *10*, 186–196.

Orlowski, A. (2005, October 18). Wikipedia founder admits to serious quality problems [Newsbrief]. *The Register*. Retrieved January 4, 2008, from http://www.theregister.co.uk/2005/10/18/wikipedia_quality_problem/

Pan American Health Organization. (1998). United States of America. *Health conditions in the Americas*. Retrieved June 21, 1999, from http://www.paho.org/english/country.htm.

Paniagua, F. A. (2005). *Assessing and treating culturally diverse clients: A practical guide* (3rd ed.). Thousand Oaks, CA: Sage.

Parker, E. A., Eng, E., Laraia, B., Ammerman, A., Dodds, J., Margolis, L., & Cross, A. (1998). Coalition building for prevention. In R. C. Brownson, E. A. Baker, & L. F. Novick (Eds.), *Community-based prevention: Programs that work*. Gaithersburg, MD: Aspen.

Parker, R. C. (1997). *Web design and desktop publishing for dummies* (2nd ed.). Hoboken, NJ: Hungry Minds.

Partnership for a Drug Free America. (2006). *The partnership's 'fried egg' TV message*. Retrieved April 13, 2008, from http://www.drugfree.org/General/Articles/article98f123-9734-4b0f-bebc-947adfcbc784&PrintPage=true

Partnership for Prevention. (2001). *Healthy workforce 2010: An essential health promotion sourcebook for employers, large and small*. Washington, DC: Author. Retrieved August 7, 2008, from http://www.prevent.org/images/stories/Files/publications/Healthy_Workforce_2010.pdf

Partnership for Prevention. (2008a). *The community health promotion handbook: Action guides to improve community health*. Washington, DC: Author. Retrieved July 15, 2008, from http://www.prevent.org/content/view/142/173/

Partnership for Prevention. (2008b). *Investing in health: Proven health promotion practices for workplaces*. Washington, DC: Author. Retrieved August 7, 2008, from http://www.prevent.org/images/stories/2008/investinginhealth_finalfinal.pdf

Payne, C. A. (1999). The challenges of employing performance monitoring in public health community-based efforts. *Journal of Community Health, 24*(2), 159–170.

PCMag.com. (n.d.). "Podcast." Retrieved January 4, 2008, from http://www.pcmag.com/encyclopedia_term/0,2542,t=podcast&i=49433,00.asp

Penner, L. A., & Finkelstein, M. A. (1998). Dispositional and structural determinants of volunteerism. *Journal of Personality and Social Psychology, 74*(2), 525–537.

Perlino, C. M. (2006, September). *The public health workforce shortage: Left unchecked, will we be protected?* [American public health association issue brief]. Retrieved August 22, 2008, from http://www.apha.org/NR/rdonlyres/8B9EBDF5-8BE8-482D-A779-7F637456A7C3/0/workforcebrief.pdf

Perry, C. L., Williams, C. L., Veblen-Mortenson, S., Toomey, T. L., Komro, K. A., Anstine, P. S., McGovern, P. G., Finnegan, J. R., Forster, J. L., Wagenaar, A. C., & Wolfson, M. (1996). Project Northland: Outcomes of a community wide alcohol use prevention program during early adolescence. *American Journal of Public Health, 86,* 956–964.

Powell, K. B. (1999). Correlates of violent and nonviolent behavior among vulnerable inner-city youths. In J. G. Sebastian & A. Bushy (Eds.), *Health behavior and health education: Theory, research, and practice* (2nd ed., pp. 60–84). Gaithersburg, MD: Aspen.

Prochaska, J. O., Redding, C. A., & Evers, K. E. (1997). The transtheoretical model and stages of change. In K. Glanz, F. M. Lewis, and B. K. Rimer (Eds.), *Health behavior and health education: Theory, research, and practice* (2nd ed., pp. 60–84). San Francisco: Jossey-Bass.

Public Health Functions Steering Committee. (1994). *Public health in America*. Washington, DC: U.S. Public Health Services. Retrieved August 14, 2008, from http://www.health.gov/phfunctions/public.htm

Purnell, L. D. (1998). Mexican-Americans. In L. D. Purnell and B. J. Paulanka (Eds.), *Transcultural health care: A culturally competent approach* (pp. 163–188). Philadelphia: F. A. Davis.

Raskin, M. S. (1994). The Delphi Study in field instruction revisited: Expert consensus on issues and research priorities. *Journal of Social Work Education, 3*(1), 75–89.

Reardon, T. R. (1999, September 23). *Pass Norwood-Dingell patient protection bill.* American Medical Association (Released statement). Retrieved November 15, 1999, from http://www.ama-assn.org/advocacy/statemnt/990923.htm

Robert Wood Johnson Foundation. (2008). *About RWJF.* Retrieved August 14, 2008, from http://www.rwjf.org/about/

Rodman, J., Weill, K., Driscoll, M., Fenton, T., Hill, A., Salem-Schatz, S., & Palfrey, J. (1999). A nationwide survey of financing health-related services for special education students. *Journal of School Health, 69*(4), 133–139.

Rosenstock, I. M., Strecher, V. J., & Becker, M. H. (1988). Social learning theory and the health belief model. *Health Education & Behavior, 15*(2), 175–183.

Schrock, K. (2006). Critical Evaluation of a Weblog. *Kathy Schrock's Guide for Educators* [Online manual]. Retrieved from http://www.discoveryschool.com/schrockguide/

Seelye, H. N., & Seelye-James, A. (1996). *Culture clash: Managing in a multicultural world.* Lincolnwood, IL: NTC.

Simons-Morton, B. G., Greene, W. H., & Gottlieb, N. H. (1995). *Introduction to health education and health promotion* (2nd ed.). Long Grove, IL: Waveland Press.

Skolnik, R. (2008). *Essentials of global health.* Sudbury, MA: Jones & Bartlett.

Slonim, A. B., Callaghan, C., Daily, L., Leonard, B. A., Wheeler, F. C., Gollmar, C. W., & Young, W. F. (2007, April). Recommendations for integration of chronic disease programs: Are your programs linked? *Prevention of Chronic Disease.* Retrieved April 20, 2008, from http://www.cdc.gov/pcd/issues/2007/apr/pdf/06_0163.pdf

Smith, G. I. (2005). On construct validity: Issues of method and measurement. *Psychological Assessment, 17*(4), 396–408.

Smith, K. C., & Wakefield, M. (2005). Textual analysis of tobacco editorials: How key are media gatekeepers for framing the issues? *American Journal of Health Promotion, 19*(5), 472–480.

Snyder, M. (1993). Basic research and practical problems: The promise of a "functional" personality and social psychology. *Personality and Social Psychology Bulletin, 19*(3), 251–264.

Sotomayor, M., Pawlik, F., Dominguez, A. (2007). Building community capacity for health promotion in a Hispanic community. *Preventing Chronic Diseases, 4*(1), A16.

Spector, R. E. (1996). *Cultural diversity in health and illness* (4th ed.). Norwalk, CT: Appleton and Lange.

Spector, R. (2004). *Cultural diversity in health and illness* (6th ed.). Upper Saddle River, NJ: Pearson Prentice Hall.

Steptoe A., & Wardle, J. (2001). Locus of control and health behaviour revisited: A multivariate analysis of young adults from 18 countries. *British Journal of Psychology, 92*(4), 659–672.

Still, O., & Hodgins, D. (1998). Navajo Indians. In L. D. Purnell and B. J. Paulanka (Eds.), *Transcultural health care: A culturally competent approach* (pp. 423–447). Philadelphia: F. A. Davis.

Stith, S. M. (2007). *Prevention of intimate partner violence.* Binghamton, NY: Haworth Press.

Strack, R. W., Magill, C., & McDonagh, K. (2003). Engaging youth through Photovoice. *Health Promotion Practice, 5*(1), 49–58.

Strecher, V. J., & Rosenstock, I. M. (1997). The health belief model. In K. Glanz, F. M. Lewis, and B. K. Rimer (Eds.), *Health behavior and health education: Theory, research, and practice* (2nd ed., pp. 41–59). San Francisco: Jossey-Bass.

Sullivan, D. (2005, January 28). Search engine sizes. *Search Engine Watch.* Retrieved January 17, 2008, from http://www.searchenginewatch.com/2156481

Swartz, M. (1990). Infant mortality: Agenda for the 1990s. *Journal of Pediatric Health Care 4,* 169–174.

Synique. (2008). *Transformational leadership.* Retrieved August 1, 2008, from http://www.changingminds.org/disciplines/leadership/styles/transformational_leadership.htm

Technorati. (2006). *State of the blogosphere* [Special Report]. Retrieved January 3, 2008, from http://www.technorati.com/weblog/2006/11/161.html

Teixeira, C. (2007). Health educators: Working for wellness. *Occupational Outlook Quarterly, Summer,* 30–36. U.S. Department of Labor. Retrieved April 20, 2008, from http://www.nchec.org/forms/OOQ_health_educators.pdf

Tonkin, E. (2006). Making the case for a Wiki. *Ariadne, 42*(12), 43–44.

Trochim, W. M. (2006). *Research methods knowledge base.* Retrieved July 12, 2008, from http://www.socialresearchmethods.net/kb/qualapp.php

Tsui, A. B. M., & Law, D. Y. K. (2007). Learning as boundary-crossing in school–university partnerships. *Teaching and Teacher Education, 23*, 1289–1301. Retrieved August 1, 2008, from http://www.hku.hk/curric/amytsui/TATE882.pdf

U.S. Administration on Aging. (2008). *Media advocacy toolkit.* Retrieved August 23, 2008, from http://www.aoa.gov/press/more/media_advocacy/media_advocacy.aspx

U.S. Census Bureau. (2008a, June). Poverty: 2007 highlights. *Current population survey.* Retrieved December 29, 2008, from http://www.census.gov/hhes/www/poverty/poverty07/pov07hi.html

U.S. Census Bureau. (2008b, June). USA statistics in brief. *Statistical abstract of the United States: 2008* (127th ed.). Washington, DC: Author. Retrieved September 4, 2008, from http://www.census.gov/compendia/statab/brief.html

U.S. Department of Agriculture, Food Safety and Inspection Services. (2007). *News and events.* Retrieved April 12, 2008, from http://www.fsis.usda.gov/News_&_Events/Recall_049_2007_Release/index.asp

U.S. Department of Health and Human Services. (n.d.). *Be a healthy person.* Retrieved August 14, 2008, from http://www.healthypeople.gov/BeHealthy/

U.S. Department of Health and Human Services. (n.d.). *Leading health indicators: Priorities for action.* Washington, DC: U.S. Government Printing Office. Retrieved July 25, 2008, from http://www.healthypeople.gov/LHI/LHIPrioritiesforAction.pdf

U.S. Department of Health and Human Services. (n.d.). *Special populations.* Retrieved August 23, 2008, from http://www.healthfinder.gov/justforyou/

U.S. Department of Health and Human Services. (n.d.). *Steps to a healthier U.S. initiative.* Rockville, MD: Author. Retrieved August 1, 2008, from http://www.healthierus.gov/steps/

U.S. Department of Health and Human Services. (1980). *Promoting health/preventing disease: Objectives for the nation.* Washington, DC: U.S. Government Printing Office.

U.S. Department of Health and Human Services. (1990). *Healthy people 2000: National health promotion disease prevention objectives.* Washington, DC: U.S. Government Printing Office.

U.S. Department of Health and Human Services. (1998). *Report to the vice president of the United States: Status of implementation of the Consumer Bill of Rights and responsibilities in the Department of Health and Human Services.* Released November 2, 1998. Retrieved November 15, 1999, from http://aspe.os.dhhs.gov/health/vpreport.htm

U.S. Department of Health and Human Services. (2000, November). *Healthy people 2010: Understanding and improving health* (2nd ed.). Washington, DC: U.S. Government Printing Office. Retrieved August 2, 2008, from http://www.healthypeople.gov/Document/pdf/uih/2010uih.pdf

U.S. Department of Health and Human Services. (2001, February). *Healthy people in healthy communities.* Washington, DC: U.S. Government Printing Office. Retrieved July 25, 2008, from

http://www.healthypeople.gov/Publications/HealthyCommunities2001/
healthycom01hk.pdf

U.S. Department of Health and Human Services. (2004a, October 18). *Health status of adolescents and young adults. Improving the health of adolescents and young adults: A guide for states and communities.* Retrieved August 30, 2008, from http://www.nahic.ucsf.edu/downloads/niiah/ch2.pdf

U.S. Department of Health and Human Services. (2004b). *Successful strategies for recruiting, training, and utilizing volunteers: A guide for faith and community-based service providers* [Manual]. Retrieved January 3, 2008, from http://www.ncadistore.samhsa.gov/catalog/productDetails.aspx?ProductID=17055

U.S. Department of Health and Human Services. (2007a, July 15). *About the office of global health affairs.* Retrieved August 14, 2008, from http://www.globalhealth.gov/office/index.html

U.S. Department of Health and Human Services. (2007b, September). *The guide to clinical preventive health services 2007* [AHRQ Pub. No. 07-05100]. Washington, DC: U.S. Government Printing Office. Retrieved August 8, 2008, from http://www.ahrq.gov/clinic/pocketgd07/pocketgd07.pdf

U.S. Department of Health and Human Services. (2007c, April). *Healthy People 2010: Midcourse review.* Washington, DC: U.S. Government Printing Office. Retrieved August 2, 2008, from http://www.healthypeople.gov/data/midcourse/html/execsummary/progress.htm

U.S. Department of Health and Human Services. (2007d, September 20). *Maternal, infant, and child health. Healthy people 2010 progress review.* Retrieved August 30, 2008, from http://www.healthypeople.gov/Data/2010prog/focus16/

U.S. Department of Health and Human Services. (2008a, January). *Health risks in the United States: Behavioral risk factor surveillance system 2008.* Washington, DC: U.S. Government Printing Office. Retrieved July 25, 2008, from http://www.cdc.gov/nccdphp/publications/aag/pdf/brfss.pdf

U.S. Department of Health and Human Services. (2008b, March). *What we do.* Retrieved August 8, 2008, from http://www.hhs.gov/about/whatwedo.html/

U.S. Department of Labor. (2008). *Career voyages.* Retrieved August 30, 2008, from http://www.nlm.nih.gov/medlineplus/healthoccupations.html

U.S. Food and Drug Administration. (2007). *Experimental study of health claims on food packages.* Retrieved June 14, 2008, from http://www.cfsan.fda.gov/~comm/crnutri4.html

U.S. Food and Drug Administration, Center for Food Safety and Applied Nutrition. (n.d.). *2008 intramural research portfolio.* Retrieved from http://www.cfsan.fda.gov/~dms/cfsres08.html

U.S. Health Resources and Services Administration. (n.d.). *Guidelines for medically underserved area and population designation.* Retrieved July 29, 2008, from http://www.bhpr.hrsa.gov/shortage/muaguide.htm

U.S. Public Health Service. (1979). *Healthy people: The surgeon general's report on health promotion and disease prevention.* Washington, DC: U.S. Government Printing Office.

UNICEF. (2008a, August 17). *World Water Week 2008 focuses on sanitation, health and hygiene.* Retrieved August 20, 2008, from http://www.unicef.org/media/media_45228.html

UNICEF. (2008b, August 18). *Zambia: Early childhood development in focus.* Retrieved August 20, 2008, from http://www.unicef.org/media/media_45248.html

United Nations. (2006). *Violence against children.* Retrieved August 21, 2008, from http://www.unviolencestudy.org/

United Nations. (2007a, December). *Social indicators.* Retrieved February 29, 2008, from http://www.unstats.un.org/unsd/demographic/products/socind/statistics.htm

United Nations. (2007b). *World population prospects: The 2006 revision.* New York: Author. Retrieved August 11, 2008, from http://www.esa.un.org/unpp

United Nations. (2009). *World population prospects: The 2008 revision.* New York: Author. Retrieved May 1, 2009, from http://www.un.org/esa/population/

United Nations Development Programme. (2005). *Human development report 2005 summary.* Retrieved August 20, 2008, from http://www.hdr.undp.org/en/media/hdr05_summary.pdf

United Nations Development Programme. (2006). *Human development report 2006.* Retrieved August 20, 2008, from http://www.hdr.undp.org/en/reports/global/hdr2006/

United Nations Development Programme. (2007/2008). *Human development report 2007–2008 summary.* Retrieved August 20, 2008, from http://www.hdr.undp.org/en/media/HDR_20072008_Summary_English.pdf

United Nations Development Programme. (2008, July 16). *UNDP promotes small arms control in Mozambique.* Retrieved August 22, 2008, from http://www.content.undp.org/go/newsroom/2008/july/undp-promotes-small-arms-control-in-mozambique.en

United Nations Development Programme Azerbaijan. (2007). *Azerbaijan human development report 2007.* Retrieved August 21, 2008, from http://www.hdr.undp.org/en/reports/nationalreports/europethecis/azerbaijan/nhdr2007gendereng.pdf

United Nations Environmental Program. (2004). *Annual report: 2003.* Retrieved August 13, 2008, from http://www.unep.org/annualreport/2003/

USAID. (2008). *IDP and humanitarian protection—March 2008.* Retrieved August 22, 2008, from http://www.usaid.gov/our_work/humanitarian_assistance/disaster_assistance/sectors/mods/docs/idp_protection_03-2008.pdf

Verhoef, L., Depoortere, E., Boxman, I., Duizer, E., van Duynhoven, Y., Harris, J., Johnsen, C., Kroneman, A., Le Guyader, S., Lim, L., Maunula, L., Meldal, H., Ratcliff, R., Reuter, G., Schreier, E., Siebenga, J., Vainio, K., Varela, C., Vennema, H., & Koopmans, M. (2008, February). Emergence of new norovirus variants on spring cruise ships and prediction of winter epidemics. *Emerging Infectious Diseases, 14*(2), 238. Retrieved February 26, 2008, from http://www.cdc.gov/EID/content/14/2/238.htm

W. K. Kellogg Foundation. (n.d.). *Who we are.* Retrieved August 14, 2008, from http://www.wkkf.org/default.aspx?tabid=78&NID=68&LanguageID=0

W. K. Kellogg Foundation. (2004, January). *Logic model development guide.* Battle Creek, MI: Author. Retrieved January 18, 2009, from http://www.wkkf.org/Pubs/Tools/Evaluation/Pub3669.pdf

Waldram, J. B. (2004). *Revenge of the Windingo: The construction of the mind and mental health of North American aboriginal peoples.* Toronto: University of Toronto Press.

Walker, A. (2008). Using Photovoice and participatory action research to identity factors which impede and provide health among orphans in Sierra Leone. Unpublished doctoral dissertation, Texas Woman's University.

Wallerstein, N. (1992). Powerlessness, empowerment and health. Implications for health promotion programs. *American Journal of Health Promotion, 6,* 197–205.

Walter, S. L. (1999). *Plan a literacy program.* Retrieved February 20, 2009, from http://www.sil.org/lingualinks/literacy/planaliteracyprogram/

Wang, C. C. (2006). Youth participation in Photovoice as a strategy for community change. *Journal of Community Practice, 14*(1/2), 147–161.

Wang, C. C., & Burris, M. (1997). Photovoice: Concept, methodology, and use for participatory needs assessment. *Health Education and Behavior, 24*(3), 369–387.

Wang, W. L., Lee, H. L., & Fetzer, S. J. (2006). Challenges and strategies of instrument translation. *Western Journal of Nursing Research, 28*(3), 310–321.

Ward, M. (1998, March). Embracing volunteerism. *School Foodservices and Nutrition,* 24–31.

Ward, S. E., & Koontz, N. (1999). Putting advocacy into action. *Eta Sigma Gamma Monograph, 17*(2), 36–40.

Watkins, K. (2007). Fighting climate change: Human solidarity in a divided world. *Human development report 2007/2008.* New York: United Nations Development Programme.

Webster's New Millennium Dictionary of English (2007). "Blog." Retrieved January 4, 2008, from Dictionary.com Web site: http://www.dictionary.reference.com/browse/blog

Weil, M., & Reisch, M. (2005). *The handbook of community practice.* Thousand Oaks, CA: Sage.

Weiler, R. M., Dorman, S. M., & Pealer, I. N. (1999). The Florida school violence policies and programs study. *Journal of School Health, 69*(7), 273–279.

Weiner, J., Aguirre, A., Ravenell, K., Kovath, K., McDevit, L., Murphy, J., Asch, D. A., & Shea, J. (2004). Designing an illustrated patient satisfaction instrument for low-literacy populations. *American Journal of Managed Care, 10*(part 2), 853–860.

Weinreich Communications. (1999). *What is social marketing?* Retrieved September 22, 1999, from http://www.socialmarketing.com/whatis.html.

Weinstein, N. D., & Sandman, P. M. (1992). A model of precaution adoption process: Evidence from home radon testing. *Health Psychology 11*(3), 170–180.

Wenger, E., McDermott, R., & Snyder, W. M. (2002). *Cultivating communities of practice.* Boston: Harvard Business School Press.

Westerinen, A. (2003). *What is policy and what can it be?* Retrieved August 17, 2008, from http://www.policy-workshop.org/2003/web/policy2003/common/AndreaPresentation.pdf

Wikipedia. (n.d.). *Wikipedia: Size comparisons.* Retrieved January 4, 2008, from http://www.en.wikipedia.org/wiki/Wikipedia:Size_comparisons

Woodhouse, L. D., Auld, M. E., Livingood, W. C., & Mulligan, L. A. (2006). Survey of accredited master of public health (MPH) programs with health education concentrations: A resource for strengthening the public health workforce. *Health Promotion Practice, 7*(2), 258–265.

World Bank. (2008). *Overview: Social capital.* Washington, DC: Author. Retrieved July 30, 2008, from http://www.go.worldbank.org/C0QTRW4QF0

World Health Organization. (1947). Constitution of the World Health Organization. *Chronicle of the World Health Organization, 1,* 1–2.

World Health Organization. (1999). *Health for all.* Retrieved August 11, 1999, from http://www.who.org/aboutwho/en/healthforall.htm

World Health Organization. (2004). *Global health and infectious disease: Tropics disease report.* Retrieved August 21, 2008, from http://www.who.int/tdr/topics/social-research/globalization.htm

World Health Organization. (2006a, April). *Migration of health workers* [Fact sheet No. 301]. Retrieved August 18, 2008, from http://www.who.int/mediacentre/factsheets/fs301/en/index.html

World Health Organization. (2006b). *Working together for health: World health report 2006.* Geneva, Switzerland: Author.

World Health Organization. (2008a). *Global burden of disease: 2004 update.* Retrieved March 25, 2009, from http://www.who.int/healthinfo/global_burden_disease/2004_report_update/en/index.html

World Health Organization. (2008b). *Millennium development goals.* Retrieved August 22, 2008, from http://www.who.int/topics/millennium_development_goals/en/

World Health Organization. (2008c, May). *Report on the expert consultation on positive synergies between health systems and global health initiatives.* Geneva, Switzerland: Author. Retrieved August 22, 2008, from http://www.who.int/healthsystems/hs_&_ghi.pdf

World Health Organization. (2008d). *Strengthening health systems through primary health care.* Retrieved August 22, 2008, from http://www.who.int/healthsystems/en/index.html

World Health Organization. (2008e, November). *Top ten causes of death* (Fact Sheet No. 310). Retrieved from http://www.who.int/mediacentre/factsheets/fs310/en/index.html

World Health Organization. (2008f). *The WHO agenda.* Retrieved August 14, 2008, from http://www.who.int/about/agenda/en/index.html

World Health Organization. (2008g). *World impact assessment.* Retrieved August 1, 2008, from http://www.who.int/hia/evidence/doh/en/index.html

Wright, K. B. (2005). Researching Internet-based populations: Advantages and disadvantages of online survey research, online questionnaire authoring software packages, and web survey services. *Journal of Computer-Mediated Communication, 10*(3), article 11. Retrieved from http://www.jcmc.indiana.edu/vol10/issue3/wright.html

Zeng, Q., Eunjung, K., & Tse, T. (n.d.). *A text corporal-based estimation of the familiarity of health terminology.* Retrieved August 10, 2008, from http://www.lhncbc.nlm.nih.gov/lhc/docs/published/2005/pub2005041.pdf

Zweigenhaft, R., Armstrong, J., Quintis, F., & Riddick, A. (1996). The motivations and effectiveness of hospital volunteers. *The Journal of Social Psychology, 136*(1), 25–34.

Index